Immunology of

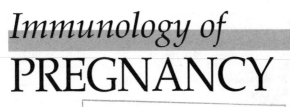

PREGNANCY

Edited by

Gérard Chaouat, M.D., Ph.D.

Director of Research
Laboratory of Cellular and Molecular Biology
  of Reproduction
Antoine Béclère Hospital
Clamart, France

CRC Press

Boca Raton   Ann Arbor   London   Tokyo

Library of Congress Cataloging-in-Publication Data

Immunology of pregnancy/edited by Gérard Chaouat.

    p. cm.

    Includes bibliographical references and index.

    ISBN 0-8493-8868-6

    1. Pregnancy—Immunological aspects. 2. Pregnancy—Complications-
-Immunological aspects. 3. Maternal—fetal exchanges. I. Chaouat,
Gérard.

    [DNLM: 1. Pregnancy—immunology. WQ 200 1327]

RG557.I47 1992

612.6'3—dc20

DNLM/DLC

for Library of Congress   92-20057

                                                             CIP

Developed by Telford Press

INTRODUCTION

Reproductive Immunology is burgeoning, and with its expansion there have arisen some controversies in the field that are very important. (For a review of these, see David A. Clark's comprehensive and quite objective review article, "Controversies in Reproductive Immunology" in *CRC — Critical Reviews in Immunology,* 11, 3, 1991.)

Immunology is viewed by some as being imperialistic, i.e., setting up strongholds in almost every field that it can. This view does not make exception in the field of Reproductive Immunology. Indeed, the discovery that cytokines have pleiotropic effects has set the pace for studies of integrated functions of various systems, and the reproductive tract is no exception to this rule. For example, in most cases there are indeed interactions between the immune system, on the one hand, and the endocrine central nervous system, on the other. Progesterone-dependent immunoregulatory factors have been identified, cloned, or purified. A monoclonal antibody against it is shown to be abortifacient. Interferons, or IL-6, are shown to act on corpus luteum maintenance; whereas an intracerebral injection of IL-1 is indeed abortifacient.

Yet the field of Reproductive Immunology has had, in general, a variable reputation, going up and down like a scenic railway, among serious immunologists who make up the bulk of this scientific community. It was sometimes considered as an unpopular field by them and one where known theories had failed in giving a general explanation of the functioning of the immune system. It is surprising to some, including the Editor of this book, that the studies go on, thriving and attempting to teach lessons in the field of Immunology. It was also perceived, though not wrongly, as a projecting hypothesis that, however attractive it might have sounded for the explanation of some clinical syndromes, a masters student in genetics might have found difficult to sustain. Furthermore, it was linked for a while with events and experiments that were associated with remnants of the Lyssenkist period, a period now that is definitely bygone and hopefully will remain thus. As a consequence, the scientific content of some of its congresses was not to the standard that it **could** have reached, and the **real** necessity to maintain links with Eastern Europe did not necessarily justify the fact that some meetings indeed were plagued with experiments that had a flavor acquainted with Stalinian style remnants.

This undiplomatic and personal assessment is made by this Editor, but one must realize that over the past 25 years a gradual change has appeared, and the fact that after a purgatory status in Berlin, the field is now back to a symposium-like status in Budapest, as it was in the Toronto, Kyoto, and Paris IUIS meetings. This change is brought by the now massive arrival of the fields of Cellular Immunology and Molecular Biology in Reproduction. We do not any longer deal with riddles that were not necessarily intriguing or experiments that failed to be convincing outside our own social circle, and sometimes not even convincing to us, but we now work with **defined** effects of purified or recombinant cytokines in precise *in vitro* or *in vivo* systems, whose pitfalls and borders are beginning to be understood.

Regulatory events have been studied at genomic levels, and the field has even now its own and unique MHC molecule with the recent discovery of HLA-G. Although it must be confessed that the progress has perhaps been more impressive in the studies of the maternal-fetal relationship (the scope of this book) than in the immunology of gametes. The trend seems obviously to contaminate this topic, too.

The subject of this treatise is restricted mostly to maternal-fetal inter-actions. It, thus, covers the various aspects of what Medawar used to call in 1953 the ''riddle of the fetal allograft''. Some, like Jan Klein, whom I greatly esteem, thought once that where was NO problem in having the mother accept a histoincompatible fetus. To quote the few words he devoted to the field in one of his several remarkable books, he thought that the success of pregnancy could be explained solely by the fact that there was a neutral barrier between the mother and the fetus. Fortunately enough, in his more recent *Natural History of the Major Histocompatibility Complex,* (John Wiley & Sons, New York, 1986, 1990), a magistral book to be recommended to anyone devoted to Immunology, he describes quite well the MHC class I expression on the placenta of rodents as well as other species. Thus, the placental neutral barrier theory, i.e., the existence of a neutral boundary between the mother and fetal tissues, is confronted with a classical problem that was recognized in the 1950s.

The aim of this book is to provide the reader with a state-of-the-art knowledge of some immunoregulatory events that might explain these phenomena and their action in both a normal and pathological situation. It also attempts to cover other important aspects currently being developed, such as contraceptive vaccines and the present status of immune abortions.

The book will not devote much space to already alluded bygone theories, because they may cause confusions that are already quite widespread, especially among some clinicians who believe these hypotheses are backed by a solid scientific background. Nor will it review systemic regulatory events, i.e., maternal-antipaternal alloantibodies or paternal antigen-specific suppressor T cells in the peripheral blood of the mother, not to mention anti-idiotypic antibodies. It will also not devote space to the TLX gene product theory, at least in its original form. It is hoped that this book will serve the newcomer, as well as the current researcher in the field, by providing them with basic information of which they should be aware, and dismissing as irrelevant the ones they do not necessarily need to consider. The choice of subject matter and the selection of topics do not reflect the opinions of the distinguished authors of this book, nor does the personal bias expressed in this Introduction reflect anyone's views but my own.

Dr. G. Chaouat

THE EDITOR

Dr. Gérard Chaouat is Directeur de Recherches for the Centre National de la Recherches Scientifique (CNRS) at the Laboratoire de Biologie Celiulaire et Moléculaire de la Relation Materno Fetale, at the Maternité Baudelocque, Hôpital Antoine Béclére, Clamart, France.

After graduating from the Paris Medical School in St. Louis, France in 1973 with a M.D. degree, he was appointed Interne des Hôpitaux. He joined research in Unité Institut National de la Santé et de la Recherche Medicale (INSERM) U23 at the St. Antoine Hospital under the leadership of Dr. Guy André Voisin. During his studies in Science for his M.Sc. degree, he demonstrated the presence of enhancing maternal antibodies during allopregnancy in mice, elutable from the placenta.

In 1974 to 1975, he had the opportunity to benefit from a British Medical Research Council (MRC) grant and learn cellular immunology in the Department of Immunology at the Wellcome Research Institute, Beckenham, Kent, U.K. under Dr. James Howard, working both on T cell independent antigens and T suppressor mechanisms. Upon return, he was recruited as a CNRS agent and obtained his Ph.D., dealing with the role of enhancing antibodies and T cell-mediated suppression of maternal-antipaternal activity in fetal acceptance. In 1980 to 1981, he spent 18 months at the National Institute of Allergy and Infectious Diseases, National Institutes of Health, Bethesda, Maryland as a visiting scientist. Upon returning to France, he devoted most, though not all, of his research interests to local immunoregulatory events in the fetomaternal relationship and was appointed Directeur de Recherches in 1985. A member of the editorial board of several journals, he is also Councillor of the Board of the International Society for Immunology of Reproduction. He has published more than 150 papers and regularly presented his work in international immunology, reproductive immunology, and biology of reproduction in various scientific meetings.

CONTRIBUTORS

David T. Armstrong, Ph.D.
Department of Obstetrics and
 Gynecology
University of Adelaide
Adelaide, Australia
 and
Departments of Physiology,
 Obstetrics, and Gynecology
University of Western Ontario
London, Ontario, Canada

Malcolm G. Baines, Ph.D.
Department of Microbiology and
 Immunology
McGill University
Montreal, Quebec
Canada

**Judith N. Bulmer, M.B.Ch.B.,
 Ph.D., MRCPath**
Division of Pathology
University of Newcastle upon
 Tyne
Newcastle upon Tyne, England

Gérard Chaouat, M.D., Ph.D.
Department of Obstetrics and
 Gynecology
University of Paris XI
Clamart, France

**David A. Clark, M.D., Ph.D.,
 F.R.C.P.C.**
Department of Medicine/Obstetrics
 and Gynecology
McMaster University
Hamilton, Ontario
Canada

Robert L. Gendron, Ph.D.
Department of Microbiology and
 Immunology
McGill University
Montreal, Quebec
Canada

Thomas J. Gill, III, M.D.
Department of Pathology
University of Pittsburgh
School of Medicine
Pittsburgh, Pennsylvania

Hong-Nerng Ho, M.D.
Department of Obstetrics and
 Gynecology
National Taiwan University
 Hospital
Taipei, Taiwan

Gholam Reza Jalali, M.Sc.
Immunopathology Department
St. Mary's Hospital Medical
 School
London, England

Christian Jaulin
Department of Immunology
INSERM Unit 277
Institut Pasteur
Paris, France

Hideharu Kanzaki, M.D.
Department of Gynecology and
 Obstetrics
Kyoto University
Kyoto, Japan

Miljenko Kapovic
University of Rijeka
Rijeka, Yugoslavia

Radslav Kinsky, D.Vet., Ph.D.
INSERM Unit 262
Paris, France

Philippe Kourilsky
Department of Immunology
INSERM Unit 277
Institut Pasteur
Paris, France

Heinz W. Kunz, Ph.D.
Department of Pathology
University of Pittsburgh School of
  Medicine
Pittsburgh, Pennsylvania

Elizabeth Menu, Ph.D.
INSERM Unit 262
Clinique University of
  Baudelocque
Paris, France

Takahide Mori, M.D.
Department of Gynecology and
  Obstetrics
Kyoto University
Kyoto, Japan

**James F. Mowbray, M.A.,
  F.R.C.P.**
Immunopathology Department
St. Mary's Hospital Medical
  School
London, England

Raj Raghupathy, Ph.D.
National Institute of Immunology
New Delhi, India

**Christopher W. G. Redman,
  F.R.C.P.**
Nuffield Department of Obstetrics
  and Gynaecology
John Radcliffe Hospital
Oxford, England

Fumitaka Saji, M.D., D.M.Sc.
Department of Obstetrics and
  Gynecology
Osaka University Medical School
Osaka, Japan

Ian L. Sargent, Ph.D.
Nuffield Department of Obstetrics
  and Gynaecology
John Radcliffe Hospital
Oxford, England

Roger F. Searle, Ph.D.
Department of Immunology
The Medical School
University of Newcastle upon
  Tyne
Newcastle, England

**Julia Szekeres-Bartho, M.D.,
  Ph.D.**
Institute of Microbiology
University Medical School
Pécs, Hungary

**Gursaran Prashad Talwar,
  D.Sc., F.A.M.S., F.A.Sc.,
  F.N.A.**
National Institute of Immunology
New Delhi, India

M. N. Thang
INSERM Unit 245
St. Antoine Hospital
Paris, France

Jennifer L. Underwood, M.A.
Immunopathology Department
St. Mary's Hospital Medical
  School
London, England

Thomas G. Wegmann, Ph.D.
Department of Immunology
University of Alberta
Edmonton, Alberta
Canada

TABLE OF CONTENTS

The Roots of the Problem: "The Fetal Allograft"

Gerárd Chaouat

Laboratory of Cellular and Molecular Biology of Reproduction
Antoine Béclère Hospital
Clamart, France

In outbred species, the fetus is semiallogeneic for the mother; indeed, the antigenic composition is different for each conceptus, hence more for each subsequent litter.

Recent developments in *in vitro* fertilization and embryo transfer in humans, as well as domestic or wild animals, now allow the transfer of fully allogeneic embryos until offspring delivery. This is indeed seen in the human species, with surrogate mothers, and, anonymous or not, sperm and oocyte donors. In some cases, xenogeneic pregnancy has been achieved with (as will be discussed later on) or without the creation of interspecies chimeras, challenging the "riddle" for an immunologist by realizing fully xenogeneic offspring. Indeed, it has been possible to transfer Grant's Zebra embryo into mare surrogate mothers, an elegant experiment by Allen et al.[1]

Immunology is a field biased for awhile toward the so-called "externally oriented"—e.g., rejection of nonself vs. acceptance of self—a trend baffled by the discovery of "natural autoantibodies." Students learn that class I major histocompatibility complex (MHC) plus class II MHC grafts

8868-6/93/$0.00 + $.50

are rejected within 12 to 14 days at first set; class II disparate transplants are rejected within usually 40 to 45 days; whereas, on similar MHC background, minor histocompatibility divergent transplants elicit rejection within 40 to 110 days. The second set of rejection is even more rapid, occurring within 7 to 8 days for MHC alone or MHC plus minor histoincompatible tissues. A second allograft with the same minor H differences can, in some cases, trigger a much stronger rejection reaction even than one observed during the first transplant of an MHC-only incompatible organ (the Simonsen's immunization factor).

Yet, the fetus not only manages to survive, it thrives quite well in the face of a potentially hostile maternal immune system. Sir Peter Medawar observed that this posed the immunologist at least "some immunological and endocrinological problems raised by the evolution of viviparity in vertebrates".[2] He called the enigma the "riddle of the success of the fetal allograft". In fact, at that time, allografts were artificial, and most of them were tissue or organ transplants used in clinics.

An important difference with such a case is that an embryo starts from a one-cell stage. It then develops a specialized interface, attaching, then implanting, and, then only, invading maternal tissues. A stalemate of progressive growth and acceptance is then maintained until delivery.

There is some evidence, albeit mostly indirect, that immunological events play a role, more limited than some authors would like to postulate, in delivery, seen by them in grossly oversimplified terms as a rejection phenomenon. However, most of the parturition is NOT mediated by the sole immune system. Furthermore, a transplant immediately confronts the host immune system with allo (MHC or not) antigens, and in the case of an organ transplant, there are the unavoidable passenger donor lymphocytes and an immediate vascularization. The setting up of the embryo is much more progressive, and the immunological "conflict", though seemingly provoked in some mammalian species, is taking place very gradually.

Let us, nevertheless, consider the ongoing pregnancy with a placenta fully organized, and, in many cases though not all, thoroughly embedded in the decidua. This represents the paradigm of the Medawar paradox.

As a first working hypothesis, Medawar envisaged that the uterus was an immunologically privileged site, equivalent to the anterior chamber of the eye, the hamster cheek pouch, where any tissue can be grafted without eliciting rejection. However, allografted tissues are normally rejected inside a nonpregnant as well as a pseudopregnant or a pregnant uterus, although the reaction is slightly delayed, the delay being mostly due to local steroid production.[3] Furthermore, extrauterine pregnancies do not fail for maternal immunological reactions, indeed some abdominal pregnancies have been carried to "term" even in the human species via Caesarean delivery.

The second theory postulated that the placenta was devoid of MHC antigens, and acted as a neutral antigenic barrier between the mother and the fetus. Such an antigenic negativity, with regard for MHC only, is true for implantation up to day 9.5 in mice, being MHC negative from blastocyst stage, as are both spermatozoa and oocytes themselves. In fact, from blastocoel stage, the extracellular cell mass (ECM) remains MHC negative in all species to various stages, depending upon the species, while the inner cell mass (ICM) allows MHC expression of class I or class II on the relevant cell populations. The differentiating ECM status varies between species, even in rodents.

In mice, postimplantation, the so-called extraplacental cone remains still totally MHC negative until it differentiates into the labyrinth (inner part of the rodent placenta) and the spongiotrophoblast. Interestingly, the labyrinth remains MHC negative, whereas the spongiotrophoblast, the outer part of the placenta, directly confronting the maternal circulation, becomes MHC class I positive, expressing H-2 K, H-2 D, and, in the relevant strains, H-2 L in mice. Similarly, polymorphic class I RT1a antigens are expressed in the rat.[4,5] Such a distribution is exactly the opposite one would expect if the placenta was avoiding maternal recognition of the conceptus by building a neutral antigenic barrier.

It has been convincingly shown that in mice, those class I MHCs act as a "paternal strain immunoadsorbent", i.e., MHC class I antigens are in direct contact with the maternal circulation, and maternal-antipaternal alloantibodies bind to these,[6] being then quickly degraded.[7]

No class II expression is seen under physiological circumstances. This fact, observed in rodents, holds true also for human, equine, or porcine species. In fact, in mice, induction of class II by various drugs on both spongiotrophoblast and labyrinth results in abortion, and these abortions can be prevented by anti-Ia antibody treatment, proving a cardinal role for class II repression in fetal survival.[8]

In the rat, the situation is quite comparable to mice except that there is evidence for expression of a monomorphic-like antigen system named Pa1 and Pa2 (pregnancy associated) on spongiotrophoblast, with evidence of genomic imprinting on maternal MHC expression.[9]

In humans, ALL cells of the outer cellular layer of the placenta in contact with maternal blood (the so-called syncytiotrophoblast) are TOTALLY MHC class I and II negative.[10-12] The underlying cytotrophoblast is weak, or not class I positive, and although there is one single report dealing with the induction of class II *in vitro*, the consensus holds for MHC class II negativity.

The downregulation of polymorphic MHC class I in various trophoblasts seems dependent upon hypermethylation of DNA and the action of specific regulatory elements (similar to KBF1) acting on the interferon consensus sequence and NF kappa b KBF1.[13]

In humans, extravillous cytotrophoblasts do express a class I truncated antigen. This molecule was first thought to be HLA-A, -B, or -C, because it reacted with the monoclonal antibody W6 32.[14] In fact, W6 32 reacts with a conserved portion of classical MHC molecules. As for placental MHC, immunoprecipitation has shown that it does *not* exhibit variations from one individual to the other, hence it is suspected to be a monomorphic HLA.[15] This assumption has been proved since the material has been cloned[16,17] by two independent groups and christened HLA-G. Its expression is apparently absolutely restricted to placenta. Such a conservation in evolution (it has analogies with Pa), as well as restricted expression, suggests an immunoregulatory role in defense of the fetoplacental unit.

Indeed, cells transfected so as to express HLA-G are much less sensitive to natural killer (NK) cell-mediated lysis than the HLA-A, -B, or -C transfected control ones.[18]

It is suggested that HLA-G might confuse, trap, or defuse the T cell receptor complex, though no studies yet have been conducted to elucidate in detail the mechanisms of such an action.

The third theory of Medawar purported nonspecific immunosuppression during pregnancy. Indeed, a wide variety of pregnancy-associated materials, of fetal or maternal origin, have been found in human serum to have profound *in vitro* immunosuppressive activities. In fact, most of them when thoroughly purified, lost such activity. Such materials are still referred to in the literature as pregnancy-associated (seric) "blocking factors".

The range of studied molecules encompass HCG, alpha-fetoprotein, SP1, PAP, a variety of steroids, etc. For all of them, it is now suggested that the active moiety was a carried-over contaminant.[19] In the same vein, it has been suggested that the placenta expresses an antigen, named TLX, whose recognition during pregnancy would elicit a specific maternal antibody response. Since activated lymphocytes (maternal?) would express TLX, those antibodies would block their expansion and therefore control maternal antipaternal cellular reactivity.[20]

The problems with those theories, not to mention difficulties in explaining how lymphocytes would present the so-called TLX in a nonimmunogenic form vs. placenta, and difficulties in its purification/identification (TLX has evolved from dimorphic to widely polymorphic, etc.) is that, like the aforementioned immunosuppressive materials, anti-TLX immunity or blocking factors would result in a nonspecific immunosuppression. In fact, ANY activated lymphocyte, irrespective of its specificity, should express TLX or be sensitive to such factors, and, as such, be repressed during pregnancy. In short, the picture should look like acquired immunodeficiency syndrome (AIDS) or SCID mice in a normal environment. However, it is well known that maternal antiviral immunity is not affected by pregnancy,[21] whereas rejection of paternal-strain allografts, albeit alightly enhanced, occurs in primiparous, or even biparous or multiparous animals, even in congenic mating combinations where one deals with an "optimized for memory" system.

This holds true even if one deals with enhancement-prone tumor systems, like the sarcoma SA1, which is optimally enhanced only in multiparous mice. The author's objective opinion is NOT to consider it as representative of a normal situation.[22] Furthermore, one can observe only a flare of some tumors in humans, as well as depressed immunity to *Pneumococcus* SIII and a few viruses and tumors not generally immunodepressive.

The last hypothesis was that specific maternal antipaternal suppressors or regulatory mechanisms were operating during pregnancy. Historically, the first specific mechanism one could suggest is enhancement, since Kaliss and Dagg, who described the enhancement phenomenon, found evidence of antipaternal antibodies during allopregnancy.[23]

Indeed, enhancing antibodies are produced in some strains of mice, and can be eluted from the placenta.[22,24,25] In "producer" strains of mice,[23] where such a response is seen, the alloantibody at seric level is of restricted IgG1 non-complement-fixing isotype,[26] as seen at placental level.

Conversely, one can demonstrate in mice, as well as humans, specific maternal-antipaternal suppressor cells studied in detail *in vitro*,[25,27-35] or, in rodents, by *in vivo* transfer assay systems. Those cells are induced by placental products seen in mice[36] and humans.[37-39] However, pregnancy is perfectly normal in antipaternal-immunized rodent individuals, which reject in a secondary fashion a paternal strain allograft.[40-42] This occurs even in the CBA/J strain, a quasi-perfect strain to study the role of these phenomena, since allopregnancy induces in CBA/J both enhancing antibodies and suppressor cells.[42]

It has, in fact, been shown that the fetus and the placenta were NOT harmed by previous antipaternal-strain immunization of the mother, be it during pregnancy or even before mating. In such cases, cells of paternal-strain origin (a leukemia has been used by T. Wegmann for immunization and clearance monitoring during pregnancy) are cleared from maternal circulation; whereas, this does not occur in the first part of a normal first pregnancy. Thus, according to Wegmann, "Pregnant mice are not primed but can be primed to paternal alloantigens".

Similarly, fourth parity CBA/J mice preimmunized against paternal-strain lymphocytes develop perfectly normal antipaternal CTLs, and reject in a second-set rejection reaction fashion even such a target as sarcoma SA1.[42] Furthermore, not only is the fetus unharmed, but, in fact, in such a preimmunized mother, mean litter size and placental weight are larger than that observed in normal individuals. Similar observations were made by Beer et al.,[43] confirming the concept of "hybrid vigor". They observed that in nonimmunized animals, the litter size and mean placental weight was larger in allogeneic pregnancies than in syngeneic ones. Furthermore, they confirmed that litter size was larger in multiparous than primiparous animals. (In the human, it is well known that, statistically, the mean placental weight is larger in multiparous women than primigravidae.)

Beer et al.[43] also made the paradoxical observation that if one renders the future mother tolerant (at birth, using the classical Medawar neonatal tolerance-inducing protocol) to the antigens of her (future) offspring, the litter size observed later was smaller than the one seen in nonimmunized individuals.[44]

Further dismissal of the humoral (i.e., antibody-mediated) enhancement theory come from observations that pregnancy is perfectly normal in agammaglobulinemic women. In a series of experiments, Mattson and co-workers[44] used anti-μ-depleted B cell mice. Quite interestingly, the placental weight and litter size of such mice is normal. Similarly, they obtained a normal pregnancy common in CD8+ T cell-depleted rats,[45] and we have NOT observed abortions using anti "I-J" antisera, a maneuver that reduced Sal enhancement in classical systems.[46,46a] It follows from the above that systemic regulatory mechanisms are probably NOT essential for successful pregnancy.

The same reasoning that applies for alloantibody production dismisses a necessary role for anti-idiotypic antibodies, whose presence is documented in murine and human pregnancies.[47,48] Nevertheless, at this stage, it is worth signaling that a monoclonal antibody has been produced against a putative suppressor T cell factor named J6B7. This factor has been cloned, its production by T cells is **progesterone dependent**, and monoclonal antibodies raised against it have been shown to be abortifacient in mice. It is important to state here that these antibodies do demonstrate cross-reactivity with lipomodulin[49-51]—an antibody that does not interfere with embryo development *in vitro*.[52] This is a very important control lacking in many polyclonal or monoclonal suppressor factor systems, since a wide variety of polyclonal antibodies, antisera, and even normal sera (some rabbit sera are abortifacient per se in mice due to natural antibodies), are in fact abortifacient because they are teratogens. This is essentially because most cytokines have pleiotropic activities. With this caveat, which will be discussed later, it is the present consensus that systemic regulatory events are not necessary for successful pregnancy. Therefore, the trend has moved towards the observation of local events in the 1980s since the pioneering work of Rossant, followed later by Croy and Clark, with the *Mus musculus/Mus caroli* system.

Mus caroli is a Japanese mouse which has long been segregated from the European/North American *Mus musculus* wild mice—the species from which stems almost all laboratory mice. It is possible to mate a male *Mus musculus* mouse with a *Mus caroli* female, and to obtain a viable, though sterile, offspring. Transfer of *musculus* eggs into *caroli* are always successful, whereas there is almost a constant time schedule for failure of *caroli* embryos in *musculus* uterus. In such a case, eventually cotransferred adjacent *musculus* embryos do survive, whereas all *caroli* embryos die with almost the same program. They are, at day 9.5, surrounded by a dense lymphocytic infiltrate, embryo death with massive CTLs and NK infiltration being observed by day 10 or 11, and the embryos are all completely resorbed by day 13.

It is possible to construct interspecies chimeras. This has been elegantly demonstrated by Rossant and colleagues.[53] Injection chimeras permit selection of the ECM (the future placenta) and ICM (the future embryo) of the strain selected. It is possible to check the injection result later using appropriate enzyme markers. It was observed that *caroli* embryos CAN survive until delivery, provided they are "using" a *musculus* placenta. Conversely, it suffices that an important part of the placenta is of *caroli* origin to provoke death and resorption of *musculus* embryos.[53] This model was the first one allowing the description of immunologically mediated abortions.[53-55] Although this assertion is now debated, one of the great merits of this model, which had other important spin-offs for developmental biology, was to put the focus on local immunoregulatory events.

These may differ from species to species. One of the best examples is oTP1-trophoblastin. In humans, luteolysis is exerted by HCG (human chorionic gonadotrophin hormone). Such a material, however, is lacking in ovine species. The substance that biologically replaces HCG has been isolated and named trophoblastin and, later on, oTP1. It has been purified and sequenced, as well as cloned, and five isoforms are known in goat. The surprise was that this material shows great homology with interferon alpha 2. In fact, it shows antiviral and cytostatic activities comparable to bona fide interferons. Yet, it is secreted **constitutionally** from ovine trophectoderm. It is probably one of the best examples of immunoendocrine interactions available.[55-58] The material is now available in recombinant form either from yeast or *Escherichia coli*. It displays immunosuppressive activity on both PHA-driven lymphocyte proliferation assays and mixed lymphocyte reaction (MLR) per cell-mediated lypholysis (CML) but also triggers (paradoxically, as expected from an interferon), enhanced NK activity.[59,60] However, ovine trophectoderm is, at the stage when it is secreted, most probably resistant to cell-mediated lysis, as observed in mice.[61] Thus, this material could play an important role in the protection of the embryo at the preimplantation stage in ovine species. Indeed, it inhibits a local graft-versus-host (GVH) reaction in mice,[60] and is immunosuppressive of both CD4 and CD8 functions in goat, in *in vitro* assays (unpublished observations). Since then, similar materials have been traced in the pig,[62] and it has been proposed that such nonimmune, pregnancy-related, alpha-like interferons be allowed the special denomination of interferons omega. As stated above, this is one example of immunoendocrine interactions.

No such materials are (yet?) found in mice, where the placenta seems to secrete gamma interferons constitutionally at the preimplantation stage. In the human,[63] the known levels of placental interferons are quite low (below 50 units per milliliter), which is not comparable to the 45,000 units per milliliter observed at peak secretion in sheep and goats.[61] However, care must be taken with interpretation of these human results, since they were obtained with antibodies and probes for classical interferons. The search must go on with interferon omega probes, since such an interleukin 2 (IL-2)-independent pathway has great importance.[64]

An immunoendocrine pathway regulating luteolysis has been described in human. Human placenta secretes high levels of IL-6, and this regulates HCG production. Interestingly enough, the IL-6 production itself is under the control of tumor necrosis factor (TNF),[65] known to be produced by several cells, especially granulated metrial glands in the decidua.

Another mediator involved in pre- and periimplantation events is PAF aceter. The "immunorepulsion" process observed long ago in the uterus by Fauve et al.[66] is in fact a programmed one. If one looks at the uterus of pregnant or pseudopregnant rats and sees that they are pseudopregnant after fallopian tube ligature, one can see that the T cells wane off from the fallopian tube. Such a process is progesterone dependent (it is prevented by RU-43086) and, moreover, PAF dependent. Injection of an anti-PAF aceter compound, known to be anti-implantable and abortifacient in very early pregnancy, perturbs this lymphocyte pattern.[67] Once pregnancy is established (in most species as discussed above) the invasive placenta confronts the mother with paternal MHC antigens, not to mention minor H histocompatibility antigens, as well as developmental and sex-linked ones.[68]

In the human, one must realize that the syncytiotrophoblast is a weak barrier. Indeed, there is small, albeit significant, cellular traffic from both sides in the placental area. For example, small maternal cells gain access into fetal circulation; this is probably the explanation of a certain degree of infant hyporesponsiveness to maternal HLA antigen, a phenomenon being studied at present in detail by van Rood and co-workers in The Netherlands. This is also one of the possible routes of entry of human immunodeficiency virus (HIV) during pregnancy, causing prenatal AIDs. Conversely, fetal cells of various types gain access into the maternal circulation. This is peculiarly evident for fetal erythrocytes, as exemplified by the well-known RH⁻ anti-RH⁺ hemolytic disease. Other *in utero* hemolytic diseases are also known (such as the Kelly syndrome), leading to pregnancy loss. Not only do fetal erythrocytes gain access into the maternal circulation, but cytotrophoblasts enter it via the phenomenon christened "trophoblast deportation" into maternal circulation. This occurs in all species, irrespective of the placentation model, e.g., in pigs, rodents, primates, equids, and ovine. Furthermore, there are regularly microbreaches into syncytio- and cytotrophoblast, and a few maternal cells can be spotted on some (few, indeed, but this does exist) embedded sections of placental beds in the second and third part of pregnancy in humans if one makes regular tissue sections. They thus gain access quite easily in humans to the class I MHC-positive cytotrophoblast, and even a layer underneath to the embryonic fibroblasts (EF), a target for allograft rejection via CTLs and NK cells as well as ADCC cells. Such cellular traffic has, incidentally, excited high hopes of detection and enrichment for fetal cells, in the effort to achieve polymerase chain reactions (PCR) and *in situ* hybridization for prenatal diagnosis, a topic outside the scope of this chapter, but which may soon yield noninvasive prenatal diagnosis techniques. This cell trafficking results in maternal-antipaternal sensitization, as exemplified by the use of sera from multiparous women for tissue typing. Indeed, 16 to 20% of primiparous women, and 60 to 80% in their third pregnancy develop anti-paternal HLA *cytotoxic antibodies*. These call for a protective mechanism at the fetomaternal interface. Indeed, the placenta expresses CD55 and CD46 markers, e.g., complement regulatory proteins [69]

The DAF (decay accelerating factor) and MCP (membrane complement protein) are expressed at the trophoblast surface. These have, incidentally, been discovered as a spin-off of the search for the "TLX antigens". Their presence at the trophoblast outer poles, in contact with maternal circulation, ensures that cytotoxic antibodies cannot lyse the trophoblasts.

One has still to explain which factors are responsible for the statistical decrease of maternal NK immunity observed earlier by Brent et al. and attributed to a serum factor,[70] as well as the total lack of antipaternal CTLs in a normal pregnancy, and the immunity of placenta to CTLs even after deliberate maternal antipaternal immunization. One has also to propose an explanation for the enhancement of placental weight in such a situation.

The survival of the placenta depends for the most part on its own intrinsic properties, secretion of soluble factors, recruitment of decidual associated suppressor T cells, and eliciting an immunoendocrine regulatory pathway involving elicitation of progesterone receptors on activated CD8+ cells.

Following implantation, specific antipaternal T cells accumulate in the decidua in a hormone-dependent fashion.[71] However, a novel type of suppressor cell was discovered in the 1980s by Clark et al.[72-74] who observed that a soluble suppressor activity could be recovered from the uterus by draining lymph nodes, the production of such a factor correlating with successful pregnancy. This phenomenon is detailed in Chapter 6, by Clark. The suppressor moiety has been identified as transforming growth factor (TGF)-beta 2 in the supernatant, using specific neutralizing antibodies.[75,76] The placenta itself is resistant to CTL- and NK-mediated lysis, first, by intrinsic properties.[77,78] In fact, most murine embryonic cells are resistant to many cellular lytic processes until midgestation.[61] The reason for the intrinsic resistance of placenta to the mediated lysis of NK, CTL, and lymphokine-activated killer (LAK) cells is still unclear. It could be attributed to HLA-G, or to lack of triggering of the apoptosis program for cell death.

This resistance is, however, not absolute. For example, murine placental cells can be lyzed by CTLs cultured in Opti MEM medium, a medium which elicits a stronger CTL activity than the one obtained using normal culture media.[79] These CTLs, incidentally, have some LAK cell-like killing characteristics, and LAK cells do lyze trophoblast cells *in vitro*.[80] However, freshly explanted trophoblast cells are resistant to LAK cells and Opti MEM cultured CTLs, and one needs to culture the cells for at least 24 hours.[79] The reasons for the need of such a process, which introduces somehow some artifacts, remain unclear.

Soluble suppressor factors have been isolated from both murine and human placenta. Freshly explanted murine trophoblasts or placental explants isolated under defined conditions, excluding the use of trypsin, have been used to show that cells recovered under these conditions elaborate a potent suppressor factor able to suppress MLR/CML, CTL, and NK activity at the effector stage.[81-93] Similar activities can be traced in the supernatant of human choricarcinomas. These also secrete a suppressor inducer factor, inducing suppressor cells *in vitro* as well as *in vivo* in mice.[37-39] This is reviewed in detail in Chapter 9 by Saji.

Finally, although normal T cells do not express progesterone receptors, it was discovered that alloactivated T cells do. This has been described in detail by Szekeres Bartho and co-workers.[94-98]

The immunosuppressive factor J6B7 is also, as stated previously, produced upon Pg action by activated T lymphocytes. It plays a role in pregnancy success, having been quantified by enzyme-linked immunosorbent assay (ELISA) in spleen and draining lymph nodes during pregnancy[51] and at the fetal-maternal interface, and since an antibody against it is abortifacient.[49,50] These local mechanisms having now been reviewed, can easily be seen to afford, in synergy, a considerable protection to the embryo against potential rejection by the maternal immune system.

Then, of course, the proof that there is an immunologic component in pregnancy would stem from immunologic abortions, whereas at this stage one still requires an explanation for the enhanced placental weight in immunized animals. The reader is referred to Chapters 12 and 14 by Baines and Mowbray, respectively. The most salient feature of most animal models is that they provide systems to study the effect of alloimmunization as a treatment for abortion, and as a result of alloimmunization one observes an increase in placental weight. This observation suggests strongly that T cell soluble factors are involved as growth factors for optimal placental growth, a theory named "immunotrophism" by Tom Wegmann.

Finally, the understanding of this placental cytokine network will have important implications for studying transplacental transmission of HIV and other viruses in general during pregnancy,[99,100] since it is now clear that syncytiotrophoblasts and choriocarcinoma can be infected by HIV via a placental CD4, and this is regulated by local cytokines and enhancing or neutralizing anti-HIV antibodies.

REFERENCES

1. **Allen, W. R., Kydd, J. H., and Antczack, D. F.,** Successful application of immunotherapy to a model of pregnancy failure in equids, in *Reproductive Immunology,* Clark, D. A., Croy, B. A., Eds., Elsevier, Amsterdam, 1986, 253–261.
2. **Medawar, P. B.,** Some immunological and endocrinological problems raised by the evolution of viviparity in vertebrates, *Symp. Soc. Exp. Biol.,* 7, 320–338, 1953.
3. **Beer, A. E. and Billingham, R. E.,** Host responses to intra-uterine tissue, cellular and fetal allografts, *J. Reprod. Fertil. Suppl.,* 21, 59, 1974.
4. **Philpott, K. L., Rastan, S., Brown, S., and Mellor, A. L.,** Expression of H-2 class I genes in murine extra-embryonic tissues, 64, 479–486, 1988.

5. **Billington, W. D. and Burrows, F. J.,** The rat placenta expresses paternal class I MHC antigens, *J. Reprod. Immunol., 9,* 155–160, 1986.

6. **Wegmann, T. G.,** *Immunoregulation and Fetal Survival,* Gill, T. J., III and Wegmann, T. G., Eds., Oxford University Press, New York, 1987.

7. **Wegmann, T. G., Mossman, T. R., Carlson, G., Olingk, O., and Singh, B.,** The ability of the murine placenta to absorb monoclonal anti-fetal H-2 K antibody from the maternal circulation, *J. Immunol., 122,* 270–277, 1979.

8. **Athanassakis Vassiliadis, I. and Papamettheakis, J.,** Modulation of class II antigens on fetal placenta leads to fetal abortion, in *Biologie Cellulaire et Moléculaire de la Relation Materno Fetale,* Chaouat, G. and Mowbray, J., Eds., Editions INSERM/John Libbey, Paris, 1991, 69–81.

9. **Kanbour-Sharir, A., Zhang, X., Rouleau, A., Armstrong, D. T., Kunz, H. W., MacPherson, T. A., and Gill, T. J., III,** Gene imprinting and major histocompatibility complex class I antigen expression in the rat placenta, *Proc. Natl. Acad. Sci. U.S.A., 87,* 444–448, 1990.

10. **Faulk, W. P. and Temple, A.,** Distribution of beta 2 macroglobulin and HLA in chorionic villi of human placenta, *Nature, 262,* 799–802, 1976.

11. **Faulk, W. P. and Hunt, J. S.,** Human trophoblast antigens, *Immunol. Allergy Clin. N. Am. Reprod. Immunol.,* 10:1, 27–48, 1990.

12. **Hunt, J. S., Fishback, J. L., Andrews, G. K., and Wood, G. W.,** Expression of class I HLA genes by trophoblast cells: analysis by in situ hybridization, *J. Immunol., 140,* 1293–1299, 1988.

13. **Le Bouteiller, P., Boucraut, J., Fauchet, R., and Pontarotti, P.,** Transfected HLA class I genes human cell line escape the negative *cis* regulatory control exerted on endogenous class I genes, in *Biologie Cellulaire et Moléculaire de la Relation Materno Fetale,* Chaouat, G. and Mowbray, J., Eds., Editions INSERM/John Libbey, Paris, 1991, 41–51.

14. **Sunderland, C. A., Redman, C. W. G., and Stirrat, G. M.,** HLA A, B, C, antigens are expressed on the nonvillous trophoblasts of the early human placenta, *J. Immunol., 127,* 2614–2615, 1981.

15. **Ellis, S. A., Sargent, I. L., Redman, C. W. G., and McMichael, A. J.,** Evidence for a novel HLA antigen found on human extravillous trophoblast and choriocarcinoma cell line, *Immunology, 59,* 595–601, 1986.

16. **Kovatts, S., Main, E. K., Libbrach, C., Stublebline, M., Fischer, S. J., and De Mars, R.,** A class I antigen, HLA-G, expressed in human trophoblasts, *Science, 248,* 220–223, 1990.

17. **Ellis, S. A.,** HLA-G: At the interface, *Am. J. Reprod. Immunol., 23,* 84–86, 1990.

18. **Kovatts, S., Librach, C., Fisch, P., Main, E. K., Sondel, P. M., Fischer, S. J., and De Mars, R.,** The role of nonclassical MHC class I on human trophoblast, in *Biologie Cellulaire et Moléculaire de la Relation Materno Fetale,* Chaouat, G. and Mowbray, J., Eds., Editions INSERM/John Libbey, Paris, 1991, 13–21.

19. **Stimson, W. H.,** The influence of pregnancy associated serum proteins and steroids on maternal immune response, in *Immunology of Reproduction,* Wegmann, T. G. and Gill, T. J., III, Eds., Oxford University Press, New York, 1983, 281–288.

20. **Faulk, W. P. and McIntyre, J. A.,** Immunological studies of trophoblast markers, subsets and functions, *Immunol. Rev., 75,* 139–175, 1983.

21. **Head, J. R. and Billingham, R. E.,** Immunobiological aspects of the feto maternal relationship, in *Clinical Aspects of Immunology,* 4th ed., Lachman, P. and Peters, D., Eds., Blackwell Scientific, Oxford, 1981, 243–282.

22. **Voisin, G. and Chaouat, G. A.,** Demonstration, nature and properties of antibodies eluted from the placenta and directed against paternal antigens, *J. Reprod. Fertil. Suppl.,* 21, 89, 1974.

23. **Kaliss, N. and Dagg, N. K.,** Immune responses engendered in mice by multiparity, *Transplantation,* 2, 415–420, 1964.

24. **Chaouat, G., Voisin, G. A., Daeron, M., and Kanellopoulos, J.,** Anticorps facilitants et cellules suppressives dans la réaction immunitaire maternelle anti-foetale, *Ann. Immunol. (Inst. Pasteur),* 128, 21–24, 1977.

25. **Chaouat, G., Voisin, G. A., Escalier, D., and Robert, P.,** Facilitation reaction (enhancing antibodies and suppressor cells) and rejection reaction (sensitized cells) from the mother to the paternal antigens of the conceptus, *Clin. Exp. Immunol.,* 35, 13–24, 1979.

26. **Bell, S. C. and Billington, W. D.,** Major antipaternal allo antibody induced by pregnancy is noncomplement fixing IgG1, *Nature (London),* 288, 387–388, 1980.

27. **Smith, G.,** Maternal regulator cells during murine pregnancy, *Clin. Exp. Immunol.,* 44, 90–98, 1981.

28. **Chaouat, G. and Voisin, G. A.,** Regulatory T cell subpopulations in pregnancy. I. Evidence for suppressive activity of the early phase of MLR, *J. Immunol.,* 122, 1383–1388, 1979.

29. **Chaouat, G. and Voisin, G. A.,** Regulatory T cell subpopulations in pregnancy. II. Evidence for suppressive activity of the late phase of MLR, *Immunology,* 39, 239, 1980.

30. **Chaouat, G. and Voisin, G. A.,** Regulatory T cells in pregnancy. III. Evidence for the involvement of two T cell subsets, *Immunology,* 44, 393–399, 1981.

31. **Chaouat, G. and Voisin, G. A.,** Regulatory T cells in pregnancy. IV. Genetic characteristics and mode of action of early MLR suppressive population, *J. Immunol.,* 127, 1335–1336, 1981.

32. **Chaouat, G. and Voisin, G. A.,** Regulatory T cells in pregnancy. V. Allo-pregnancy induced T cell suppressor factor is H-2 restricted and bears Ia determinants, *Cell. Immunol.,* 62, 186–195, 1981.

33. **Baines, M. G., Millar, K. G., and Pross, H. F.,** Allograft enhancement during normal murine pregnancy, *J. Reprod. Immunol.,* 2, 141–148, 1980.

34. **Engleman, E. G., McMichael, A. J., and McDevitt, H. O.,** Suppression of the mixed lymphocyte reaction in man by a soluble T cell factor: specificity of the factor for both the responder and the stimulator, *J. Exp. Med.,* 147, 1037–1045, 1978.

35. **Smith, G.,** Maternal regulator cells during murine pregnancy, *Clin. Exp. Immunol.,* 44, 90–98, 1981.

36. **Chaouat, G., Chaffaux, S., and Voisin, G. A.,** Immunoactive products of placenta. I, *J. Reprod. Immunol.,* 2, 127–136, 1980.

37. **Hamaoka, T., Majusaki, N., Itoh, S., Tsuji, Y., Izumi, Y., Fujiwarah, M., and Ono, S.,** Human trophoblast and tumor cell derived immunoregulatory factor, in *Reproductive Immunology,* Isojima, S. and Billington, W. D., Eds., Elsevier, Amsterdam, 1983, 133–146.

38. **Canepa, S.,** Proprietes Immunologiques in Vitro de Surnageants de Cultures de Choriocarcinomes Humains, DERBH Universite Paris, 1985.
39. **Chaouat, G., Menu, E., David, F., Szekeres Bartho, J., Kinsky, R., Dang, D. C., Kapovic, M., Ropert, S., and Wegmann, T. G.,** Lymphokines, cytokines and immunoregulators involved in pregnancy success or perinatal AIDS, *Period. Biol.,* 93(1), 49–54, 1991.
40. **Mitchison, N. A.,** The effect on the offspring of maternal immunisation in mice, *J. Genet.,* 5, 406–411, 1953.
41. **Lanman, J. T., Dinenstein, J., and Fikring, S.,** Homograft immunity in pregnancy. Lack of harm to fetus from sensitization of the mother, *Ann. N.Y. Acad. Sci.,* 99, 706–718, 1962.
42. **Monnot, P. and Chaouat, G.,** Systemic active suppression is not necessary for successful allopregnancy, *Am. J. Reprod. Immunol.,* 6, 5–8, 1984.
43. **Beer, A. E., Scott, J. R., and Billingham, R. E.,** Histocompatibility and maternal immunological status as determinants of feto-placental size and litter weight in rodents, *J. Exp. Med.,* 142, 180–198, 1975.
44. **Mattson, R., Mattson, A., and Sulila, P.,** Allogeneic pregnancy in B cell depleted CBA/Ca mice. Effects on fetal survival and maternal lymphoid organs, *Dev. Comp. Immunol.,* 9, 709–713, 1985.
45. **Mattson, R. and Holmdal, R.,** Maintained allopregnancy in rats depleted of T cytotoxic/suppressor cells by OX8 monoclonal antibody treatment, *J. Reprod. Immunol.,* 1987.
46. **Kinsky, R. K., Duc, H. T., Chaouat, G., and Voisin, G. A.,** Involvement of suppressor cells in active enhancement of allografted tumors. *In vivo* (adoptive transfer) and *in vitro* (MLR) evaluation. Synergy with enhancing antibodies, *Cell. Immunol.,* 58, 107, 1981.
46a. **Kinsky, R. K. et al.,** unpublished data.
47. **Chaouat, G., Kinsky, R. G., Duc, H. T., and Robert, P.,** The possibility of anti-idiotypic activity in multiparous mice, *Ann. Immunol. (Inst. Pasteur),* 130, 601–605, 1979.
48. **Suciu-Foca, N., Reed, E., Rohowsky, C., Kung, P., and King, D. W.,** Anti-idiotypic antibodies to anti-HLA receptors induced by pregnancy, *Proc. Natl. Acad. Sci. U.S.A.,* 80, 830–834, 1983.
49. **Beaman, K. D. and Hoversland, R. C.,** Induction of "spontaneous" abortion by blocking antigen specific suppression, *J. Reprod. Fertil.,* 82, 135–139, 1988.
50. **Lee, C. K., Ghoshal, K., and Beaman, K. D.,** Cloning of a cDNA coding for a T cell molecule with putative immunoregulatory role, *Mol. Immunol.,* 27, 1131–1137, 1990.
51. **Hoversland, R. C. and Beaman, K. D.,** Embryo implantation associated with increase in T cell suppressor factor in the uterus and spleen of mice, *J. Reprod. Fertil.,* 88, 135–139, 1990.
52. **Hoversland, R. C. and Beaman, K. D.,** The lack of effect of a monoclonal antibody against murine T cell suppressor factor on murine embryo development *in vitro, Am. J. Reprod. Immunol.,* 26, 84–88, 1991.
53. **Rossant, J., Croy, B. A., Clark, D. A., and Chapman, V. M,.** Interspecific hybrids and chimeras in mice, *J. Exp. Zool.,* 288, 223–233, 1983.

54a. **Rossant, J., Mauro, V. M., and Croy, B. A.,** Importance of trophoblast genotype for survival of interspecific murine chimeras, *J. Embryol. Exp. Morphol.,* 69, 141, 1982.

54b. **Clark, D. A., Croy, B. A., Rossant, J., and Chaouat, G.,** Immune presensitisation and local intrauterine defences as determinants of success or failure of murine interspecies pregnancies, *J. Reprod. Fertil.,* 77, 633–643, 1986.

55. **Croy, B. A., Rossant, J., and Clark, D. A.,** Effects of alterations in the immunocompetent status of *Mus musculus* females on the survival of transferred *Mus caroli* embryos, *J. Reprod. Fertil.,* 74, 479–489, 1985.

56. **Charpigny, G., Reinaud, P., Huet, J. C., Guillomot, M., Charlier, M., Pernollet, J. C., and Martal, J.,** High homology between a trophoblastic protein (trophoblastin) isolated from ovine embryos and alpha interferon, *FEBS Lett.,* 228(1), 12, 1988.

57. **Charlier, M., Hue, D., Martal, J., and Gayle, P.,** Cloning and expression of cDNA encoding ovine trophoblastin. Its identity with class II interferons, *Gene,* 77, 341–348, 1989.

58. **Imakawa, K., Anthony, R. V., Kazemi, M., Marotti, K. R., Polites, H. G., and Roberts, R. M.,** Interferon-like sequence of ovine trophoblast protein secreted by embryonic trophectoderm, *Nature,* 330, 377, 1987.

59. **Martal, J., Chene, G., Charlier, M., Guillomot, M., Reinaud, P., Bertin, J., Danet, G., Zouari, K., and Charpigny, G.,** Trophoblastin, oTP, embryonic interferons, in *Placental Communications: Biochemical, Morphological and Cellular Aspects,* Cedard, L. et al., Eds., Colloque INSERM/John Libbey, Paris, 1990, 125.

60. **Fillion, C., Chaouat, G., Reinaud, P., Charpigny, J. C., and Martal, J.,** Immunoregulatory effects of trophoblastin (oTP): all 5 isoforms are immunosuppressive of PHA driven lymphocyte proliferation, *J. Reprod. Immunol.,* 19, 237–249, 1991.

61. **Croy, B. A. and Rossant, J.,** Mouse embryonic cells become susceptible to CTL mediated lysis after midgestation, *Cell. Immunol.,* 104, 355–365, 1987.

62. **Lefevre, F., Martinat-Botte, F., Guillomot, M., Zouari, K., Charley, B., and La Bonnardiere, C.,** Interferon-gamma gene and protein are spontaneously expressed by the porcine trophectoderm early in gestation, *Eur. J. Immunol.,* 20, 2485, 1990.

63. **Chard, T.,** Interferon as a fetoplacental signal in human pregnancy, in *Placental Communications: Biochemical, Morphological and Cellular Aspects,* Cedard, L. et al., Eds., Colloque INSERM/John Libbey, Paris, 1990, 117.

64. **Iwano, Y., Hansen, T. R., Kazemi, M., Malathy, P. V., Johnson, D., Roberts, R. M., and Imakawa, K.,** Suppression of T-lymphocyte blastogenesis by ovine trophoblast protein-1 and human interferon-alpha may be independent of interleukin-2 production, *Am. J. Reprod. Immunol.,* 20, 21–26, 1989.

65. **Neki, R., Matsusaki, N., Masuhiro, K., Taniguchi, T., Shimoya, K., Jo, T., Li, Y., Takagi, T., Saji, F., and Tanizawa, T.,** Analysis of the mechanism of tumor necrosis factor alpha induced release of human chorionic gonadotrophin from normal human trophoblasts, in *5th Annu. Meet. Japan Society for Basic Reproductive Immunology and Japan Society for Medical Reproductive Immunology: Joint Meeting 1990,* Honjo, K. and Kasahura, S., Eds., Japan Society for Basic Reproductive Immunology/Japan Society for Medical Reproductive Immunology, Tokyo, 1990, 108–114.

66. **Fauve, R., Hevin, B., Jacob, H., Gaillard, J., and Jacob, F.,** Anti-inflammatory effect of murine malignant cells, *Proc. Natl. Acad. Sci. U.S.A.,* 71, 4052–4056, 1974.

67. **Kachkache, M., Acker, G. M., Chaouat, G., Noun, A., and Garabedian, M.,** Hormonal and local factors control the immunohistochemical distribution of immunocytes in the rat uterus before conceptus implantation: effects of ovariectomy, fallopian tube section and RU 486 injection, *Biol. Reprod.,* 45, 860–868, 1991.

68. **Heyner, S.,** Antigens of trophoblast and early embryo, in *Immunological Aspects of Infertility and Fertility Regulation,* Dhindsa, D. S. and Schumacher, G. F. B., Eds., Elsevier, Amsterdam, 1980, 183–203.

69. **Purcel, D. F. J., Brown, M. A., Russel, S. M., Clark, C. J., McKenzie, I. F. C., and Deacon, N. J.,** The cDNA cloning of human CD46, an antigen system incorporating TLX and MCP. Existence of multiple alternative splice variants, *J. Reprod. Immunol. Suppl.,* 207, 1989.

70. **Barret, D. S., Rayfield, L. S., and Brent, L.,** Suppression of natural cell mediated cytotoxicity in man by maternal and neonatal serum, *Clin. Exp. Immunol.,* 47, 742–748, 1982.

71. **Clark, D. A., Brierley, J., Barwatt, D., and Chaouat, G.,** Hormone induced preimplantation LyT2+ murine uterine suppressor cells persist after implantation and may reduce the spontaneous abortion rates in CBA/J mice, *Cell. Immunol.,* 123, 334–343, 1989.

72. **Clark, D. A., McDermott, M., and Sczewzuk, M. R.,** Impairment of host-versus-graft reaction in pregnant mice. II. Selective suppression of cytotoxic cell generation correlates with soluble suppressor activity and successful allogeneic pregnancy, *Cell. Immunol.,* 52, 106–118, 1980.

73. **Clark, D. A.,** Maternal immune response to the fetus, *EOS-Rev. Immunol. Immunofarmacol.,* 2, 114–117, 1985.

74. **Clark, D. A., Chaput, A., and Tutton, B.,** Active suppression of host-versus-graft reaction in pregnant mice. VII. Spontaneous abortion of CBA × DBA/2 fetuses in the uterus of CBA/J mice correlates with deficient non-T suppressor cell activity, *J. Immunol.,* 136, 1668–1771, 1986.

75. **Clark, D. A., Flanders, K. C., Banwatt, D., Millar-Book, W., Manuel, J., Stedronska-Clark, J., and Rowley, B.,** Murine pregnancy decidua produces a unique immunosuppressive molecule related to transforming growth factor beta-2, *J. Immunol.,* 144(12), 3004–3008, 1990.

76. **Clark, D. A., Lea, R. G., Denburg, J. et al.**, Transforming growth factor beta related factor in mammalian pregnancy decidua: homologies between the mouse and human in successful pregnancy and in recurrent unexplained abortion, in *Biologie Cellulaire et Moléculaire de la Relation Materno Fetale,* Chaouat, G. and Mowbray, J., Eds., Editions INSERM/John Libbey, Paris, 1991, 131–141.

77. **Zuckerman, F. A. and Head, J. R.**, Murine trophoblasts resist cell mediated lysis. I. Resistance to allospecific cytotoxic T lymphocytes, *J. Immunol.,* 139(9), 2856–2865, 1987.

78. **Zuckerman, F. A. and Head, J. R.**, Murine trophoblasts resist cell mediated lysis. II. Resistance to natural cell mediated cytotoxicity, *Cell. Immunol.,* 116, 274, 1988.

79. **Drake, B. L. and Head, J. R.**, Murine trophoblast cells can be killed by allospecific cytotoxic T lymphocytes generated in Gibco OPTI MEM medium, *J. Reprod. Immunol.,* 15, 71, 1989.

80. **Drake, B. L. and Head, J. R.**, Murine trophoblast cells are susceptible to lymphokine activated killer (LAK) cell lysis, *Am. J. Reprod. Immunol.,* 16(3), 114, 1988.

81. **Chaouat, G. and Kolb, J. P.**, Immunoactive products of murine placenta. II. Afferent suppression of maternal cell mediated immunity by supernatants from short term enriched cultures of murine trophoblast enriched maternal cell populations, *Ann. Immunol. Inst. Pasteur,* 135C, 205, 1984.

82. **Kolb, J. P., Chaouat, G., and Chassoux, D. J.**, Immunoactive products of placenta. III. Suppression of natural killing activity, *J. Immunol.,* 132, 2305–2312, 1984.

83. **Chaouat, G. and Kolb, J. P.**, Immunoactive products of placenta. IV. Impairment by placental cells and their products of CTL function at the effector stage, *J. Immunol.,* 135, 215–221, 1985.

84. **Chaouat, G. and Kolb, J. P.**, Immunoactive products of placenta. IV. Impairment by placental cells and their products of CTL function at effector stage, *J. Immunol.,* 135, 215–221, 1985.

85. **Culouscou, J. M., Remacle Bonnet, M. M., Pommier, G., Rancer, J., and Depieds, R. C.**, Immunosuppressive properties of human placenta: study of supernatants from short term syncytiotrophoblast cultures, *Cell. Immunol.,* 9, 33, 1986.

86. **Hamaoka, T., Majusaki, N., Itoh, S., Tsuji, Y., Izumi, Y., Fujiwarah, M., and Ono, S.**, Human trophoblast and tumor cell derived immunoregulatory factor, in *Reproductive Immunology,* Isojima, S. and Billington, W. D., Eds., Elsevier, Amsterdam, 1983, 133.

87. **Skibin, A., Segal, S., and Quastel, R.**, Suppression of lymphocyte activation by a soluble factor from human placental membranes, in *6th Congress of Immunology,* National Council of Canada, Toronto, 1986, 6–21.

88. **Saji, F., Koyama, M., Kameda, T., Negoro, T., Nakamuro, R., and Tanizawa, O.**, Effect of a soluble factor secreted from human trophoblast cells on *in vitro* lymphocyte reactions, *Am. J. Reprod. Immunol.,* 13(4), 121, 1987.

89. **Tsuji, S., Lee, Y., Nakagawa, S., Satomi, S., and Isojima, S.,** IL-2 receptor-inhibiting substance in the sedimented fraction (105,000 g) of culture medium of choriocarcinoma cell line, in 6th Int. Congress of Immunology, National Research Council of Canada, Toronto, 1986, 6, 14, and 21.

90. **Menu, E., Kaplan, L., Andreu, G., Denver, L., and Chaouat, G.,** Immunoactive products of human placenta. I. An immunoregulatory factor obtained from explant cultures of human placenta inhibits CTL generation and cytotoxic effector activity, *Cell. Immunol.,* 119, 341, 1989.

91. **Menu, E., David, V., Bensussan, A., and Chaouat, G.,** Immunoactive products of human placenta. II. Direct inhibition of non-MHC specific, non-MHC restricted cytolytic activity of human alpha beta, but not gamma delta positive T cell clones, *J. Reprod. Immunol.,* 16, 137, 1989.

92. **Menu, E., Jankovic, D. L., Theze, J., David, V., and Chaouat, G.,** Immunoactive products of human placenta. III. Characterization of an inhibitor affecting lymphocyte proliferation, *Reg. Immunol.,* 3, 254–259, 1991.

93. **Menu, E., Kinsky, R., Hoffman, M., and Chaouat, G.,** Immunoactive products of human placenta. IV. Immunoregulatory factors obtained from cultures of human placenta inhibit local and general murine graft-versus-host reactions (GVHR), *J. Reprod. Immunol.,* 20, 195–204, 1991.

94. **Szekeres-Bartho, J., Kilar, F., Falkay, G., Csernu, V., Torok, A., and Pacsa, A. S.,** Progesterone treated lymphocytes release a substance inhibiting cytotoxicity and prostaglandin synthesis, *Am. J. Reprod. Immunol.,* 9, 15–24, 1985.

95. **Szekeres Bartho, J., Autran, B., Debre, P., Andreu, G., Denver, L., Blot, P., and Chaouat, G.,** Immunoregulatory effects of a suppressor factor from healthy pregnant women's lymphocytes after progesterone induction, *Cell. Immunol.,* 122, 281, 1989.

96. **Szekeres Bartho, J., Reznikoff Etievant, M., Varga, P., Pichon, M. F., Varga, Z., and Chaouat, G.,** Lymphocytic progesterone receptors in human pregnancy, *J. Reprod. Immunol.,* 16, 239, 1989.

97. **Szekeres Bartho, J., Weill, B. J., Mike, G., Houssin, D., and Chaouat, G.,** Progesterone receptors in lymphocytes of liver transfused patients, *Immunol. Lett.,* 22, 259, 1989.

98. **Szekeres Bartho, J., Szekeres, G., Debre, P., Autran, B., and Chaouat, G.,** Reactivity of lymphocytes to a progesterone receptor specific monoclonal antibody, *Cell. Immunol.,* 125, 273, 1990.

99. **David, F. J. E., Autran, B., Tran, H. C., Menu, E., Raphael, M., Debre, P., Barre-Sinoussi, F., Wegmann, T. G., Hsi, B., and Chaouat, G.,** Human placental cells are CD4 positive and permissive to HIV infection, *Clin. Exp. Immunol.,* 88, 10–16, 1992.

Chapter 2

Immunogenetics of Reproduction

Thomas J. Gill III
Department of Pathology
University of Pittsburgh School of Medicine
Pittsburgh, Pennsylvania

Hong-Nerng Ho
Department of Obstetrics and Gynecology
National Taiwan University Hospital
Taipei, Taiwan

Heinz W. Kunz
Department of Pathology
University of Pittsburgh School of Medicine
Pittsburgh, Pennsylvania

1. INTRODUCTION

The reproductive process is critical to all biological systems, and its stabilization is a central force in evolution. The biological mechanisms that control it also influence future growth and development—both normal and abnormal. The program regulating this complex process is embedded in the genome, and it is closely related to the development of biological individuality. The factors influencing the latter process are controlled to a large extent

8868-6/93/$0.00 + $.50

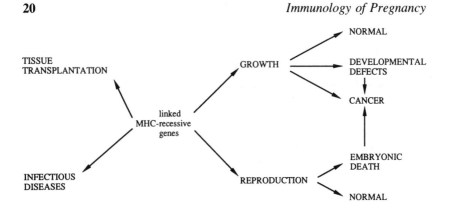

Figure 1. Schematic representation of the hypothesis showing the relationship between MHC-linked recessive lethal genes and reproduction, developmental defects, and susceptibility to cancer. The MHC genes that affect tissue transplantation and resistance to infectious diseases are the ones involved in the immunological aspects of the maternal fetal interaction. (Reprinted from Gill, T. J., III, in *Immunological Obstetrics,* Coulam, C. et al., Eds., W. W. Norton, New York, in press. With permission.)

by the genes of the major histocompatibility complex (MHC), and these genes and the segment of the chromosome carrying them have been conserved throughout evolution from the sponge to the human.[15] Their functions in transplantation and in resistance to infectious diseases have been studied extensively, and in recent years their role, and that of the genes linked to them, in implantation and in the development of the embryo has been systematically explored.

The immunogenetic factors influencing reproduction fall into two broad categories: those regulated by the genes of the MHC itself and those regulated by the MHC-linked genes. The hypothesis delineating the unique role of this segment of the chromosome in a broad range of crucial biological functions is illustrated in Figure 1.[13] First, the role of the MHC genes themselves may be considered a part of the general problem of tissue transplantation. This area focuses on three questions: (1) the study of the monomorphic class I antigens found in relatively large amounts in the placenta—the Pa antigen in the rat, and the W6/32-positive antigen and HLA-G antigen in the human; (2) the control of the expression of the MHC antigens in the placenta; and (3) the lack of immunological rejection of the placenta. Second, the MHC-linked genes play a role more closely associated with developmental genetics. These gene have been shown both in experimental animals and in humans to be involved in the pathogenesis of recurrent spontaneous abortions, developmental defects (congenital anomalies), and susceptibility to cancer.[12,16,23-25,33,36]

2. PLACENTAL MHC ANTIGENS AND THEIR EXPRESSION

2.1. Monomorphic Class I Antigens

The class I antigens encoded by the MHC have frequently been referred to as classical or nonclassical transplantation antigens. This differentiation is based on their role in tissue rejection, in which the classical class I antigens cause acute rejection and the nonclassical antigens cause chronic rejection. This system has been studied in detail in the mouse and, to a lesser extent, in the rat. The characteristics of the nonclassical class I antigens[9,20] are very low polymorphism; variation in the size of the heavy chain, generally due to a premature stop codon; presence in a large chromosomal region which is subject to expansion and contraction; more restrictive tissue distribution; fewer genes transcribed relative to the number present; unusual membrane linkages, for example, phosphatidyl inositol linkage; and a donor role in gene conversion. These nonclassical genes also appear to be present in the human based on studies at the molecular level, but their cell surface expression has not been studied in any detail.[6,7,11,30,31]

The Pa antigen in the rat has many of the characteristics of a nonclassical class I antigen in contrast to the A^a antigen, which is a very strong classical class I transplantation antigen. These antigens have been identified as separate entities by a variety of experimental approaches, including serology, electron microscopy, gene cloning, and transfection.[17,26,38,39] The Pa antigen does not have any serologically definable alleles, and all strains studied have been either Pa^+ or Pa^-. All Pa^- females make anti-Pa antibody when mated with Pa^+ males, and all of the antibody can be removed by absorption with any Pa^+ strain. A Pa^+ female mated with a Pa^- male or a Pa^+ female mated with a Pa^+ male do not make any antibody response. The molecular mass of the Pa antigen is 45,000, and it is the same on the trophoblast and on the lymphocytes.[42] Molecular analysis using digestion with *Xba*I and high-stringency conditions showed that Pa^+ strains have a unique 1.8-kb band and Pa^- strains have a unique 1.7-kb band.[38] Thus, the Pa gene is present in both Pa^+ and Pa^- strains, but it is not expressed in the Pa^- strains. In humans, there are class I antigens, or genes encoding them, that are similar to the Pa antigen system: the antigen detected by the W6/32 antibody on extravillous trophoblast[22,40] and the HLA-G gene that has been cloned from the placenta.[32]

2.2. Regulation of MHC Antigen Expression

The placenta is a microcosm of different—and in some cases unique—regulatory mechanisms affecting MHC antigen expression. These mecha-

TABLE 1.
Mechanisms Controlling MHC Antigen Expression in the Rat Placenta

Gene imprinting
  · Paternal (not maternal) allele-specific class I antigens (RT1.A) and the Pa
    antigen are expressed in the basal trophoblast cells

Constitutive suppression
  · All class II antigens
  · Allele-specific class I antigens and the Pa antigen in the labyrinthine
    trophoblast

Inducible suppression
  · Allele-specific class I antigens on the membrane of the basal trophoblast cells
    in allogeneic pregnancies

nisms may be classified into three general types, and they are summarized in Table 1.

First, gene imprinting occurs such that placental development depends primarily on the paternal genome, and fetal development primarily on the maternal genome.[46] This difference in genetic control is also reflected in the expression of the *A* and *Pa* genes in the placenta of the rat.[26,28] Studies involving both natural matings and embryo transfers in various combinations of the WF(*u*) and DA(*a*) strains of inbred rats showed that the maternal class I antigens are not expressed in the placenta (Table 2). In the natural mating (female × male) WF × DA, A^u is not expressed and in the DA × WF mating, A^a and Pa are not expressed. These observations were confirmed in embryo transfer studies (embryo [female × male] → pseudopregnant female): in the WF × DA → WF transfer, the A^u antigen was not expressed, and in the DA × WF → WF transfer, the Pa and A^a antigens were not expressed.[27,28]

Second, no class II antigens are expressed anywhere in the placenta of the rat,[26] mouse,[3,45] or human.[2,8] No class I antigens are expressed in the labyrinthine trophoblast of the rat[26] or the mouse[48] placentas. This lack of expression may be due to the methylation of the class II genes,[26] and this hypothesis is currently being tested in our laboratory.

Third, there is inducible downregulation of the classical class I transplantation antigens on the trophoblast membrane in allogeneic, but not in syngeneic, pregnancies: the A^a antigen on the placenta of the WF × DA mating and the A^u antigen on the placenta of the DA × WF mating are not expressed (Table 2).[26,28] This downregulation was not seen, however, in embryo transfer studies in which the female was made pseudopregnant by mechanical stimulation and the embryo was transferred at the 2-cell (24 hour) stage (Table 2). In the DA × DA → WF and WF × DA → WF transfers, there was no downregulation of the A^a antigen, and in the DA × WF →

TABLE 2.
Gene Imprinting and MHC Class I Antigen Expression in the Placenta of the Rat from Natural Matings and from Embryo Transfers in the WF (A^u Pa^-) and DA (A^a Pa^+) Strains

Type of Mating	Combination	Antigenic Disparity (Mother → Fetus)	Location	Antigen Expression			Comments
				Pa	A^a	A^u	
Natural	WF × DA	$u \rightarrow a$	M	+	0	0	Downregulation of A^a on M
			C	+	+	0	Suppression of maternal Ag
	DA × WF	$a \rightarrow u$	M	0	0	0	Downregulation of A^u on M
			C	0	0	+	Suppression of maternal Ag
	DA × DA	$a \rightarrow a$	M	+	+	0	No downregulation of A^a
			C	+	+	0	
	WF × WF	$u \rightarrow u$	M	0	0	+	No downregulation of A^u
			C	0	0	+	
Embryo transfer	DA × DA → DA	$a \rightarrow a$	M	+	+	0	Control
			C	+	+	0	
	DA × DA → WF	$u \rightarrow a$	M	+	+	0	No downregulation of A^a
			C	+	+	0	
	WF × DA → WF	$u \rightarrow u/a$	M	+	+	0	No downregulation of A^a
			C	+	+	0	Suppression of maternal Ag
	DA × WF → WF	$u \rightarrow a/u$	M	0	0	0	No downregulation of A^u
			C	0	0	+	Suppression of maternal Ag

Note: M, Membrane; C, Cytoplasm; Ag, Antigen.

Reprinted from Gill, T. J., III et al., in *Molecular and Cellular Immunobiology of the Maternal Fetal Relationship*, Chaouat, G., Ed., Editions INSERM, Paris, 1991. With permission.

WF transfer, there was no downregulation of the A^u antigen. These observations support the hypothesis that the uterine environment of the natural mating, including the presence of seminal fluid, is critical for interaction with the embryo in the immediate postfertilization period in order to induce downregulation of the classical class I transplantation antigens on the trophoblast membrane in allogeneic matings.

Preliminary support for this hypothesis comes from *in vitro* fertilization experiments.[20] The amount of Pa and A^a antigens on the trophoblast membrane and in the trophoblast cytoplasm of the DA $\times$ DA $\rightarrow$ DA embryo transfer is approximately the same regardless of whether the embryos were fertilized *in vivo* or *in vitro*. By contrast, there was a 40 to 80% decrease in the amount of these antigens on the membrane and in the cytoplasm of the trophoblast in the DA $\times$ DA $\rightarrow$ WF embryo transfer when the embryo was fertilized *in vitro*, compared to the transfer in which it was fertilized *in vivo*. Beside providing a unique experimental system in which to study the control of class I antigen expression, these observations may have important implications for *in vitro* fertilization in humans.

2.3. Lack of Immune Rejection of the Placenta

A number of different hypotheses about the success of the placental allograft have been generated and are being tested in different laboratories. Many of these hypotheses focus on the elicitation of "blocking antibodies" by antigens on the surface of the placenta; the production of local suppressor factors in the decidua that abrogate the immune response; the resistance of trophoblast cells to attack by antibodies or by sensitized cells; and immunosuppression by the hormonal milieu of pregnancy. Our own hypothesis emphasizes the lack of MHC class II antigen expression in the placenta and the consequent abrogation of the inductive arm of a destructive immune response. Expression of allogeneic class I antigens by itself appears to be tolerated in some tumor systems,[4] and it does not appear to affect pregnancy, at least the first pregnancy, in embryo transfer studies.[27,28] Hence, it does not appear as if the class I antigens play the key role in the immunogenicity of the placenta. In any event, future experiments should sort out which of these various hypotheses, or parts thereof, may explain the resistance of the placenta to immune rejection.

3. MHC-LINKED GENES

The region linked to the MHC has been the subject of study in a variety of species in recent years,[9,10,34] and it has been shown to influence the reproductive process and susceptibility to cancer in both rats and humans.[13,23-25,33,36] Similar reproductive and developmental defects also occur in mice bearing various *t*-haplotypes.[1,29,35,44]

Experimental studies in the rat have demonstrated the existence of genes linked to the MHC that influence a broad range of growth processes. This region has been designated the growth and reproduction complex (*grc*), and it has been studied in detail from the phenotypic to the molecular levels. The function of the genes in this region does not appear to be materially influenced by the MHC genes themselves or by nonMHC genes.[16,33,36,37] The effects of the *grc*⁻ phenotype—compared to the normal phenotype (*grc*⁺)—on body weight, gonadal development, and the development of cancer following exposure to diethylnitrosamine (DEN) are summarized in Table 3. Both male and female *grc*⁻/*grc*⁻ rats are smaller (developmental defects); the males are sterile (reproductive defect); the females have reduced fertility (reproductive defect); and males are highly susceptible to DEN-induced carcinogenesis. The heterozygotes (*grc*⁻/*grc*⁺) behave as do the normal rats (*grc*⁺/*grc*⁺); hence, the genetic defect in the *grc*⁻/*grc*⁻ animals is recessive. Recent studies have shown that the same pattern is true for the development of breast cancer in female rats following exposure to dimethylbenzanthracene (DMBA).[37] The basis of the growth defects and the susceptibility to chemical carcinogens appears to be the deletion of approximately 70 kb of DNA in the MHC-linked region that may carry genes important for growth and also tumor suppressor genes.[5,47]

The evidence for the existence of similar genes in humans comes from an analysis of data in the literature on the sharing of HLA antigens in recurrent spontaneous abortions,[14,18,41] and from extensive studies on recurrent spontaneous abortions (reproductive defect)[24] and gestational trophoblastic tumors (susceptibility to cancer)[25] in an ethnically homogeneous population of Chinese in Taiwan. A recent study[23] tested the major prediction of this model in humans: relatives of the index couples with recurrent spontaneous abortions should have an increased prevalence of recurrent spontaneous abortions, cancer, and congenital anomalies compared to the relatives of normally fertile couples because the genes underlying these diseases should be segregating with a higher prevalence in this population. This prediction has been borne out by epidemiological studies, and they are summarized in Table 4. Thus, both experimental studies in rats and clinical studies in humans provide strong support for the critical role of MHC-linked genes in growth, reproduction, and susceptibility to cancer.

The mechanisms underlying the action of these MHC-linked genes could involve complementation of recessive lethal genes (or gene deletions) on the same chromosome, complementation of recessive lethal genes on two different chromosomes, or lethal epistatic interaction.[21] The latter mechanism involves the synergistic interaction between genes on two different chromosomes to give a mortality higher than that expected from the additive effects of the genes.[43] This mechanism was discovered in the rat[19,43] and has been shown to occur in the human.[49] The evidence for lethal epistatic interaction in both species is summarized in Table 5.

TABLE 3.
Reproductive Defects and Susceptibility to Cancer in Rats Having Deletions of Genes Linked to the MHC (*grc⁻*)

Phenotype	Relative Body Weight[a]	Gonad Wt/Body Wt (%)[a]		Precancerous Change[b] GTT-Positive Foci/cm² (6 months)[b]	Cancer[b]	
		Testes	Ovaries		Hepatocellular Carcinoma (10–12 months) (%)[b]	Other Malignant Tumors (12 months) (%)[b]
grc⁺/grc⁺	1.00	0.39	0.013	1	3	0
grc⁺/grc⁻	1.00	0.39	0.013			
grc⁻/grc⁻	0.70	0.07	0.013	18	70	25

[a] Data from References 16 and 33.
[b] Following exposure of males to the chemical carcinogen diethylnitrosamine.[36]

TABLE 4.

HLA Sharing in Normally Fertile Couples and Couples Experiencing Recurrent Spontaneous Abortions; Prevalence of Recurrent Spontaneous Abortions, Congenital Anomalies, and Cancer in Their First-, Second-, and Third-Degree Relatives

	Patient Population	
Parameter	Normally Fertile (%)	Spontaneous Aborters (%)
Index couple		
HLA sharing	22	44
(≥3 of A, B, DR, DQ loci)		
First-degree relatives		
RSA[a]	0.16	1.39
Cancer	3.77	7.49
Congenital anomalies	0.71	0.54[b]
Second-degree relatives		
RSA	0.31	1.21
Cancer	0.82	3.02
Congenital anomalies	0.23	0.88
Third-degree relatives		
RSA	0.03	0.20
Cancer	0.85	0.96[b]
Congenital anomalies	0.25	0.55

[a] RSA, Recurrent spontaneous abortions.
[b] NS, not significant. All other differences between normally fertile couples and recurrent spontaneous aborters are significant at $p \leq 0.05$.

Data from References 23 and 24.

4. CONCLUSION

The data summarized in this paper provide cogent evidence for the central role of genetic factors, at least some of which are linked to the MHC, in controlling the immunogenic profile of the placenta with its attendent role in the reproductive process and in influencing reproductive and developmental capabilities. The close association between the latter role and the influence of these genes on susceptibility to cancer present a new paradigm in both developmental and cancer genetics: the same genes—possibly in various combinations or with mutations—can influence critically the entire growth process, both normal and abnormal. The phenotypic defects extend from the most immediate and severe (fetal loss) through a variety of gradations of less severe defects (congenital anomalies) to the least dramatic, but no less lethal, effect of providing a predisposition (possibly a "first hit") for the develop-

TABLE 5.
Lethal Epistatic Interaction in Rats and Humans

Species	MHC-Linked Recessive Lethal Gene	NonMHC Recessive Lethal Gene	Mortality (%)[a]
Rat	*grc/grc*	+/+	25
		Tal/+[b]	0
	grc/grc	*Tal/*+	<u>70</u>
		H^{re}/+[b]	0
	grc/grc	H^{re}/+	<u>68</u>
Human	HLA/HLA[c]	+/+	<u>62</u>
		C3/C3[d]	8
	HLA/HLA	C3/C3	<u>86</u>

[a]   Lethal epistatic interaction underlined.
[b]   *Tal* is the tail anomaly lethal gene, and H^{re} is the hood restriction gene. Both are recessive
      lethal genes.
[c]   Indicates sharing ≥1 HLA antigen.
[d]   C3 Allele of transferrin.

Reprinted from Gill, T. J., III, in *Immunological Obstetrics,* Coulam, C. et al., Eds., W. W.
Norton, New York (in press). With permission.

ment of cancer, either spontaneously or following exposure to a xenobiotic
agent.

ACKNOWLEDGMENTS

The work in this paper was supported by grants from the National
Institutes of Health (HD 08662, HD 09880, and CA 18659), Beaver County
Cancer Society, Tim Caracio Memorial Cancer Fund, Pathology Research
and Education Foundation, and the National Science Council of the Republic
of China (NSC77-0412-B-002-162, NSC78-0412-B-002-106, and NTUH-
77011-A06).

REFERENCES

1. **Bennett, D.,** T/t Locus, its role in embryogenesis and its relation to classical
   histocompatibility systems, *Prog. Allergy,* 29, 35, 1981.
2. **Brami, C. J., Sanyal, M. K., Dwyer, J. M., Johnson, C. C., Kohorn,
   E. I., and Naftolin, F.,** HLA-DR antigen on human trophoblast, *Am. J.
   Reprod. Immunol.,* 3, 165, 1983.

3. **Chatterjee-Hasrouni, S. and Lala, P. K.,** MHC Antigens on mouse trophoblast cells: paucity of Ia antigens despite the presence of H-2K and D, *J. Immunol.,* 127, 2070, 1981.

4. **Cole, G. A., Cole, G. A., Clements, V. K., Garcia, E. P., and Ostrand-Rosenberg, S.,** Allogeneic H-2 antigen expression is insufficient for tumor rejection, *Proc. Natl. Acad. Sci. U.S.A.,* 84, 8613, 1987.

5. **Cortese Hassett, A. L., Locker, J., Rupp, G., Kunz, H. W., and Gill, T. J., III,** Molecular analysis of the rat MHC. II. Isolation of genes that map to the *RT1.E-grc* region, *J. Immunol.,* 142, 2089, 1989.

6. **Ellis, S. A., Palmer, M. S., and McMichael, A. J.,** Human trophoblast and the choriocarcinoma cell line BeWo express a truncated HLA class I molecule, *J. Immunol.,* 144, 731, 1990.

7. **Ellis, S. A., Strachan, T., Palmer, M. S., and McMichael, A. J.,** Complete nucleotide sequence of a unique HLA class I C locus product expressed on human choriocarcinoma cell line BeWo, *J. Immunol.,* 142, 3281, 1989.

8. **Faulk, W. P., Sanderson, A. R., and Temple, A.,** Distribution of MHC antigens in human placental chorionic villi, *Transplant. Proc.,* 9, 1379, 1977.

9. **Flaherty, L., Elliott, E., Tine, J., Walsh, A., and Waters, J.,** Immunogenetics of the *Q* and *TL* regions of the mouse, *Crit. Rev. Immunol.,* 20, 131, 1990.

10. **Gazit, E., Gothelf, Y., Gil, R., Orgad, S., Pitman, T. B., Watson, A. L. M., Yang, S. Y., and Yunis, E. J.,** Alloantibodies to PHA-activated lymphocytes detect human Qa-like antigens, *J. Immunol.,* 132, 165, 1984.

11. **Geraghty, D. E., Wei, X., Orr, H. T., and Koller, B. H.,** Human leukocyte antigen F (HLA-F). An expressed HLA gene composed of a class I coding sequence linked to a novel transcribed repetitive element, *J. Exp. Med.,* 171, 1, 1990.

12. **Gill, T. J., III,** The borderland of embryogenesis and carcinogenesis. Major histocompatibility complex-linked genes affecting development and their possible relationship to the development of cancer, *Biochim. Biophys. Acta,* 738, 93, 1984.

13. **Gill, T. J., III,** MHC-linked genes affecting reproduction, development and susceptibility to cancer, in *Immunological Obstetrics,* Coulam, C., Faulk, W. P., and McIntyre, J. A., Eds., W. W. Norton, New York, (in press).

14. **Gill, T. J., III,** Immunogenetics of spontaneous abortions in humans, *Transplantation,* 35, 1, 1983.

15. **Gill, T. J., III, Smith, G. J., Wissler, R. W., and Kunz, H. W.,** The rat as an experimental animal, *Science,* 245, 269, 1989.

16. **Gill, T. J., III and Kunz, H. W.,** Gene complex controlling growth and fertility linked to the histocompatibility complex in the rat, *Am. J. Pathol.,* 96, 185–202, 1979.

17. **Gill, T. J., III, Misra, D. N., and Kunz, H. W.,** Expression on the trophoblast of an independent molecule bearing the Pa antigen, *Transplantation,* 47, 745, 1989.

18. **Gill, T. J., III, Ho, H.-N., Kanbour, A., Macpherson, T. A., Misra, D. N., and Kunz, H. W.,** Immunogenetic factors influencing the survival of the fetal allograft, in *Early Pregnancy Loss: Mechanisms and Treatment,* Beard, R. W. and Sharp, F., Eds., Peacock Press, Ashton-under-Lyne, England, 1988, 277–286.

19. **Gill, T. J., IV, Gill, T. J., III, Kunz, H. W., Musto, N. A., and Bardin, C. W.,** Genetic and morphometric studies of the heterogeneity in the testicular defect of the H^{re} rat and the interaction between H^{re} and *grc* genes, *Biol. Reprod.,* 31, 595, 1984.

20. **Gill, T. J., III, Kanbour-Shakir, A., Armstrong, D. T., and Kunz, H. W.,** Gene imprinting of class I antigens in the placenta of the rat, in *Molecular and Cellular Immunobiology of the Maternal Fetal Relationship,* Chaouat, G., Ed., Editions INSERM, Paris, 1991, 31–38.

21. **Gill, T. J., III,** Genetic factors in fetal losses, *Am. J. Reprod. Immunol.,* 15, 133, 1987.

22. **Grabowska, A., Carter, N., and Loke, Y. W.,** Human trophoblast cells in culture express an unusual major histocompatibility complex class I-like antigen, *Am. J. Reprod. Immunol.,* 23, 10, 1990.

23. **Ho, H.-N., Gill, T. J., III, Hsieh, C.-Y., Yang, Y.-S., and Yee, T.-Y.,** The prevalence of recurrent spontaneous abortions, cancer and congenital anomalies in the families of couples having recurrent spontaneous abortions or gestational trophoblastic tumors, *Am. J. Obstet. Gynecol.,* 165, 461, 1991.

24. **Ho, H.-N., Gill, T. J., III, Hseih, R.-P., Hseih, H.-J., and Yee, T.-Y.,** Sharing of human leukocyte antigens (HLA) in primary and secondary recurrent spontaneous abortions, *Am. J. Obstet. Gynecol.,* 163, 178, 1990.

25. **Ho, H.-N., Gill, T. J., III, Klionsky, B., Ouyand, P.-C., Hsieh, C.-Y., Seski, J., and Kunschner, A.,** Differences between Caucasian and Chinese populations in HLA sharing and gestational trophoblastic tumors, *Am. J. Obstet. Gynecol.,* 161, 942, 1989.

26. **Kanbour, A., Ho, H.-N., Misra, D. N., Macpherson, T. A., Kunz, H. W., and Gill, T. J., III,** Differential expression of MHC class I antigens on the placenta of the rat, *J. Exp. Med.,* 166, 1861, 1987.

27. **Kanbour-Shakir, A., Kunz, H. W., Gill, T. J., III, Armstrong, D. T., and Macpherson, T. A.,** Morphologic changes in the rat uterus following natural mating and embryo transfer, *Am. J. Reprod. Immunol.,* 23, 78, 1990.

28. **Kanbour-Shakir, A., Zhang, X., Rouleau, A., Armstrong, D. T., Kunz, H. W., Macpherson, T. A., and Gill, T. J., III,** Gene imprinting and major histocompatibility complex class I antigen expression in the rat placenta, *Proc. Natl. Acad. Sci. U.S.A.,* 87, 444, 1990.

29. **Klein, J. and Figueroa, F.,** Evolution of the major histocompatibility complex, *Crit. Rev. Immunol.,* 6, 295, 1986.

30. **Koller, B. H., Geraghty, D. E., DeMars, R., Durick, L., Rich, S. S., and Orr, H. T.,** Chromosomal organization of the human major histocompatibility complex class I gene family, *J. Exp. Med.,* 169, 469, 1989.

31. **Koller, B. H., Geraghty, D. E., Shimizu, Y., DeMars, R., and Orr, H. T.,** HLA-E. A novel class I gene expressed in resting T lymphocytes, *J. Immunol.,* 141, 897, 1988.

32. **Kovats, S., Main, E. K., Librach, C., Stubbleline, M., Kisher, S. J., and DeMars, R.,** A class I antigen, HLA-G, expressed in human trophoblasts, *Science,* 248, 220, 1990.

33. **Kunz, H. W., Gill, T. J., III, Dixon, B. D., Taylor, F. H., and Greiner, D. L.,** The growth and reproduction complex in the rat: genes linked to the major histocompatibility complex which affect development, *J. Exp. Med.,* 152, 1506, 1980.

34. **Kunz, H. W., Cortese Hassett, A. L., Inomata, T., Misra, D. N., and Gill, T. J., III,** The *RT1.G* locus in the rat encodes a Qa/TL-like antigen, *Immunogenetics,* 30, 181, 1989.

35. **Lyon, M. F.,** The *t*-complex and the genetical control of development, *Symp. Zool. Soc. London,* 47, 455, 1981.

36. **Melhem, M., Rao, K. N., Kunz, H. W., Kazanecki, M., and Gill, T. J., III,** Genetic control of susceptibility to diethylnitrosamine carcinogenesis in inbred ACP (*grc*⁺) and R16 (*grc*) rats, *Cancer Res.,* 49, 6813, 1989.

37. **Melhem, M. F., Kunz, H. W., and Gill, T. J., III,** Genetic control of susceptibility to DEN and DMBA carcinogenesis in rats, *Am. J. Pathol.,* 139, 45, 1991.

38. **Radojcic, A., Kunz, H. W., and Gill, T. J., III,** Expression and analysis of the rat placental class I cDNA clone encoding the Pa antigen, *Immunogenetics,* 31, 326, 1990.

39. **Radojcic, A., Stranick, K. S., Locker, J., Kunz, H. W., and Gill, T. J., III,** Nucleotide sequence of a rat class I cDNA clone, *Immunogenetics,* 29, 134, 1989.

40. **Redman, C. W. G., McMichael, A. J., Stirrat, G. M., Sunderland, C. A., and Ting, A.,** Class I major histocompatibility complex antigens on human extravillous trophoblast, *Immunology,* 52, 457, 1984.

41. **Reznikoff-Etievant, M. F., Durieux, I., Huchet, J., Salmon, C. H., and Netter, A.,** Recurrent spontaneous abortions, HLA antigen sharing and anti-paternal immunity, in *Reproductive Immunology—Materno-Fetal Relationship,* Vol. 154, Chaouat, G., Ed., Colloque INSERM, Paris, 1987, 187.

42. **Saito, M., Misra, D. N., Kunz, H. W., and Gill, T. J., III,** Major histocompatibility complex class I antigens expressed on rat trophoblast cells, *Am. J. Reprod. Immunol.,* 22, 26, 1990.

43. **Schaid, D. J., Kunz, H. W., and Gill, T. J., III,** Genic interaction causing embryonic mortality in the rat: epistasis between the *Tal* and *grc* genes, *Genetics,* 100, 615, 1982.

44. **Silver, L. M.,** Mouse *t* haplotypes, *Annu. Rev. Genet.,* 19, 179, 1985.

45. **Singh, B., Raghupathy, R., Anderson, D. J., and Wegmann, T. G.,** The placenta as an immunological barrier between mother and fetus, in *Immunology of Reproduction,* Wegmann, T. G. and Gill, T. J., III, Eds., Oxford University Press, New York, 1983, 229–250.

46. **Surani, M. A. H.,** Evidence and consequences of differences between maternal and paternal genomes during embryogenesis in the mouse, in *Experimental Approaches to Mammalian Embryonic Development,* Rossant, J. and Pedersen, R. A., Eds., Cambridge University Press, Cambridge, 1986, 401–435.

47. **Vardimon, D., Locker, J., Kunz, H. W., and Gill, T. J., III,** Molecular analysis of the rat MHC. III. Physical mapping of the MHC and *grc* by pulse field gel electrophoresis, *Immunogenetics,* 35, 166, 1992.

48. **Wegmann, T. G.,** The presence of class I MHC antigens at the maternal-fetal interface and hypotheses concerning the survival of the murine fetal allograft, *J. Reprod. Immunol.,* 3, 267, 1981.

49. **Weitkamp, L. R. and Schacter, B. Z.,** Spontaneous abortion, neural tube defects and natural selection, *N. Engl. J. Med.,* 313, 925, 1985.

Immunological Aspects of Human *In Vitro* Fertilization and Embryo Transfer

David T. Armstrong
Departments of Physiology, Obstetrics, and Gynecology
University of Western Ontario, London, Ontario, Canada
and
Department of Obstetrics and Gynecology
University of Adelaide
Adelaide, Australia

Gerárd Chaouat
Laboratory of Cellular and Molecular Biology of Reproduction
Antoine Béclère Hospital
Clamart, France

1. INTRODUCTION

The high rate of implantation failure and early embryonic loss in the human, as well as in many animal species, is still unexplained. Among the various theories that have been proposed to account for this failure is the possibility that the early embryo is susceptible to immune attack, and that

8868-6/93/$0.00 + $.50

failure of production of immunosuppressive factors by the developing conceptus and/or the decidua is a contributing cause in embryo loss at pre- and periimplantation stages.[8] The preimplantation human embryo,[11,37] as well as embryos of several animal species (rabbit;[15] cow, sheep, and pig;[25,27] and mouse[41]), have been reported to produce substances with immunosuppressive properties in culture. The report of a correlation between the *in vitro* release of immunosuppressive activity from early human conceptuses produced by *in vitro* fertilization (IVF) and ability of the conceptuses to establish successful pregnancies following embryo transfer (ET)[14] has stimulated research aimed at identifying the active factor(s) and at determining the feasibility of identifying embryos with the greatest developmental potential by screening IVF culture media for the factor(s). The present review examines the current status of immunomodulatory factor(s) produced by human preimplantation embryos with respect to their identity and putative role(s) in enhancing the success of pregnancy through IVF.

2. SECRETION OF IMMUNOSUPPRESSIVE ACTIVITY BY IVF EMBRYOS

Smart et al.[37] first reported the release of immunosuppressive activity from human embryos produced by IVF, using a rosette inhibition test in which human lymphocytes were incubated with ovum or embryo culture media. Both insemination phase medium (collected after the 24- to 26-h period during which oocytes are exposed to spermatozoa) and growth phase medium (collected after a further 24-h culture period following removal of the ova to fresh medium without spermatozoa) were tested. Although results were not analyzed statistically, a higher rosette inhibition titer (RIT, indicative of higher concentration of putative immunosuppressive activity[29]) was reported for growth phase media from embryos that underwent cleavage to 2- to 8-cell stages than for those that failed to cleave in the growth medium.

In a series of short communications by Daya and Clark, immunosuppressive activity of media in which human embryos were cultured at various stages after IVF was assessed on the basis of ability to inhibit mitogen-stimulated proliferation of peripheral blood lymphocytes (PBL). In the first of this series,[11] culture fluids from 61 ova were tested, representing 42 (68%) that had cleaved to at least the two-cell stage, and 19 (39%) remaining at the one-cell stage after exposure to sperm. Of those that cleaved, 55% exhibited suppressive activity, whereas only 5% of those that failed to cleave possessed such activity.

In a more detailed report, although involving fewer embryos, 12 of 28 ova (43%) that cleaved during the 30- to 32-h culture period after removal from the insemination media released suppressive activity into the growth medium, compared to only 1 of 14 ova that failed to cleave in culture.[12] In this and subsequent studies by these authors, suppression was scored as "positive" for ovum culture media for which numerical values of concanavalin A (Con A)-stimulated ^{3}H-thymidine incorporation by test lymphocytes fell below that observed for control media (cultured without ova or embryos), and negative for media for which incorporation was equal to or greater than that observed for control media. In many instances, media were scored as suppressive "even though the value given by the suppressive supernatant might be only 1 to 2% suppression".[7] In fact, in the report of Daya and Clark,[12] the range in suppressive activities of the 12 supernatants scored as suppressive was from about 2 to 28%, with a mean of only 11.2 ± 3.0%. The 16 supernatants that did not possess suppressive activity had a mean stimulatory activity (enhancement of Con A-stimulated proliferation) of 24 ± 3.5%, with a range from 4 to 52%.

Based on these results, which the authors interpreted as indicative of production of immunosuppressive activity by the recently fertilized ovum, the authors proposed that failure to produce this activity might correlate with the high proportion of embryos that fail both after IVF and ET and after fertilization by normal means *in vivo*. In further research aimed at testing this hypothesis,[14] including a multicenter trial involving considerably larger numbers of observations,[7] statistically significant correlations between the presence or absence of immunosuppressive activity in IVF culture media and the success or failure of the embryos to establish pregnancies were reported. Only embryos with supernatants that were immunosuppressive, as defined above, resulted in pregnancies after ET. Pregnancy was achieved in 22 of 61 patients who received at least one embryo with a suppressive supernatant; whereas of 19 patients receiving only negative embryos, none became pregnant. It should be pointed out that in the study of Clark et al.,[7] it was the insemination phase media, i.e., media harvested at the end of the first 24-h culture of ova with spermatozoa, that were assayed for suppressive activity. This is in contrast to the previous studies by the same group, in which the data presented were for growth-phase media. The authors rationalize this difference on the basis of kinetic data presented for a very limited number of embryos whose media were assayed after three successive days of culture. Two patterns of secretion were observed. In one, a small amount of suppressive activity was released during the first 24 h of culture, i.e., in the insemination-phase medium, followed by a larger amount of activity during the second 24 h, in growth-phase medium. In the other pattern, suppression was greatest during the first 24 h of culture, with none observed during the second and third 24-h periods. Based on these results, the authors concluded that "testing the first 24-h medium provided the best chance of detecting suppressive activity under the test conditions".[7]

Subsequent studies of a similar nature by Armstrong et al.[4] and Segars et al.[35] resulted in different conclusions. In agreement with the observations of Daya and Clark, Armstrong et al.[4] found high variability among supernatants in their effects on PBL proliferation, using phytohemagglutinin (PHA) rather than Con A as the mitogen. They examined both insemination-phase and growth-phase media. Both inhibitory and stimulatory activities were present in media obtained from each of these culture periods. Detectable levels of suppressive activity were present in some, but not all, insemination-phase media examined. Levels in growth-phase media were more highly variable, ranging from 83% inhibition to 30% enhancement of ^{3}H-thymidine incorporation. In contrast to the findings of Clark et al.,[7] no relationship was evident between the presence of inhibitory activity and success of pregnancy. In fact, the most "successful" pregnancy of the series (triplets), occurred from transfer of 4 embryos, of which none had secreted detectable suppressive activity.

Segars et al.[35] examined human IVF and embryo culture media for immunosuppressive activity, using inhibition both of Con A-stimulated ^{3}H-thymidine incorporation into PBL, and of one-way mixed lymphocyte response (MLR) as indices of immunosuppression. In their studies, more conservative criteria of immunosuppression were used, because of the "5% to 10% inherent variability in the MLR and Con A assays"; thus they considered inhibitions of only 20% or greater as indicative of "immunologically significant" suppression. Using these criteria, the authors failed to detect significant suppression by either insemination-phase media or growth-phase media during the first 24 h postfertilization. These investigators extended the period of culture to include further stages of embryo growth up to the blastocyst stage (144-h culture). Five of seven embryos that developed to normal blastocysts during the period from 24- to 144-h postfertilization produced significant levels of immunosuppressive activity, varying from 28 to 61% suppression of MLR and 27 to 39% suppression of Con A-stimulated lymphoproliferation. Embryos that developed only to morulae followed by degeneration during this period did not produce significant immunosuppression.

3. CELLULAR SOURCE OF REPORTED IMMUNOSUPPRESSIVE ACTIVITIES

In the initial report of Daya and Clark,[12] the culture media examined were those in which cleavage occurred after the fertilized ova were removed from the insemination medium, and therefore would not have been expected to contain substances of sperm or cumulus cell origin. On the other hand, in their more recent reports from this laboratory in which a correlations were observed between the presence of immunosuppressive activity and success of pregnancy, the assays were performed on media obtained at the end of the first 24 h in culture, i.e., the insemination-phase media. The latter cultures contained spermatozoa as well as cumulus cells, both of which could have contributed to the activity measured. Clark et al.[7] found immunosuppressive activity in supernatants of washed human spermatozoa of similar molecular weight (on high-performance liquid chromatography [HPLC] analysis) as that from IVF embryos, and concluded that spermatozoa were a possible source of the activity being measured.

In the studies of Armstrong et al.,[4] control media examined included IVF culture medium alone, as well as medium in which spermatozoa and cumulus cells were cultured alone and together, but without oocytes. Low levels of suppressive activity were found in medium from sperm cultures, and considerably higher levels were found in cumulus cell cultures, raising the possibility that both sperm and cumulus cells may have contributed to the activity present in IVF culture media. Particularly in view of the high levels of activity found in cumulus cell cultures, the authors suggested that variability in numbers of cumulus cells adhering to ova after transfer from the insemination media to the growth media could be the cause of the high variability in immunosuppressive activity observed among embryos.

Human embryos at later stages of development, i.e., at blastocyst stage, were found to produce considerably greater amounts of immunosuppressive activity than those at earlier stages, including the first and second 24-h culture periods following insemination *in vitro*.[35] Thus, it would appear that all the immunosuppressive activity associated with IVF embryos is not of sperm or cumulus cell origin, and that cells of the blastocyst, possibly trophoblast cells, are also a source of activity. This would appear to be in agreement with several studies with laboratory and farm animal species, in which trophoblast tissue from preimplantation blastocysts (from IVF) produced immunosuppressive material(s) (murine,[41] ovine and porcine,[27] and bovine[9]).

4. CHEMICAL NATURE OF IMMUNOSUPPRESSIVE MATERIAL

Attempts to identify immunosuppressive molecules produced by human embryos have not yet led to conclusive results. Daya and Clark[13] have employed HPLC to fractionate human IVF supernatants obtained from both insemination-phase and embryo-growth-phase cultures. Two low-molecular-weight fractions, corresponding to 3700 and 1200 Da, were found to have immunosuppressive activity. In a later study employing similar analytical techniques,[7] high-molecular-weight (>100 kDa) peaks of activity were also seen, in addition to the two peaks at 3700 and 1200 Da. These high-molecular-weight peaks were attributed to molecules present in the adult human serum used in the culture media, and lacking in the human cord serum used in the previous studies. They were present in IVF media whether or not the embryos were successful in establishing pregnancies. On the other hand, the authors claimed that the two low-molecular-weight compounds were present only in media from embryos that resulted in pregnancies, supporting their belief that it is these low-molecular-weight compounds that are responsible for the immunosuppression that is of relevance to the success of pregnancy.

In addition to the peaks of suppressive activity, HPLC peaks of stimulatory activity were evident in supernatants from embryos that failed to establish pregnancies.

Of considerable interest in the report of Clark et al.[7] was the observation that low-molecular-weight HPLC peaks of immunosuppressive activity were also found in supernatants from 24-h cultures of spermatozoa alone. This observation, and the fact that compounds in this size range apparently were present in IVF supernatants from embryos that established pregnancies but absent in those of embryos that failed, has led these authors to focus further attention on substances of this size present in embryo culture media, as well as on polyamine compounds (spermine, spermidine) known to be present in semen. Lea et al.[23] performed HPLC analyses on pooled IVF culture media from inhibitory and from stimulatory supernatants, and analyzed the resulting HPLC fractions in Con A-stimulated lymphoproliferation assays. Confirming previous findings, they observed peaks of suppressive activity in the 1000- to 5000-Da range in pooled suppressive supernatants; these peaks had significantly more suppressive activity than the same HPLC fractions from pooled supernatants that were stimulatory.

Previous authors had shown that the immunosuppressive activity of human seminal plasma was attributable largely to polyamines such as spermine, which are converted by monoamine oxidases in fetal calf serum to products such as spermine dialdehyde and acrolein that have potent nonspecific cytotoxic activity on a variety of cells.[2,40] Since polyamines such as spermine can associate as complexes,[3] Lea et al.[23] suggested that such complexes might elute from HPLC columns as molecules larger than 202 Da (the molecular weight of spermine), and therefore spermine complexes might be responsible for the immunosuppressive activity of the peaks which they found in the 1000- to 5000-Da range.

Since the conversion of spermine to cytotoxic products depends on enzymes in noninactivated fetal calf serum, the authors compared the immunosuppressive activity of IVF culture media in lymphoproliferation assays performed in the presence of noninactivated fetal calf serum with that in assays performed with heat-inactivated calf serum, and with human serum, which contains considerably lower levels of monoamine oxidase activity. When fetal calf serum was heat inactivated or replaced with human serum, significantly lower suppressive activity was observed. Further, the addition of inhibitors of monoamine oxidase (hydroxylamine, aminoguanidine) prevented or decreased the magnitude of suppression seen with either unfractionated or HPLC-fractionated IVF culture media. The addition of aminoguanidine to assays in which HPLC fractions of a solution of spermine hydrochloride were tested similarly prevented the ability of these fractions to suppress Con A-stimulated lymphoproliferation. Taken together, these observations suggest that the immunosuppressive activity reported previously in human embryo and sperm culture media may be an artifact of the peculiar culture conditions in which the lymphoproliferation assays were performed, resulting from conversion of polyamines such as spermine in the IVF media to cytotoxic products by enzymes in the noninactivated bovine serum.

A further argument that the suppressive activity in the IVF media could be due to polyamine(s) was that after 66-h culture in the presence of suppressive IVF media, lymphocytes exhibited 30% loss of viability, cited by the authors as ''typical of polyamine-mediated cytotoxicity''.[23] This statement appears to be at variance with conclusions of earlier investigations from the same laboratory, in which incubation of lymphocytes with embryo culture medium for 3 d was found to have no effect on cell viability.[13] Thus, there may be some question whether the embryo-associated immunosuppression reported in the earlier studies from this laboratory[11,12] was due to the same molecular species as those reported in the later studies, in which the active components appear to be similar to polyamines, and may be of sperm rather than embryo origin.

Studies with mouse sperm and embryo culture media, reported by Porat and Clark,[32] provide additional support for the concept that polyamines of embryo and seminal origin may be responsible for the immunosuppressive activity detected. Supernatants prepared from cultured epididymal sperm were highly inhibitory to Con A-stimulated proliferation of mouse lymph node cells. Embryo culture media from the second 24-h period after IVF (growth phase, during which cleavage occurred) of oocytes from young fertile CBA/J mice inseminated with sperm from young fertile males, also were uniformly suppressive, although the inhibition was not as complete as seen with sperm supernatants. In contrast, oocytes from old females failed to cleave in culture following insemination with sperm from fertile young males and did not produce suppressive activity; instead of inhibiting, supernatants from these cultures stimulated lymphoproliferation by 10 to 25%. Oocytes from young females, cultured without spermatozoa, were either stimulatory or only mildly inhibitory, indicating that either residual spermatozoa attached to fertilized ova, or cleaving embryos, and not the oocytes themselves, were the likely source of the immunosuppressive activity. On HPLC fractionation, culture media from both mouse sperm and cleaving embryos produced peaks of immunosuppressive activity with molecular weights in the 1- to 7-kDa range, similar to those reported by Lea et al.[23] for cleaving human ova and sperm. Two additional peaks of suppressive activity in both embryo and sperm supernatants had molecular weights of 100 kDa and 0.3 to 0.4 kDa, and a fifth peak at 20 to 30 kDa was seen in sperm supernatants. The suppressive activities of the 1- to 7-kDa and 0.3- to 0.4-kDa fractions of both embryo and sperm supernatants were not seen when the lymphoproliferation assays were carried out in the presence of amine oxidase inhibitors and human instead of bovine serum, suggesting that the suppressive activity in these low-molecular-weight fractions was due to polyamines, similar to the conclusions reached for human sperm and embryo culture media by Lea et al.[23]

Other compounds with known immunosuppressive properties have been reported in culture media from preimplantation-stage embryos of humans and animals. Prostaglandin E_2 (PGE$_2$), a potent immunosuppressive molecule[18] which downregulates interleukin-2 receptors on T lymphocytes,[34] has been found in culture media from rabbit,[16] mouse,[28] and pig[24,39] blastocysts. Holmes et al.[20] have recently reported PGE$_2$ in culture media from human embryos produced by IVF. All stages examined, from 4-cell to hatched blastocysts, produced PGE$_2$, the greatest amounts being from late blastocysts. Cumulus cell complexes cultured without spermatozoa also produced large amounts of this prostaglandin, but they were apparently not the source of the PGE$_2$ produced by cleaving embryos, since the authors stated that care was taken to completely denude embryos of adherent cumulus cells at the time of examination for fertilization. These findings raise the possibility that the immunosuppressive activity reported by Armstrong et al.[4] in cumulus cell cultures could have been due in part to PGE$_2$.

Van Vlasselaer and Vanderputte[41] tested mouse blastocyst culture supernatant for immunosuppressive activity, using one-way and two-way MLR. Day 3.5 blastocysts cultured in multiwell plates exhibited trophoblast outgrowth and the resulting supernatant medium was highly effective in dose-dependent suppression of both types of MLR. In contrast, no suppressive activity was produced by blastocysts cultured in round-bottomed microtiter plates, under which conditions trophoblast outgrowth did not occur. Later-stage trophoblast cells, from day 7.5 ectoplacental cones and from day 14.5 placentas, also produced immunosuppressive activity, indicating trophoblast cells as the most likely source of the immunosuppressive activity. Addition of anti-progesterone antiserum to ectoplacental cone supernatants abolished their immunosuppressive activity at titers that also reduced the suppressive activity of authentic progesterone. Progesterone has immunosuppressive activity at physiological concentrations at the placenta:endometrium interface[36] and mouse blastocysts have been shown previously to secrete progesterone after, but not before, trophoblast attachment and outgrowth has begun.[6] The findings of Van Vlasselaer and Vanderputte[41] therefore argue strongly in favor of progesterone as the immunosuppressive factor produced by trophoblast cells of mouse blastocysts in their studies, but would seem to exclude progesterone as the compound responsible for the immunosuppression produced by embryos at earlier preimplantation stages of development. Since cumulus cells and granulosa cells are known to undergo luteinization and to secrete progesterone *in vitro,* progesterone may have contributed, along with PGE$_2$, to the immunosuppression observed with culture media from human cumulus cells.[4]

5. SUSCEPTIBILITY OF THE PREIMPLANTATION EMBRYO TO IMMUNOLOGICAL ATTACK

Among the numerous explantations that have been offered to account for the high preimplantation embryo losses that occur in women, especially those undergoing IVF and ET, immunological rejection by the maternal immune system remains one of the more widely cited proposals. Since trophoblast and decidual tissues at postimplantational stages of gestation have been shown to produce immunosuppressive molecules which act locally to protect the normally semiallogeneic fetus from immune rejection, several authors have extrapolated this concept to include the preimplantation period. Indeed, immunosuppressive activity produced as early as the first 24 h after fertilization has been suggested to be correlated with successful establishment of pregnancy following IVF and ET.[7] However, there are several theoretical reasons why this seems unlikely. First, the theory for immunosuppression by the preimplantation embryo postulates that the early embryo is susceptible to immune lysis. Such a mechanism would require the sensitization of cytotoxic lymphocytes (CTLs) to paternal antigens some time prior to conception. A primary immune reaction in an unsensitized mother would require at least 6 to 8 d to occur. It would also be expected that anti-paternal CTL and possibly alloantibodies be detectable either in the peripheral blood or uterine secretions of women having experienced one or several unsuccessful embryo transfers. There is no evidence for either.

A second reason to doubt the importance of immunosuppression by the preimplantation embryo as a means of protection from immunological rejection is that most T cell recognition, especially by CTL, is major histocompatibility complex (MHC) restricted. MHC expression would be required for the preimplantation embryo to be a target for presensitized CTLs. The data on this are limited for humans, but the available evidence indicates HLA-B, -C, and -DR negativity on IVF products.[17] In rodents, the evidence is clearly that MHC antigens are absent from the early embryo and are poorly inducible until the mid-somite stage.[30]

The cellularity of the fallopian tube and uterine lumen would seem to make the odds of an encounter between the embryo and appropriately sensitized T cell, or even a natural killer (NK) cell much too low to account for the 80 to 90% of transferred embryos that are normally lost in human IVF-ET programs. Furthermore, it has been demonstrated recently[10] that the early mouse embryo is not susceptible to cell-mediated lysis by NK cells, CTLs, or even lymphokine-activated killer (LAK) cells. Thus, there is no need to protect the preimplantation-stage embryo from the consequences of attack by CTLs, MHC restricted or not.

6. PHYSIOLOGICAL SIGNIFICANCE OF PREIMPLANTATION EMBRYO-DERIVED IMMUNOSUPPRESSIVE ACTIVITY

As discussed above, there have been several reports of polyamines, probably spermine, in human IVF and sperm culture media, and correlations have been shown between the presence of polyamines and successful establishment of pregnancies from transfer of the resulting embryos. Polyamine synthesis is a characteristic of rapidly proliferating cells,[19,22] including embryos,[1] and blockade of polyamine synthesis in mouse embryos has been reported to block development at the 16-cell stage, resulting in failure of blastocoele formation and further development.[1] In considering the physiological significance of polyamines in embryo culture media, Lea et al.[23] have offered several suggestions. First, polyamine synthesis may be a reflection of normal cleavage, and those embryos that are deficient in polyamine synthesis may exhibit developmental arrest before the blastocyst stage, as reported for mouse embryos,[1] and therefore are unable to implant. Second, polyamines may actually be necessary to stimulate embryo cleavage, in the manner of growth factors both *in vitro* before transfer, and *in vivo,* after transfer. In support of this is the report of Alexandre[1] that the addition of low levels of spermine to mouse embryos in which polyamine synthesis has been inhibited was able to partially restore the arrested embryo growth. Also, Porat and Clark[32] were able, by addition of spermine to the embryo culture medium, to partially overcome the developmental block in embryos resulting from IVF of oocytes from old infertile CBA mice, which did not produce immunosuppressive activity *in vitro.* A third possible role of polyamines in embryo survival, suggested by Lea et al.,[23] is related to their conversion to cytotoxic products by monoamine oxidase. Decidual tissue and endometrium possess amine oxidase activity,[21] which could result in localized conversion of polyamines of embryo or sperm origin to cytotoxic products which could inhibit activation of maternal effector cells by interleukin-2, thereby preventing fetal rejection by the latter cells.

Another possible explanation for the apparent increased embryo viability associated with the presence of immunosuppressive compounds in IVF medium is that such compounds may be indicative of biochemical changes in the oocyte that are associated with oocyte maturity and developmental capacity. The fact that the compounds possess immunosuppressive activity *in vitro* may be purely coincidental, and the increased embryo survival may have nothing to do with immunosuppression or immune rejection. Sheep oocytes that have undergone final maturation *in vivo* within the intact follicle exhibit a very different pattern of protein synthesis than those undergoing meiotic maturation as isolated oocytes, and the ability to develop to normal blastocysts and establish successful pregnancies are correlated with the pattern of protein synthesis characteristic of cytoplasmic maturity.[42] Specific proteins are released from oocytes at the time of fertilization, which play a role in the mechanisms that prevent polyspermy, and may be necessary for the fertilized ovum to achieve full developmental potential.[26,31] Among these are specific proteases, including tissue plasminogen activator (tPA),[43] a biologically highly potent compound which could be involved in initiation of a cascade of reactions of which immunosuppression may be a component. Other compounds of early embryonic origin that have been associated with embryo survival include "early pregnancy factor" (EPF)[5] and platelet activating factor(s) (PAF),[33,38] even though the mechanism by which these compounds may promote pregnancy success is unknown. Thus, the detection in IVF or early-embryo culture medium of specific molecules, immunosuppressive or otherwise, that are correlated with pregnancy success, may simply be indicative of normality and therefore of developmental capacity of the oocytes, but not at all related to immunosuppression.

7. CONCLUDING COMMENTS

The existence of local immunosuppressive mechanisms that aid in the protection of the semiallogenic mammalian fetus against rejection by the maternal immune system is well recognized. Although there have been numerous attempts to relate early embryo losses to lack of operation of such mechanisms, unequivocal demonstration of this has not been achieved, especially for preimplantation-stage embryos. In this review, we have attempted to summarize the evidence relating to immunosuppressive factors produced by preimplantation human embryos, in the context of their possible role in the success of pregnancy resulting from IVF and ET. Although correlations between the presence of immunosuppressive factors in ovum and embryo culture medium and successful establishment of pregnancy following embryo transfer have been reported, the evidence of cause-effect is not convincing, particularly since available evidence strongly suggests that the putative immunosuppression that has been demonstrated for identified compounds in early IVF media is an artifact of the particular *in vitro* conditions used to measure the activity. We have presented arguments against embryo losses before implantation being immunologically mediated, leading us to question the importance of putative immunosuppressive products secreted by preimplantation embryos. On the assumption that reported correlations between the presence of molecules or their metabolites that have immunosuppressive activity and success of pregnancy are real and reproducible, we propose that these products of oocyte or early embryo secretion are merely indicative of biochemical or metabolic normality of the oocytes or embryos. The fact that they also possess immunosuppressive activity is incidental and irrelevant to the success of pregnancy. There is no doubt that the availability of nondestructive biochemical markers of oocyte normality indicative of developmental competence would be of enormous value in enabling us to distinguish between embryos likely to succeed and those likely to fail. Unfortunately, no such marker, immunosuppressive or otherwise, has yet been reported that is sufficiently reliable for routine clinical use in selection of IVF embryos most likely to establish normal pregnancies, either for humans or animals.

REFERENCES

1. **Alexandre, H.,** The utilization of an inhibitor of spermine and spermidine synthesis as a tool for the study of the determination of cavitation in the preimplantation mouse embryo, *J. Embryol. Exp. Morphol.,* 53, 145–162, 1979.
2. **Allen, R. D. and Roberts, T. K.,** Role of spermine in the cytotoxic effects of seminal plasma, *Am. J. Reprod. Immunol. Microbiol.,* 13, 4–8, 1987.
3. **Allen, J. C., Smith, C. J., Hussain, J. I., and Thomas, J. M.,** Inhibition of lymphocyte proliferation by polyamines requires ruminant plasma polyamine oxidase, *Eur. J. Biochem.,* 102, 153–158, 1979.
4. **Armstrong, D. T., Chaouat, G., Guichard, A., Cedard, L., Andreu, G., and Denver, L.,** Lack of correlation of immunosuppressive activity secreted by human *in vitro* fertilized (IVF) ova with successful pregnancy, *J IVF ET,* 6, 15–21, 1989.
5. **Cavanagh, A. C., Morton, H., Rolfe, B. E., and Gidley-Baird, A. A.,** Ovum factor: a first signal of pregnancy?, *Am. J. Reprod. Immunol.,* 2, 97–101, 1982.
6. **Chew, N. J. and Sherman, M. I.,** Biochemistry of differentiation of mouse trophoblast: 3B-hydroxysteroid dehydrogenase, *Biol. Reprod.,* 12, 351–359, 1975.
7. **Clark, D. A., Lee, S., Fishel, S., Mahadevan, M., Goodall, H., Moye, M. A. H., Schechter, O., Stredonska-Clark, J., Daya, S., Underwood, J., Craft, I., and Mowbray, J.,** Immunosuppressive activity in human *in vitro* fertilization (IVF) culture supernatants and prediction of outcome of embryo transfer: a multicenter trial, *J IVF ET,* 6, 51–58, 1989.
8. **Clark, D. A., Slapsys, R., Chaput, A., Walker, C., Brierly, J., Daya, S., and Rosenthal, K. L.,** Immunoregulatory molecules of trophoblast and decidual cell origin at the maternofetal interface, *Am. J. Reprod. Immunol. Microbiol.,* 10, 100–104, 1986.
9. **Croy, B. A., Betteridge, K. J., Chapeau, C., Beriault, R., Johnson, W. H., and King, G. J.,** Assessment of immunoregulation by cultured, pre-attachment bovine embryos, *J. Reprod. Immunol.,* 14, 9–25, 1988.
10. **Croy, B. A. and Rossant, J.,** Mouse embryonic cells become susceptible to CTL-mediated lysis after midgestation, *Cell. Immunol.,* 104, 355–365, 1987.
11. **Daya, S. and Clark, D. A.,** Production of immunosuppressor factor(s) by preimplantation embryo, *Am. J. Reprod. Immunol. Microbiol.,* 11, 98–101, 1986.

12. **Daya, S. and Clark, D. A.**, Immunosuppressive factor (or factors) produced by human embryos *in vitro, N. Engl. J. Med.,* 315, 1551–1552, 1986.

13. **Daya, S. and Clark, D. A.**, Identification of two species of suppressive factor of differing molecular weight released by *in vitro* fertilized human oocytes, *Fertil. Steril.,* 49, 360–363, 1988.

14. **Daya, S., Lee, S., Underwood, J., Mowbray, J., and Clark, D. A.**, Prediction of outcome following transfer of *in vitro* fertilized embryos by measurement of embryo-associated suppressor factor, in *Reproductive Immunology,* Clark, D. A. and Croy, B. A., Eds., Elsevier, Amsterdam, 1986, 277–285.

15. **Dey, S. K., Stechschulte, D. J., and Abdou, N. I.**, Modulation of the *in vitro* lymphocyte response by rabbit blastocysts, *J. Reprod. Immunol.,* 3, 141–146, 1981.

16. **Dickmann, Z. and Spilman, C. H.**, Prostaglandins in rabbit blastocysts, *Science,* 190, 997–998, 1975.

17. **Dohr, G. A., Motter, W., Leitinger, S., Desoye, G., Urdl, W., Winter, R., Wilders Truscini, M. M., Uchanska Ziegler, U., and Ziegler, A.**, Lack of expression of histocompatibility leucocyte antigen class I and class II molecules on the human oocyte, *J. Immunol.,* 138, 3766–3771, 1987.

18. **Goodwin, J. and Ceuppens, J.**, Regulation of the immune response by prostaglandins, *J. Clin. Immunol.,* 3, 295–315, 1983.

19. **Helby, O.**, Role of polyamines in the control of cell proliferation and differentiation, *Differentiation,* 19, 1–20, 1981.

20. **Holmes, P. V., Sjogren, A., and Hamberger, L.**, Prostaglandin-E_2 released by pre-implantation human conceptuses, *J. Reprod. Immunol.,* 17, 79–86, 1990.

21. **Illei, G. and Morgan, D. M. L.**, The distribution of polyamine oxidase activity in the fetomaternal compartments, *Br. J. Obstet. Gynaecol.,* 86, 873–877, 1978.

22. **Janne, J., Poso, H., and Raina, A.**, Polyamines in rapid growth and cancer, *Biochim. Biophys. Acta,* 473, 241–293, 1978.

23. **Lea, R. G., Daya, S., and Clark, D. A.**, Identification of low molecular weight immunosuppressor molecules in human *in vitro* fertilization supernatants predictive of implantation as a polyamine—possibly spermine, *Fertil. Steril.,* 53, 875–881, 1990.

24. **Lewis, G. S. and Waterman, R. A.**, Metabolism of arachidonic acid *in vitro* by porcine blastocysts and endometrium, *Prostaglandins,* 25, 871–880, 1983.

25. **Masters, R. A., Roberts, R. M., Lewis, G. S., Thatcher, W. W., Bazer, F. W., and Godkin, J. D.**, High molecular weight glycoproteins released by expanding preattachment sheep, pig and cow blastocysts in culture, *J. Reprod. Fertil.,* 66, 571–583, 1982.

26. **Moller, C. C. and Wassarman, P. M.**, Characterization of a proteinase that cleaves zona pellucida glycoprotein ZP2 following activation of mouse eggs, *Dev. Biol.,* 137, 276–286, 1989.

27. **Murray, M. K., Segerson, E. C., Hansen, P. J., Bazer, F. W., and Roberts, R. M.**, Suppression of lymphocyte activation by a high molecular weight glycoprotein released from preimplantation ovine and porcine conceptuses, *Am. J. Reprod. Immunol. Microbiol.,* 14, 38–44, 1987.

28. **Niimura, S. and Ishida, K.,** Immunohistochemical demonstration of prostaglandin E_2 in preimplantation mouse embryos, *J. Reprod. Fertil.,* 90, 505–508, 1987.

29. **Noonan, F. P., Halliday, W. J., Morton, H., and Clunie, G. J. A.,** Early pregnancy factor is immunosuppressive, *Nature,* 178, 649–651, 1979.

30. **Ozato, K., Yan, Y. S., and Orrison, B. M.,** Mouse histocompatibility class I gene expression begins at midsomite stage and is inducible in earlier stage embryos by interferon, *Proc. Natl. Acad. Sci. U.S.A.,* 82, 2427–2431, 1985.

31. **Pierce, K. E., Siebert, M. C., Kopf, G. S., Schultz, R. M., and Calarco, P. G.,** Characterization and localization of a mouse egg cortical granule antigen prior to and following fertilization or egg activation, *Dev. Biol.,* 141, 381–392, 1990.

32. **Porat, O. and Clark, D. A.,** Analysis of immunosuppressive molecules associated with murine *in vitro* fertilized embryos, *Fertil. Steril.,* 54, 1154–1161, 1990.

33. **Punjabi, U., Vereecken, A., Delbeke, L., Angle, M., Gielis, M., Gerris, J., Johnston, J., and Buytaert, P.,** Embryo-derived platelet activating factor, a marker of embryo quality and viability following ovarian stimulation for *in vitro* fertilization, *J IVF ET,* 7, 321–326, 1990.

34. **Scodras, J. M. and Lala, P. K.,** Reactivation of maternal killer lymphocytes in the decidua with indomethacin, IL-2, or combination therapy is associated with embryonic demise, *Am. J. Reprod. Immunol. Microbiol.,* 14 (Abstr. 49), 12, 1987.

35. **Segars, J. H., Niblack, G. D., Osteen, K. G., Rogers, B. J., and Wentz, A. C.,** The human blastocyst produces a soluble factor(s) that interferes with lymphocyte proliferation, *Fertil. Steril.,* 52, 381–387, 1989.

36. **Siiteri, P. K. and Stites, D. P.,** Immunologic and endocrine interrelationships in pregnancy, *Biol. Reprod.,* 26, 1–14, 1982.

37. **Smart, Y. C., Cripps, A. W., Clancy, R. L., Roberts, T. K., Lopata, A., and Shutt, D. A.,** Detection of an immunosuppressive factor in human preimplantation embryo cultures, *Med. J. Aust.,* 1, 78–79, 1981.

38. **Spinks, N. R. and O'Neill, C.,** Embryo-derived platelet-activating factor is essential for establishment of pregnancy in the mouse, *Lancet,* 1, 106–107, 1987.

39. **Stone, B. A., Seamark, R. F., Kelly, R. W., and Deam, S.,** The production of steroids and release of prostaglandins by spherical pig blastocysts *in vitro, Aust. J. Biol. Sci.,* 39, 283–293, 1986.

40. **Valleley, P. J. and Rees, R. C.,** Seminal plasma suppression of human lymphocyte responses *in vitro* requires the presence of bovine serum factors, *Clin. Exp. Immunol.,* 66, 181–187, 1986.

41. **Van Vlasselaer, P. and Vanderputte, M.,** Immunosuppressive properties of murine trophoblast, *Cell. Immunol.,* 83, 422–432, 1984.

42. **Warnes, G. M., Moor, R. M., and Johnson, M. H.,** Changes in protein synthesis during maturation of sheep oocytes *in vivo* and *in vitro, J. Reprod. Fertil.,* 49, 331–335, 1977.

43. **Zhang, X. Rutledge, J., Khamsi, F., and Armstrong, D. T.,** Release of tissue-type plasminogen activator (tPA) by activated rat eggs and a possible role of tPA in zone hardening, *Biol. Reprod.* 44 (Suppl. 1), 73, 1991.

Chapter

4

The Role of Defined Major Histocompatibility Antigens in Preventing Fetal Death*

Radslav Kinsky, Elisabeth Menu, and Gerárd Chaouat
INSERM Unit 262, Clinique Universitaire Baudelocque
Paris, France

Miljenko Kapovic
University of Rijeka
Rijeka, Yugoslavia

Christian Jaulin and Philippe Kourilsky
INSERM Unit 277, Institut Pasteur
Paris, France

Thomas G. Wegmann
University of Alberta
Edmonton, Alberta, Canada

M. N. Thang
INSERM Unit 245, St. Antoine Hospital
Paris, France

*This work was supported by grants from Institute National de la Santé et de la Recherche Medicale (INSERM) and the Medical Research Council of Canada.

1. INTRODUCTION

Recent reports indicate that transgenic mice with homozygously defective β2-microglobulin (Beta 2M) gene expression can survive beyond birth.[1] Since the Beta 2M protein is necessary for classical major histocompatibility complex (MHC) class I cell surface expression, these experiments strongly suggest that the presence of MHC class I antigen on fetal and placental cells is not an absolute requirement for fetal survival.[1] The question that remains is whether, and if so, how, maternal anti-MHC class I reactivity can be beneficial in enhancing the chances of fetal survival. By now, there is general agreement that MHC class I antigens are expressed on the outer invasive layer of the trophoblast.[2-4] In rodents, classical MHC class I antigens are expressed there.[3,4] In humans they are not, whereas unusual ones are, such as HLA-G.[5,6]

There is suggestive evidence in both mice and humans that gene products associated with the MHC may indeed enhance fetal survival, although the nature of the substances involved has not yet been well defined. For example, mice at risk for increased spontaneous fetal resorption can have normal litters if they are immunized prior to pregnancy with allogeneic spleen cells of certain strains.[7,8] Other spleen cells show no effect if they differ from the effective ones by genes linked to the MHC on chromosome 17. Another example involves couples who share MHC haplotypes because of living in a semi-inbred colony, such as the Hutterites.[9] They show significantly increased early embryonic wastage when compared to nonmatched couples within the same colony. These observations prompted us to inquire whether MHC class I and/or class II gene products can influence fetal survival; we used a newly described method of inducing murine fetal resorption, which can be applied to a variety of strain combinations. Thus, we have taken advantage of the observation that increased murine natural killer cell (NK)-mediated resorption occurs following injection of Poly (I) Poly (C12U) or other double-stranded RNAs into day 3 pregnant mice in a number of different strain combinations.[10,11] Evidence from two laboratories indicates that asialo GM1-positive NK or NK-derived cells are the effectors involved in the induced fetal death, as well as that seen in the spontaneous fetal resorption models mentioned above.[11-13] In the spontaneous CBA × DBA/2 model, De Fougerolles and Baines have shown that asialo GM1-positive cells appear in areas of putative fetal resorption, based on their correlation with fetal resorption rates.[13] More directly, they showed that fetal death could be prevented by injecting the mother with anti-asialo GM1 antibody, a finding that we have confirmed.[14,15] The Poly (I) Poly (C12U)-induced fetal resorption can be adoptively transferred via spleen cells to naive pregnant animals, and this effect can be eliminated by treating the spleen cells prior to transfer with anti-NK or anti-asialo GM1 antibody, which simultaneously eliminates their enhanced NK activity.[14,15]

Since spontaneous fetal resorption can be reduced by allogeneic spleen cell immunization, we enquired whether this is also true for Poly (I) Poly (C12U)-induced fetal resorption. We report here that this is indeed the case. Furthermore, the flexibility of the Poly (I) Poly (C12U)-induced fetal resorption model with respect to strain utilization allows us for the first time to enquire whether immunization with defined MHC class I and/or class II gene products can positively influence fetal survival. The results reported here lead us to conclude that they can indeed do so, but paternal specificity is not required, because the fetal protection effect is seen when alloimmunization is applied to inbred crosses.

2. MATERIAL AND METHODS

Mice—All mice (except CBA/J, BALB/b, and H-2 bm mutants) were obtained from the IRSC breeding center (CNRS, Villejuif, France) at the age of 8 weeks. CBA/J mice, also 8 weeks old, were obtained from Iffa Credo, L'Arbresie, France. BALB/b were obtained in our animal facility from pedigree breeders kindly furnished to us by INSERM U152 (Professor J. P. Levy), Hôpital Cochin. H-2bm[1], H-2 bm[6], and H-2 bm[12] H-2K[b] mutant mice were obtained from the U 136 INSERM (Centre d'Immunologie de Marseille Luminy, France). The CBA/J × DBA/2, C57BL/6 × H-2 bm mating experiments were performed at the Hôpital Cochin U 289 INSERM-U 262 INSERM joint animal quarters. All other matings were performed at the INSERM St. Antoine breeding center, under strict gnotobiotic conditions. Successful matings were checked daily by vaginal plug examinations and mated females were randomly separated into experimental and control groups.

Ds RNA Treatment—Poly (I) Poly (C12U) was obtained from the Johns Hopkins University as a cooperative program, and prepared as previously detailed by Zarling et al.[16] A single dose of 20 µg was administered intraperitoneally (i.p.) in 0.2 ml saline. Control mice received saline only. The same was true in the CBA × DBA/2 system, except that all experiments were carried out in the Cochin Hospital, where Poly (I) Poly (C12U) as well as Poly (I) Poly (C) (Sigma Chemicals) were delivered, both at the same doses as above, except when otherwise stated.

Assessment of fetal resorption—Experimental and control females were sacrificed on day 13 of pregnancy and living and resorbing fetuses were counted. The uterus was inspected under a magnifying glass to establish eventual morphological modifications (such as thickening, or the presence of some hitherto unnoticed microresorptions, resulting from early embryo loss).

Immunizations—Allogeneic spleen cells were injected i.p. at a dose of 10^7 live spleen cells in a volume of 0.5 ml.

Transfected L cells—Transfected L cells obtained as a kind gift from Dr. Keiko Ozato were maintained under selective pressure as already described and checked by fluorescence-activated cell sorter (FACS) for H-2 expression before use. A typical FACS profile, performed on such a screening, is shown in Figure 1, and demonstrates that these L cells (clone LS2.0) did express the transfected MHC class I gene product $H-2D^d$ immediately prior to injection, as detected by monoclonal antibody (MAb) 34-2-12.[17]

General procedure—Each experiment presented in this paper was repeated at least 3 times with qualitatively similar results.

Statistical analysis—Percentages of living and resorbing embryos and pregnant females were compared using chi square analysis.

3. RESULTS

3.1. Paternal Cell Alloimmunization Prevents Ds RNA-Induced Fetal Resorption

We initially enquired whether Poly (I) Poly (C12U)-induced fetal resorption could be influenced by a prior immunization with paternal spleen cells. To evaluate this, BALB/c females were injected i.p. with 10^7 C3H/He/J spleen cells, or saline, approximately one week prior to conception with C3H/HeJ males. They were subsequently injected with 20 μg of Poly (I) Poly (C12U) (or saline) i.p. on day 3.5 postconception as determined by vaginal plug. They were sacrificed on day 14, and examined for fetal resorption as already described. Figure 2 shows that Poly (I) Poly (C12U) raised the resorption rate from 9 to 28% ($p < 0.03$). Prior immunization with C3H/HeJ spleen cells reduced this rate to background levels (7%, $p < 0.01$). These results indicate that Poly (I) Poly (C12U)-induced fetal resorption, like the spontaneous type, can be reversed by alloimmunization with cells bearing paternal MHC antigens. Unlike the spontaneous fetal resorption model involving the CBA × DBA/2 mating,[7,8] paternal spleen cells themselves were found to be effective. Note also that the effect of Poly (I) Poly (C12U) on fetal viability, while significant, is not dramatic using that dose in this particular strain combination. As previously reported, inbred matings generally show higher death rates than outbred matings.[11] This effect will also be apparent in data to be presented below.

3.2. Paternal Cells, but Not Congenic Cells Expressing Paternal Haplotype Can Prevent Poly (I) Poly (C12U)-Induced Resorption

In order to evaluate the effect of MHC vs. genetic background on the ability of allogeneic spleen cells to prevent Ds RNA-induced resorption, we

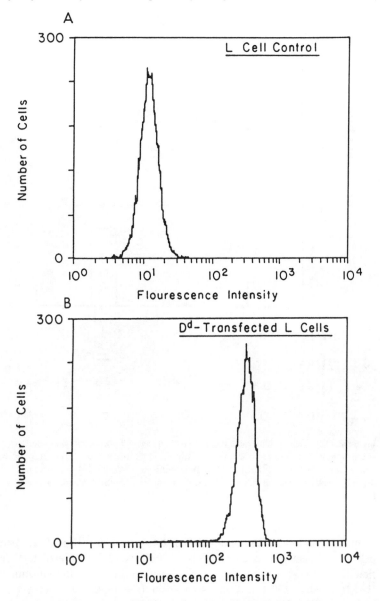

Figure 1. Typical FACS analysis of H-2^d transfected L cells using a K^d-specific monoclonal antibody (34-2-12) on a Becton-Dickinson FACS STAR machine. (Top) Control C3H.AN L cells. (Bottom) H-2D^d transfected C3H.AN L cells. FACS analysis was routinely performed to check H-2D^d positivity after *in vitro* expansion.

injected BALB/c females with either C57BL/6 or BALB/b spleen cells one week prior to conception by C57BL/6 males. Both C57BL/6 and BALB/b carry the H-2^b haplotype, but on different genetic backgrounds. As expected

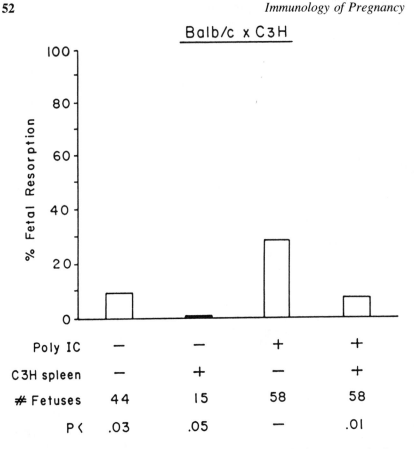

Figure 2. The effect of allogeneic (i.e., paternal) spleen cell immunization at one week prior to conception on fetal resorption induced by Poly IC administration to 3.5-day pregnant BALB/c females impregnated by C3H/HeJ males. The significance values listed were obtained by testing the null hypothesis that the values obtained do not differ from the pregnancies treated with Poly IC alone.

from the previous experiment, immunization with C57BL/6 (i.e., paternal) cells significantly reduced the Poly (I) Poly (C12U)-mediated fetal resorption (35% to 5%). However, the reduction seen upon immunization with BALB/b cells (26%) was not significant (see Figure 3). Since C57BL/6 mice differ from BALB/c mice at both MHC and background genes, while BALB/b differ from BALB/c primarily at MHC, the difference in effectiveness between the two types of immunizing cells could either be due to minor antigens, or to complex genetic interactions leading to enhanced MHC allogenicity in C57BL/6 vs. BALB/b mice. We therefore decided to evaluate whether MHC alloantigenicity in isolation might lead to prevention of Poly (I) (C)-induced fetal death. Such an opportunity is provided by mice that carry class I or class II mutations, the so-called H-2 bm mutants.

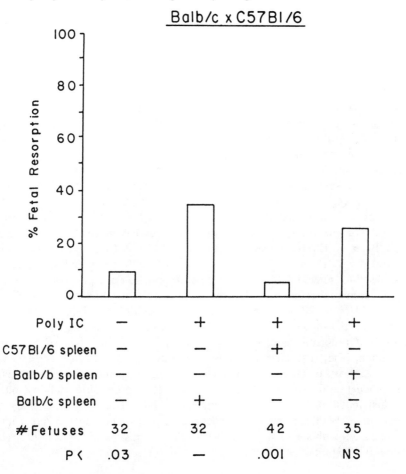

Figure 3. The effect of paternal (C57BL/6) and maternal congenic (BALB/c) cell immunization on reversing Poly IC-induced fetal resorption. All statistical comparisons are made with the group receiving Poly IC and control (maternal type) BALB/c cells only.

3.3. Immunization with Cells Bearing Immunogenic Class I or Class II MHC Mutations Can Prevent Poly (I) Poly (C12U)-Induced Fetal Resorption

In order to determine whether defined MHC class I or class II MHC antigens can influence fetal survival, we next asked whether bm mutant spleen cells[18,19] could influence the outcome of C57BL/6 × C57BL/6 matings, subjected to Poly (I) Poly (C12U)-induced fetal resorption. We deliberately chose the type of class I MHC antigen mutant that does not elicit allo-antibody response in C57BL/6 mice alloimmunized with mutant spleen cells, even when these are injected in complete Freund's adjuvant (CFA). This type of mutation does not exist for class II alloantigens, and we were therefore restricted to the bm[12] mutant. Thus, the mutant lines evaluated were H-2 bm[1], H-2 bm[6], and H-2 bm[12]; Bm[1] and bm[6] both have alterations that are restricted to a few amino acid residues in the H-2 K class I gene. Bm[1] differs from the prototype C57BL/6 at three positions (residues 152, 155, 156) while bm[6] differs at only one position (residue 119). The more extensive alteration in bm[1] is also reflected, though there is not necessarily a causal correlation, in the fact that it is far more immunogenic for C57BL/6 than bm[6].[18] Bm[12] is one of the few known MHC class II mutants. The mutation affects the class II Ia β chain, and like bm[1], is highly immunogenic for the prototype strain.[19] In order to keep the genetic situation as simple as possible, we evaluated the effects of cells from those three strains on a completely inbred mating, which also has the advantage of showing a pronounced influence of Poly (I) Poly (C12U) on fetal resorption. This is shown on Figure 4, in which unimmunized C57BL/6 × C57BL/6 matings undergo a 53% fetal resorption rate when injected with Ds RNA. This rate is reduced to 22% when bm[6] spleen cells are used to immunize the female C57BL/6 prior to conception ($p < .01$). A more dramatic reduction is obtained by prior immunization with bm[1] spleen cells (11%, $p < 0.001$), or, surprisingly enough, bm[12] (7%, $p < 0.001$). These results support the conclusion that maternal immunity against individual MHC alloantigens can prevent Poly (I) Poly (C12U)-induced fetal resorption. They also clearly indicate that paternal alloantigen specificity is not necessary to obtain this protective effect, since the mating is inbred. Reproduction of isolated laboratory strains that initially differ only by individual mutational events can accumulate additional unpredictable changes over time. We therefore sought independent confirmation that maternal immunization with single allogeneic MHC class I antigens can prevent Poly (I) Poly (C12U) fetal resorption.

3.4. L Cells Transfected with D[d] Class I Genes Can Prevent Poly (I) Poly (C12U) Fetal Resorption

One way to obtain isolated class I gene products is to use L cells expressing individual class I gene products following transfection. Figure 1 shows that, following transfection with a gene coding for H-2D[d], the C3H/An-derived L cells (clone LS2.0) expressed D[d] antigens in high density on the cell surface, as determined by its reactivity to anti-D[d]-specific MAb (34-2-12) as detected by FACS analysis, when compared to untransfected control L cells. These cells, and their controls, were used to immunize C3H/HeJ × C3H/HeJ and CH3/HeJ × BALB/cJ matings, to determine whether the D[d] alloantigen could provoke protective immunity against Poly (I) Poly (C12U)-induced fetal resorption. As can be seen in Figure 5, C3H × BALB/c matings are not significantly affected by Poly (I) Poly (C12U) at the doses used in this study when injected during pregnancy, and thus no effect was seen upon injecting the transfected L cells 7 days prior to conception. On the other

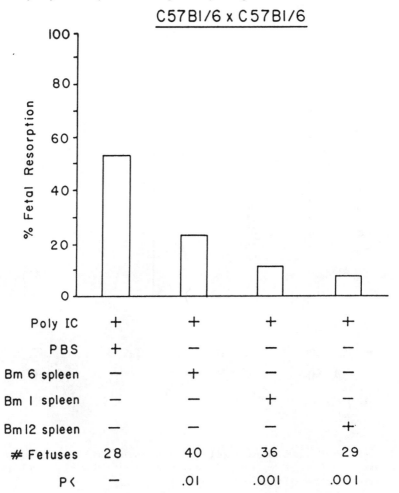

Figure 4. The effect of well-defined Bm mutant class I (Bm⁶ and Bm¹) on class II (Bm¹²) MHC antigens when given one week prior to conception on fetal resorption induced by Poly IC administration to 3.5-day pregnant C57BL/6 females mated to males of the same strain. All statistical comparisons are made to mice treated with Poly IC alone (first column).

hand, C3H × C3H matings show increased fetal resorption when subjected to Poly (I) Poly (C12U) treatment, even after being injected with control L cells. This can be prevented by injecting L cells that have been transfected with D^d alloantigen and as a result show D^d antigen expression on the cell surface (37% vs. 9%, $p < 0.001$) (Figure 5). Along with the H-2 bm mutants (Figure 4), these results implicate isolated class I MHC alloantigen in preventing Poly (I) Poly (C12U)-induced fetal death, while at the same time confirming that there is no necessity for paternal alloantigen specificity in achieving this effect.

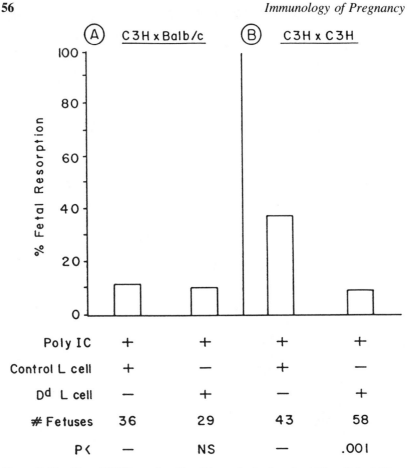

Figure 5. The effect of H-2D^d transfected L cell immunization in outbred (A) and inbred (B) on reversing Poly IC-induced fetal resorption. In both cases, the statistical comparison is made with the group receiving Poly IC and control L cells alone.

4. DISCUSSION

The experiments reported here allow a number of novel conclusions concerning the effect of maternal immunity on the survival of the fetal allograft. First of all, it is clear that, as reported before,[11] outbred pregnancies are relatively resistant to Ds RNA damage to the fetoplacental unit, which appears to be due to NK cell activation. The current experiments provide a likely explanation for this, which is that the natural alloreactivity seen in outbred matings due to the expression of paternal MHC class I alloantigen on the placenta usually automatically provides resistance to the effect of Ds RNAs. This possibly occurs because a strong anti-MHC response, perhaps in concert with other alloreactivity, alters the profile of the maternal immune response towards local and eventually systemic production of cytokines such as CSF-1, GM-CSF, and interleukin (IL)-3, and away from cytokines such as gamma interferons, IL-2, and tumor necrosis factor (TNF)-α. These particular cytokines are mentioned because they have been implicated in preventing or enhancing spontaneous fetal resorptions, respectively.[20] The details of how they interfere with or enhance NK-mediated killing of the fetoplacental unit remain to be determined. No doubt a complex cytokine network exists that produces the changes observed here. This is discussed elsewhere.[21]

Second, it is clear from a number of the experiments reported here that reactivity to paternal alloantigens at the fetomaternal interface is not essential to achieve fetal protection. It appears that the minimal requirement is a strong anti-third-party MHC reaction, irrespective of the alloantigenic status of the fetoplacental unit. This is reminiscent of the work of Toder and colleagues, who showed that CBA × DBA/2 fetuses could be rescued from spontaneous resorption by footpad (but not intraperitoneal) injection of CFA.[22] The authors also postulated that the effect could be due to a favorable but nonspecific release of cytokines at the fetomaternal interface. The work reported here adds to these observations by indicating that isolated anti-MHC class I or even class II reactivity by the mother is sufficient to reorient the immune network into a mode of response favorable for fetal survival. It is unnecessary that it be directed against the fetus. The best way to observe this effect was to set up the mating in such a way as to eliminate maternal alloresponse to the father's alloantigens, thereby preventing masking the effects of Poly (1) Poly (C12U) by the maternal antipaternal reaction, a masking phenomenon that has already been observed in certain mating combinations.[11] This should allow us in the near future to determine the type of maternal response (cells, cytokines, etc.) that is capable of rescuing the fetus from attack by the NK-like activated cells triggered by the Poly (I) Poly (C12U). If these results obtained in a somewhat artificial situation relate to the normal maternal-fetal immune interaction, they indicate that, although pregnancy can proceed in the absence of paternal class I stimulation, the fetus is far better protected from NK-mediated attack if the mother can mount an anti-class I or -class II MHC response. Somehow this response thwarts the NK-like cells from compromising the pregnancy. Since the current results suggest that this is usually occurring naturally in outbred matings, the providing of class I or class II MHC alloantigens to an inbred pregnancy simulates the hybrid vigor effect seen with outbred pregnancy, and shows that these antigens can do so in relative isolation. This no doubt has implications for explaining one aspect of the function of these antigens, as well as some proportion of their polymorphism, at least in viviparous animals. Thus, a long-standing argument as to whether they are implicated in promoting fetal survival by stimulating maternal immunity has been answered in the affirmative, at least in the experimental systems used here. The generalization of these conclusions to other systems and species must await further experimentation. We have preliminary evidence that maternal reactivity to allogeneic class I MHC peptides is also beneficial for fetal survival, but this is the subject of another communication.

SUMMARY

It is possible to induce increased fetal resorption in a number of inbred mating combinations by injecting Poly (I) Poly (C12U) 3.5-day postconception, a maneuver that appears to induce NK-like damage to the fetoplacental unit, such as occurs in spontaneous fetal resorption. We show here that alloimmunization can block this effect. In addition, responses to isolated mutant class I and class II, as well as transfected class I MHC antigens, are sufficient to restore normal fetal viability. It is not necessary that the maternal response be directed against paternal alloantigens for the protection to ensue. Indeed the protection works in inbred matings when the mother is immunized against unrelated class I or class II alloantigens. These results implicate defined MHC antigens in mediating fetal protection, and suggest that one driving force in promoting their polymorphism is their capacity to confer protection from NK-induced fetal demise.

ACKNOWLEDGMENTS

We wish to thank our colleagues, and in particular Dr. D. Green and Dr. A. Fotedar for valuable discussions.

REFERENCES

1. **Zijlstra, M., Bix, M., Simister, M. E., Loring, J. M., Rauliet, D. A., and Jaenisch, R.,** Beta 2-microglobulin deficient ice lack CD4-8 + cytolytic cells, *Nature*, 344, 742, 1990.
2. **Bulmer, J. B. and Johnson, P. M.,** Antigen expression by trophoblast populations in the human placenta and their possible immunologic relevance, *Placenta*, 6, 127, 1985.
3. **Billington, W. D. and Burrows, F. J.,** The rat placenta expresses paternal class I MHC antigens, *J. Reprod. Immunol.*, 9, 155–160, 1986.
4. **Wegmann, T. G., Mosmann, T. R., Carlson, G. A., Olignyk, O., and Singh, B.,** The ability of the murine placenta to absorb monoclonal antifetal H-2K antibody from the maternal circulation, *J. Immunol.*, 123, 1020, 1979.

5. **Kovatts, S., Main, E. K., Librach, C., Stubblebine, M., Fisher, S. J., and DeMars, R.,** A class I antigen, HLA-G, expressed in human trophoblasts, *Science,* 248, 220, 1990.

6. **Ellis, S. A.,** HLA-G: at the interface, *Am. J. Reprod. Immunol.,* 23, 84, 1990.

7. **Chaouat, G., Kiger, N., and Wegmann, T. G.,** Vaccination against spontaneous abortion in mice, *J. Reprod. Immunol.,* 5, 389, 1983.

8. **Chaouat, G., Clark, D. A., and Wegmann, T. G.,** Genetic aspects of the CBA/J × DBA/2J and B10 × B10.A models of murine spontaneous abortions and prevention by leukocyte immunization, in *Early Pregnancy Loss. Mechanisms and Treatment,* Allen, W. R., Clark, D. A., Gill, T. J., III, Mowbray, J. F., and Robertson, W. R., Eds., Royal College of Obstetrics and Gynecology Press, London, 1988, 89.

9. **Ober, C., Martin, A. O., and Simpson, J. L.,** Shared HLA antigens and reproductive performances among Hutterites, *Am. J. Hum. Genet.,* 35, 994, 1983.

10. **Chaouat, G., Menu, E., Kinsky, R., Dy, M., Minkowski, M., Delage, G., Thang, M. N., Clark, D. A., Wegmann, T. G., and Szekeres-Bartho, J.,** Lymphokines and nonspecific cellular lytic effects at the feto-maternal interface affect placental size and survival, in *Reproductive Immunology 1989.* 4th Int. Congr. of Reproductive Immunology, Elsevier, Amsterdam, 1990, 283.

11. **Kinsky, R., Delage, G., Rosin, N., Thang, M. N., Hoffmann, M., and Chaouat, G.,** A murine model of NK mediated fetal resorption, *Am. J. Reprod. Immunol.,* 23(3), 73, 1990.

12. **Gendron, R. and Baines, M.,** Infiltrating decidual natural killer cells are associated with spontaneous abortion in mice, *Cell. Immunol.,* 113, 261, 1988.

13. **De Fougerolles, R. and Baines, M.,** Modulation of natural killer activity influences resorption rates in CBA × DBA/2 matings, *J. Reprod. Immunol.,* 11(2), 147, 1988.

14. **Chaouat, G., Menu, E., Wegmann, T. G., Clark, D. A., Minkowski, M., Dy, M., and Thang, M. N.,** Explications actuelles du maintien de l'allogreffe fetal et hypotheses de travail sur le mecanisme d'effet des vaccines antiavortifs (modeles murins), *Contraception Fertil. Sexualite,* 171, 57, 1988.

15. **Chaouat, G., Menu, E., Bustany, P., Rebut-Bonneton, C., and Wegmann, T. G.,** Role du placenta dans le maintien de l'allogreffe fetale, *Reprod. Nutr. Dev.,* 28(6B), 1587, 1988.

16. **Zarling, J., Schlais, J., Eskra, L., Greene, J. J., Ts'o, P. O. P., and Carter, W. A.,** Augmentation of human natural killer activity by polyisonic acid polycytidilic acid and its nontoxic mismatched analogs, *J. Immunol.,* 124, 1852, 1980.

17. **Hedley, M. L., Ozato, K., Maryanaski, J., Tucker, P. W., and Forman, J.,** Expression of mutant H-2^d proteins encoded by class I genes which alternately process the 5' end of their transcripts, *J. Immunol.,* 143, 1026, 1989.

18. **Nathenson, S. G., Geliebter, J., Pfaffenbach, G. M., and Zeff, R. A.,** Murine major histocompatibility complex class I mutants: molecular analysis and structure-function implications, *Annu. Rev. Immunol.,* 4, 471, 1986.

19. **Mengle-Gaw, L. and McDevitt, H. O.,** Genetics and expression of mouse Ia antigens, *Annu. Rev. Immunol.,* 3, 367, 1985.

20. **Chaouat, G., Menu, E., Dy, M., Minkowski, M., Clark, D. A., and Wegmann, T. G.,** Control of fetal survival in CBA × DBA/2 mice by lymphokine therapy, *J. Fertil. Steril.,* 89, 447, 1990.
21. **Wegmann, T. G.,** The cytokine basis for cross-talk between the maternal immune and reproductive systems, *Curr. Opinion Immunol.,* 2, 765, 1990.
22. **Toder, V., Shepelovitch, J., Carp, H., Altaraz, H., and Strassburger, D.,** Cytokine function in immunopotentiated females, in *Biologie Cellulaire et Moleculaire de la Relation Materno Fetale,* Chaouat, G. and Mowbray, J., Eds., Les colloques INSERM, INSERM/John Libbey, Paris (in press).

Chapter

5

Cells of Immunological Relevance in the Human Uterus During Pregnancy

Judith N. Bulmer
Division of Pathology
University of Newcastle upon Tyne
Newcastle upon Tyne, England

1. INTRODUCTION

Considerable interest has developed in the role played by the decidualized endometrium lining the uterine cavity in the establishment and maintenance of normal pregnancy. The characteristic morphology of human decidua has been described in detail at both light- and electron-microscope levels. During pregnancy, endometrial stromal cells accumulate glycogen to form large polygonal cells with a pale vesicular nucleus. Similar stromal changes occur, particularly around vessels, in the late secretory phase of the menstrual cycle (predecidua) and after progesterone administration (pseudodecidua).[53]

The precise role of decidua has remained an enigma. Nutritional and endocrine functions have been proposed. Decidualization is, however, a feature of hemochorial placentation, in which maternal and fetal circulations are most closely apposed. Earlier workers suggested that decidua may act as a barrier separating maternal cells and extraembryonic fetal cells. However,

8868-6/93/$0.00 + $.50

in human pregnancy, the extravillous placental trophoblast shows an unusual capacity to invade maternal uterine tissues and vessels.[48] Maternal and fetal cells thus lie adjacent to one another within the placental bed. This unique coexistence of genetically disparate cells has focused attention on the possibility that decidua may have an immunoregulatory function, preventing immune rejection of fetal cells. The following short review will focus on the investigation of cell types within decidua which may play a role in maternofetal immunological interactions in normal pregnancy.

2. TECHNIQUES FOR INVESTIGATION OF IMMUNE CELLS IN HUMAN DECIDUA

Diverse approaches have been used for the study of immunologically relevant cells in human decidua. Each has advantages and disadvantages. Golander et al.[27] reported suppression of lymphocyte responses to mitogens and in the mixed lymphocyte reaction by supernatants produced by explant cultures of first-trimester human decidua. This approach involves no tissue disruption but provides no information regarding the cell types responsible for an observed activity.

Cell suspensions of decidua may be prepared by enzymatic or mechanical methods.[50] Enzyme disaggregation produces a suspension rich in infiltrating bone marrow-derived cells,[25,50] but prolonged enzyme digestion or the use of proteases may cause loss of surface antigens.[50] Unfractionated cell suspensions of human decidua have been used to investigate immunosuppressive activity, antigen-presenting capacity, and natural killer activity, but for many studies it has not been possible to attribute a given *in vitro* function to a particular cell type.

Various cell populations can be enriched or purified from cell suspensions prepared from human decidua. Glandular epithelial cells may be separated using sieves of varied mesh sizes.[36] Various density gradient centrifugation techniques have been used to separate decidual stromal cells,[38] and decidual lymphocytes.[33,37] Expression of specific cell surface antigens may be employed for positive or negative selection by panning, fluorescence-activated cell sorting, or magnetic beads.[23,52]

Cell suspensions prepared by tissue disaggregation may not be representative of the tissue under investigation since loosely bound infiltrating cells may be released more readily from the extracellular matrix. For example, Starkey et al.[55] reported that 75% of cells within enzyme-disaggregated suspensions of first-trimester human decidua were leukocytes. In contrast, CD45-positive leukocytes constituted only up to 36% of stromal cells in quantitative immunohistochemical studies of frozen sections of early pregnancy decidua.[11] This discrepancy is most probably due to the selective effects of the dispersal procedure, but may also be affected by inclusion of circulating blood elements within suspensions produced by tissue disaggregation.

Immunohistochemical studies have been extensively used to characterize leukocyte populations in nonpregnant and pregnant human endometrium (reviewed in Reference 5). The information gained by immunohistochemistry is dependent on the antibodies available. Although direct functional analysis is not possible, expression of many antigens may provide clues to function. Investigation of pathological uteroplacental tissues may also provide evidence for the functional importance of specific leukocyte populations: in ectopic pregnancies, macrophages predominate at the local implantation site[21] and increased numbers of CD3-positive T lymphocytes have been reported at the implantation site in hydatidiform moles. Thus, immunohistochemical studies may provide a firm basis for functional investigations.

3. MAJOR LEUKOCYTE POPULATIONS IN FIRST-TRIMESTER HUMAN DECIDUA

The bulk of trophoblastic invasion of maternal uterine tissues and the majority of spontaneous abortions occur in the first trimester of human pregnancy. The immune status of early pregnancy decidua has therefore stimulated considerable interest. Leukocytes form a substantial proportion of stromal cells in nonpregnant human endometrium, but they increase in number during the secretory phase of the cycle and in early pregnancy, accounting for up to 36% of stromal cells in first-trimester decidua,[11] where they fall into three major categories: granulated lymphocytes, macrophages, and T-lymphocytes. The major leukocytes, their phenotypes, and proposed functions are summarized in Table 1.

TABLE 1.
Leukocytes and Their Proposed Functions in Human Decidua

Cell Type	Phenotype	Proposed Functions
Endometrial granulated lymphocyte	CD56 + CD38 + CD2 ± CD11a ± CD3 − CD4 − CD8 − CD16 − CD57 −	Natural killer activity Antitrophoblast activity Immunosuppression Cytokine secretion
Macrophage	CD14 + CD68 + Class II MHC + CD11c + CD11b −	Immunosuppression Accessory cell function Cytokine secretion Nonspecific defense against infection
T lymphocyte	CD3 + CD8 +	Immunosuppression Cytokine secretion

3.1. Granulated Lymphocytes

Lymphocytes with an unusual antigenic phenotype account for up to 75% of stromal leukocytes in first-trimester decidua.[11] They are much less prominent in the second half of gestation. These cells were characterized initially by the detection of a large population of CD2-positive, CD7-positive cells in decidua which failed to label for other T cell antigens such as CD3, CD4, CD5, and CD8 or for the natural killer (NK) cell antigens CD16 and CD57. They also expressed CD38, a marker of immature and activated lymphoid cells.[7] The introduction of antibodies directed against CD56, expressed by large granular lymphocytes including NK cells, cast further light on the lineage of this cell which is intensely reactive for CD56[51] (Figure 1). Further immunohistochemical studies of first-trimester decidua have demonstrated two distinct populations of CD56-positive cells. Expression of CD38 overlaps with CD56 but only 50 to 60% of CD56-positive cells also express CD2.[11] There have been no separate functional studies to date of CD2-positive and CD2-negative subgroups.

CD56-positive cells are scattered singly throughout decidua basalis and decidua parietalis and also form aggregates adjacent to endometrial glands

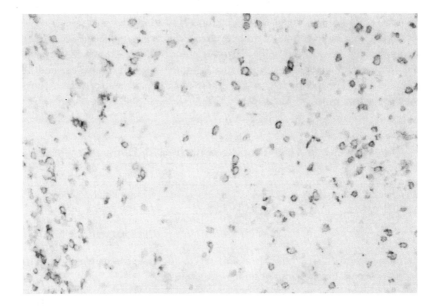

Figure 1. Frozen section of first-trimester human decidua labeled with NKH1 (anti-CD56) using an indirect immunoperoxidase technique showing abundant positive cells. Magnification × 160.

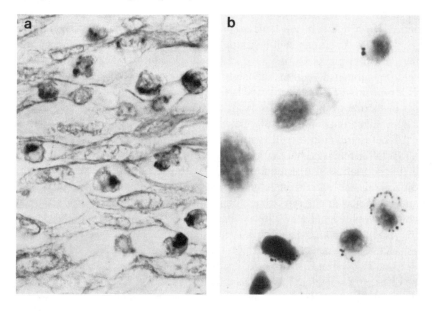

Figure 2. (A) Paraffin-embedded section of first-trimester human decidua stained with alcian blue/eosin showing many cells with cytoplasmic granules. (B) Imprint preparation of first-trimester human decidua stained with Giemsa showing endometrial granulated lymphocytes. Magnification × 100.

and arterioles. Phenotypically similar cells may be detected in premenstrual endometrium. This distribution mirrors that of the "endometrial stromal granulocytes" (Figure 2). These cells, also termed "Körnchenzellen", "K cells", and "granular endometrial stromal cells", were formerly considered to derive from stromal cells and to secrete relaxin,[18] but it is now generally accepted that they are granulated lymphocytes. Although the characteristic granules are lost when tissues are snap frozen, immunohistochemical studies of paraffin-embedded tissues and cell smears have provided conclusive evidence of a lymphoid lineage.[8] Some CD56-positive cells may be agranular: the number of granulated cells in paraffin-embedded sections is generally lower than that of CD56-positive cells in frozen sections, although direct comparison is not possible. Acquisition of cytoplasmic granules as well as antigenic heterogeneity may reflect changes in maturation, since it has been established that CD56-positive cells proliferate actively in premenstrual endometrial stroma.[44] It would be interesting to correlate CD2 expression with the presence of cytoplasmic granules.

The phenotype of endometrial granulated lymphocytes (eGL) (CD56-bright CD16-negative) resembles that of a small subpopulation, (less than 2%) of peripheral blood lymphocytes.[35] It has been suggested that these cells may represent a stage in the development of NK cells. CD56-bright CD16-negative cells are agranular and do not lyse NK targets; whereas CD16-dim and CD16-bright cells are large granular lymphocytes with potent NK activity.[41] Studies in human endometrium and decidua do not support the concept that CD56-bright CD16-negative cells are immature NK cells, since these cells are abundant within endometrial stroma and significant numbers of CD56-positive CD16-positive cells have not been detected at any stage of the menstrual cycle or pregnancy. It appears likely that these cells represent a specialized population within the endometrium.

The distribution of eGL within endometrium shows distinct spatial and temporal differences, but the stimuli which govern recruitment, proliferation, differentiation, and distribution of eGL within endometrium are unknown. Since eGL are present in large numbers within nonpregnant premenstrual endometrium, an embryo is not a prerequisite for their recruitment, although an embryonic signal may activate specific functions.

Double immunohistochemical labeling studies have shown that eGL proliferate very actively in premenstrual endometrial stroma, although cell division is lower in first-trimester decidua.[44] Nevertheless, decidual eGL may be difficult to maintain *in vitro*[52] and clones of CD56-positive CD3-negative decidual lymphocytes show a low proliferative frequency.[14]

In both late secretory phase endometrium and early-pregnancy decidua, eGL accumulate around endometrial glands and vessels. Adhesion molecules play a vital role in the regulation of lymphocyte migration;[54] varying expression of intercellular and cell-matrix adhesion molecules may influence the distribution of eGL within the endometrium. LFA-1 (CD11a) is a β_2 integrin expressed by T lymphocytes, which reacts with counter receptors ICAM-1 (CD54) or ICAM-2, which are members of the immunoglobulin family. A large proportion of CD56-positive eGL also express CD11a and CD2. In early pregnancy decidua, aggregates of CD11a-positive lymphocytes are often associated with CD54-positive decidual stromal cells. Endothelial cells in decidua also express CD54. LFA-2 (CD2) and LFA-3 (CD58) are both members of the immunoglobulin family. LFA-3 is expressed by glandular epithelium and vascular endothelium in first-trimester decidua. Thus, aggregation of eGL around glands and vessels may be due to expression of LFA-3 by glands and vessels, or of ICAM-1 by vessels, associated with CD2 and CD11a, respectively. The importance of these intercellular adhesion molecules in the distribution of eGL could be further investigated using frozen section assays and blocking antibodies.

The β_1 integrins (VLA 1 to 6) include receptors which bind to extracellular matrix components such as fibronectin, laminin, and type IV collagen. The distribution of laminin varies with menstrual cycle stage and in the first trimester of pregnancy laminin forms a capsule around decidualized stromal cells, suggesting a distribution within the external lamina.[1,22] Although the distribution of VLA antigens in decidua has not been reported, the expression of VLA antigens has been shown to vary with menstrual cycle stage.[56] This is an area worthy of further study.

3.2. Macrophages

Macrophages are present within endometrial stroma throughout the menstrual cycle, but increase both in absolute number and as a proportion of the total leukocyte population in early pregnancy, accounting for around 40% of decidual leukocytes.[11] Macrophages are scattered throughout decidua parietalis and decidua basalis, where they may lie adjacent to invasive extravillous trophoblast.[9] They express CD14 and CD68, but are generally CD11b-negative. The large majority express class II MHC antigens and the cell adhesion molecule CD11c.[6,11] Mues et al.[40] have suggested an immunoregulatory noninflammatory role for macrophages in term decidua basalis supported by expression of an antigen associated with downregulatory stages of inflammation. However, acid phosphatase, nonspecific esterase, $\alpha 1$ antitrypsin, and $\alpha 1$ antichymotrypsin activity has been detected in macrophages in first-trimester decidua, providing some support for a phagocytic role.

3.3. T Lymphocytes

T cells account for less than 20% of leukocytes in early pregnancy decidua. In nonpregnant endometrium in which CD56-positive eGL are less common, T cells account for a higher proportion of endometrial stromal leukocytes. Around 70% of decidual T cells are CD8-positive, showing a reversal of the CD4:CD8 ratio in peripheral blood.[11] Although $\gamma\delta$-bearing T cells have been reported in mouse endometrium[29], the large majority of CD3-positive cells in human endometrium and decidua express the $\alpha\beta$ heterodimer, less than 10% expressing the $\gamma\delta$ heterodimer.[12,58]

4. LEUKOCYTES IN TERM HUMAN DECIDUA

Although placental bed biopsies provide optimal material, fruitful studies may be performed on specimens obtained from the delivered placenta: decidua basalis may be retrieved from the maternal-facing surface of the placenta and a substantial thickness of decidua parietalis is attached to the reflected amniochorionic membranes.

Endometrial granulated lymphocytes decline in number in the second half of pregnancy, although scattered granulated cells may be detected in term basal plate.[18] The majority of leukocytes in term decidua are T lymphocytes and/or macrophages. Aggregates of B lymphocytes may be associated with focal necrosis or calcification, as may neutrophil polymorphs. Classical CD16-positive NK cells are rare.

Maternal macrophages in decidua basalis lie adjacent to genetically disparate invasive extravillous trophoblast. However, Khong[31] noted no difference in macrophage numbers in association with invasive trophoblast.

There was also no difference in decidual macrophages between normal pregnancy and preeclampsia. Macrophages in term decidua are phenotypically similar to those in the first trimester, expressing CD14, CD68, and usually, class II MHC antigens.

The majority of T-lymphocytes in term decidua are of the CD8-positive subset. T cells are often detected in small aggregates within both decidua parietalis and decidua basalis, but there is no obvious concentration around glands and vessels.

5. LEUKOCYTES IN NONPREGNANT ENDOMETRIUM

Macrophages, T cells, and phenotypically unusual granulated lymphocytes can all be identified within the stroma of nonpregnant endometrium. B lymphocytes, neutrophil polymorphs, and classic CD16-positive NK cells are rare, although B cells may be detected within lymphoid aggregates in the stratum basalis.

The number of leukocytes in nonpregnant endometrial stroma increases during the menstrual cycle, CD45-positive cells forming approximately 8% of stromal cells in proliferative and early secretory endometrium, increasing to 23% of stromal cells in the late secretory phase. CD14-positive macrophages account for around 33% of stromal leukocytes in proliferative endometrium. In the late secretory phase the absolute number of macrophages increases, although they form a lower proportion of the total leukocyte number.[11] T lymphocytes account for 45% of leukocytes in the proliferative phase. Their number remains stable in the secretory phase, but they account for only 21% of leukocytes as the macrophages and CD56-positive lymphocytes increase in number.

CD56-positive cells account for a substantial proportion of stromal leukocytes in proliferative endometrium, but they double in number in the late secretory phase and account for around 60% of the increased total leukocyte count. The increase in stromal leukocytes in the late secretory phase is due mainly to the increased number of CD56-positive endometrial granulated lymphocytes.

Leukocyte populations in the stratum basalis do not alter according to menstrual cycle stage. A notable feature is the presence of lymphoid aggregates that contain an admixture of T lymphocytes, B lymphocytes, and macrophages.[10] CD56-positive eGL are present in scanty numbers in stratum basalis, and these may form a source for the replenishment of precursors following loss of the stratum functionalis during menstruation.

6. INTRAEPITHELIAL LYMPHOCYTES

Although intraepithelial lymphocytes (IEL) in the gastrointestinal tract have been a source of considerable interest, endometrial IEL have received less attention. Macrophages, T cells, and CD56-positive eGL may occur in an intraepithelial position throughout the menstrual cycle and early pregnancy. The relative proportions of T cells and eGL vary. CD56-positive granulated IEL increase in number in the late secretory phase of the menstrual cycle and account for 50% of IEL in early pregnancy. The remainder of IEL are CD8-positive T cells. Comparison of cell phenotype with the number of cells with cytoplasmic granules indicates that at least a proportion of the intraepithelial T cells must be granulated.[45] The function of IEL in the gastrointestinal tract has stimulated interest. Separation of IEL from human endometrium and decidua would pose technical problems but further *in situ* analysis of IEL in endometrial and pregnancy pathology may provide clues to their function.

7. FUNCTIONAL INVESTIGATION OF HUMAN DECIDUAL LEUKOCYTES

Functional studies of decidua are the subject of other chapters. The following section provides a brief summary of proposed roles for the three major leukocyte populations in human decidua. The *in vivo* role of decidual leukocytes remains to be established, but *in vitro* studies may provide information concerning their role in normal pregnancy. Functional studies have focused primarily on first-trimester decidua; leukocytes in term decidua have received little attention. Most studies have concerned immunoregulatory function and potential antitrophoblast activity. Little attention has been directed towards the possibility that decidual leukocytes could play a vital role in defense against infection.

7.1. Granulated Lymphocytes

The increase in number of CD56-positive eGL in the late secretory phase of the menstrual cycle and in early pregnancy decidua has suggested a role in implantation and placentation. Granulated cells form a major component of decidua in other species with hemochorial placentation (reviewed in Reference 47), providing further support for a role in normal pregnancy.

In common with peripheral blood large granular lymphocytes, eGL of varying purity extracted from human decidua by density gradient centrifugation, panning, or fluorescence-activated cell sorting all show lysis of the NK-sensitive target, K562.[23,33,37,52] However, eGL are poor effectors compared with peripheral blood NK cells: this may be an inherent property of the cells but could be partly due to lengthy tissue disaggregation and purification procedures.

In all the functional studies described above, the purified CD56-positive cells must have included varying numbers of CD16-positive CD56-positive classical NK cells, either from within decidua itself, or from circulating blood within the tissue. Christmas et al.[14] produced clones of CD3-negative lymphocytes from first-trimester human decidua. Clones expressing CD16 and CD56 showed high lytic activity against NK and lymphokine-activated killer (LAK) cell targets, whereas CD16-negative clones showed low cytotoxic activity. These results have raised the possibility that NK activity reported in other studies may be due to the presence of a small CD16-positive population.

It has been suggested that the *in vivo* role of eGL may be to control trophoblast invasion of maternal uterine tissues, although there is no direct evidence for this in tissue sections. Human first-trimester cytotrophoblast resists lysis by decidual CD56-positive cells and peripheral blood NK cells, apparently lacking the appropriate NK target structure.[34] However, trophoblast can be lysed by LAK cells generated by pretreatment of NK cells with interleukin (IL) 2.[24,32] The possible activation of decidual eGL to act as LAK cells in spontaneous pregnancy loss is a source of considerable interest.

Evidence has accumulated that first-trimester human decidua can mediate immunosuppression, but the cell type responsible is not clear. In murine decidua, immunosuppression appears to be mediated by a population of small granulated non-T, non-B lymphocytes by secretion of a transforming growth factor (TGF)-β_2.[17] A similar suppressor mechanism has been suggested for human decidua[16] and the prominence of eGL in early-pregnancy decidua promoted speculation that they may function as suppressor cells. However, *in vitro* studies to date have not supported this proposal. Supernatants from purified eGL showed less suppression of lymphocyte mitogen responses than those from unfractionated decidual cell suspensions and some eGL supernatants caused stimulation of a mixed lymphocyte reaction.[13] CD56-positive eGL may contribute to decidual immunosuppression, but other mechanisms must also play an important role.

Endometrial granulated lymphocytes may also play a role in cytokine secretion. Supernatants from >90% purified eGL contain various cytokines on Western blot analysis, including IL-1, tumor necrosis factor (TNF)-α, TGF-β, and macrophage colony-stimulating factor (M-CSF). Christmas et al.[14] detected TNF-α, gamma interferon (IFN)-γ, and TGF-β production by decidual lymphocyte clones and CD3-negative clones generally produced higher levels of TGF-β. The cytokine production of purified CD56-positive eGL merits more attention in future studies.

7.2. Macrophages

Macrophages have nonspecific anti-inflammatory, protective, and phagocytic roles, but also play a vital role in the immune response as antigen-presenting cells. Expression of class II MHC antigens and CD11c has suggested an immunological role and Mues et al.[40] have suggested that the phenotype of macrophages in term decidua basalis supports a role in the inhibition of specific cellular responses.

Antigen-presenting activity has been reported in both human and mouse decidua. Fibronectin-adherent cells from first-trimester human decidua can function as accessory cells in various lymphoid responses.[20,43] The cell type responsible is not certain, although accessory cell function can be decreased with anti-class II MHC antibodies and class II MHC-positive cells have been noted in decidual cell suspensions with antigen-presenting capacity. Macrophages thus appear to be prime candidates for decidual antigen-presenting cells.

Decidual macrophages have also been implicated as suppressor cells. It is well established that supernatants produced by explant cultures of first-trimester human decidua show immunosuppressive activity, but the cell type responsible is uncertain: stromal cells, lymphocytes, macrophages, and epithelial cells have been implicated. Human decidual macrophages have been reported to produce prostaglandin E_2, which mediates immunosuppressive activity that can be partly inhibited by indomethacin and blocks activation of lymphocytes with potential antitrophoblast activity.[46] The relative contributions of the various proposed suppressor cells is not clear. Macrophages can also produce a range of cytokines, some of which may have an immunoregulatory or growth-regulatory role.[3] Receptors for macrophage (M)-colony stimulating factor (CSF), granulocyte macrophage (GM)-CSF, G-CSF, and TNF-α have been reported in the human placenta and it has been proposed that cytokines play an important role in the regulation of placental growth.[57] Although epithelial cells have been implicated as a source of M-CSF in mouse decidua,[2] macrophages could also contribute to cytokine production. Human decidua has been reported to produce IL-1, TNF-α, and G-CSF, but the precise cell of origin remains uncertain.

Decidual macrophages are equipped for phagocytic and nonspecific anti-inflammatory roles and it is possible that an important *in vivo* role is in the nonspecific defense of the fetoplacental unit against infective agents. Furthermore, the extensive invasion of maternal uterine tissues by extravillous trophoblast which occurs in normal pregnancy may lead to tissue debris requiring removal by phagocytosis.

7.3. T Lymphocytes

T lymphocytes account for only 20% of leukocytes in first-trimester decidua and, to date, have not been isolated for functional studies. Most T cells both within the stroma and in an intraepithelial position are CD8-positive and could function as suppressor cells. In murine decidua, hormone-dependent suppressor cells express T-suppressor cell surface antigens.[4] CD8-Positive T lymphocytes may also secrete cytokines, including IL-2, IL-3, IFN-γ, and GM-CSF.

T cells in first-trimester decidua do not express the IL-2 receptor but in nonpregnant endometrium expression of VLA-1 and class II MHC antigens has suggested long-term activation.[56] A report that decidual CD3-positive

T cells lack both αβ and γδ T cell receptor heterodimers[19] await confirmation and conflicts with other studies;[12,58] if confirmed, nonclassical pathways of activation must be considered.[15]

8. DECIDUAL LEUKOCYTES IN PATHOLOGICAL PREGNANCY

Functional studies of leukocytes in human decidua and endometrium are necessarily limited by availability of tissues. Investigation of pathological pregnancy may provide information concerning cell function in both normal and abnormal gestation. However, a major drawback is that many pathological pregnancy tissues remain *in utero* following fetal death. Tissues therefore often undergo secondary inflammatory changes so that in the event of any abnormal pattern of decidual leukocytes, the separation of cause and effect may present problems.

8.1. Spontaneous Abortion

Most spontaneous abortions occur during the first trimester. The introduction of immunotherapy for recurrent miscarriage has directed attention towards elucidation of the mechanisms of pregnancy loss. Non-MHC-restricted cytotoxicity may play a role in spontaneous pregnancy loss, although there are few studies to date in humans. Resorption rates in the CBA/J × DBA/2 mouse model are increased by enhancement of NK activity with polyIC and decreased with anti-asialo GM1 antibody; the implantation site of resorbing pregnancies is infiltrated with asialo GM1-positive cells.[26] Murine trophoblast is not lysed by NK cells but is susceptible to LAK cells.[28]

Human trophoblast has also been reported to be nonsusceptible to NK cells but lysed by LAK cells.[32] Accumulation of lymphocytes was noted at the implantation site of pregnancies destined to abort in an *in vitro* fertilization-embryo transfer program, but the cells were not phenotyped.[42] Michel et al.[39] reported decidual lymphocytes with small (<1 μm) granules in women destined to abort and decidual lymphocytes with large (>1 μm) granules in normal pregnancy. Despite problems with these latter studies, these results raise the possibility that granulated lymphocytes may mediate pregnancy loss in humans. Loss of the IL-2 blocking essential for normal pregnancy could lead to LAK cell generation either from the resident CD56-positive eGL population or from newly recruited peripheral blood NK cells.

8.2. Ectopic Pregnancy

In ectopic pregnancy, implantation occurs at an abnormal site. The pregnancy proceeds until rupture or hemorrhage necessitates surgical removal. Most ectopic pregnancies are in the fallopian tube and decidualization at this site is often scanty. In the absence of decidualization, class II MHC-positive, CD14-positive macrophages are the predominant leukocyte at the tubal implantation site. CD56-positive granulated lymphocytes are only prominent in foci of decidualization.[21] Intrauterine decidua in ectopic pregnancy is similar to intrauterine pregnancy containing large numbers of eGL. Investigations of ectopic pregnancy have therefore highlighted the importance of macrophages at the local implantation site. The observation that eGL are abundant in intrauterine decidua but often absent at the tubal implantation site raises the possibility that the *in vivo* role of CD56-positive eGL may be to secrete soluble mediators rather than to interact directly with other cells.

8.3. Molar Pregnancy

In hydatidiform moles the trophoblast implants normally but exhibits abnormal proliferation. Many molar pregnancies show dense decidual inflammation at the time of uterine evacuation. However, Kabawat et al.[30] have reported increased T cells in decidua associated with hydatidiform moles compared with normal pregnancy. Decidual T cells could be increased due to secondary inflammatory changes but could also secrete cytokines which may stimulate placental growth.[57] Increased T cell numbers could also reflect a cytotoxic response to the abnormal trophoblast.

Despite the problems which may be encountered in the study of pathological pregnancy tissues, notably the possibility of secondary inflammation, considerable information can be obtained provided that the limitations are recognized. Deficiency or excess of a leukocyte population provided that the limitations are recognized. Deficiency or excess of a leukocyte population in pathological pregnancy may cast light on function in normal gestation.

9. ANIMAL STUDIES: USES AND LIMITATIONS

The use of animal models with hemochorial placentation, particularly the murine model, allows considerably more scope for planning of specific experiments than is available for humans. However, care should be taken not to extrapolate too readily between human and murine systems. The implantation site in murine pregnancy may differ considerably from that of humans. For example, murine decidua basalis is deficient in macrophages and T lymphocytes,[49] whereas both leukocyte types are abundant in human decidua basalis. The extensive trophoblastic invasion of maternal uterine tissues which is an essential feature of normal human pregnancy is often absent in animal models. Furthermore, many abnormalities of human pregnancy have no counterpart in animal species. Indeed, models such as those of spontaneous pregnancy resorption may not be comparable with human recurrent miscarriage.

Nevertheless, animal studies have focused attention on non-MHC-restricted cytotoxicity as a possible mechanism of pregnancy loss. Studies of granulated metrial gland cells in rat and mouse,[47] which are proposed analogs of CD56-positive eGL in human decidua, have provided insight into their possible roles in hemochorial placentation. Studies in experimental animals demonstrating immunosuppression, accessory cell function, and cytokine activity in decidua have also focused attention on similar investigations in human pregnancy.

10. CONCLUSIONS

Considerable advances have been made in the characterization and investigation of cells with potential immunological function in human decidualized endometrium lining the uterine cavity during pregnancy. Various leukocyte populations have been purified for *in vitro* analysis but their *in vivo* role remains to be established. Experimental animals with hemochorial placentation have considerably advanced understanding of decidua in those species, but care must be taken in extrapolating to humans. Similarly, animal models of pregnancy loss have directed studies of human spontaneous abortion but for many abnormalities of human pregnancy there is no comparable disorder in experimental animal species. Studies of pathological pregnancy tissues have inherent problems but may provide valuable clues to the function of decidual leukocytes in normal pregnancy.

REFERENCES

1. **Aplin, J. D., Charlton, A. K., and Ayad, S.,** An immunohistochemical study of human endometrial extracellular matrix during the menstrual cycle and first trimester of pregnancy, *Cell Tissue Res.,* 253, 231, 1988.
2. **Arceci, R. J., Shanahan, F., Stanley, E. R., and Pollard, J. W.,** Temporal expression and localisation of colony stimulating factor 1 (CSF-1) and its receptor in the female reproductive tract are consistent with CSF-1 regulated placental development, *Proc. Natl. Acad. Sci. U.S.A.,* 86, 8818, 1989.
3. **Balkwill, F. R. and Burke, F.,** The cytokine network, *Immunol. Today,* 10, 299, 1989.
4. **Brierley, J. and Clark, D. A.,** Characterisation of hormone dependent suppressor cells in the uterus of mated and pseudopregnant mice, *J. Reprod. Immunol.,* 10, 201, 1987.
5. **Bulmer, J. N.,** Immunopathology of pregnancy, *Baillière's Clin. Immunol. Allergy,* 2, 697, 1988.
6. **Bulmer, J. N. and Johnson, P. M.,** Macrophage populations in the human placenta and amniochorion, *Clin. Exp. Immunol.,* 57, 393, 1984.

7. **Bulmer, J. N. and Sunderland, C. A.**, Immunohistological characterisation of lymphoid cell population in the early human placental bed, *Immunology*, 52, 349, 1984.

8. **Bulmer, J. N., Hollings, D., and Ritson, A.**, Immunocytochemical evidence that endometrial stromal granulocytes are granulated lymphocytes, *J. Pathol.*, 153, 281, 1987.

9. **Bulmer, J. N., Smith, J., Morrison, L., and Wells, M.**, Maternal and fetal cellular relationships in the human placental basal plate, *Placenta*, 9, 237, 1988.

10. **Bulmer, J. N., Lunny, D. P., and Hagin, S. V.**, Immunohistochemical characterization of stromal leukocytes in nonpregnant human endometrium, *Am. J. Reprod. Immunol. Microbiol.*, 17, 83, 1988.

11. **Bulmer, J. N., Morrison, L., Longfellow, M., Ritson, A., and Pace, D.**, Granulated lymphocytes in human endometrium: further histochemical and immunohistochemical studies, *Hum. Reprod.*, 6, 791, 1991.

12. **Bulmer, J. N., Morrison, L., Longfellow, M., and Ritson, A.**, Leucocytes in human decidua: investigation of surface makers and function, in Chaouat, G., Ed., *Maternofetal Relationship: Molecular and Cellular Biology*, Libbey Eurotext, Paris, 1989.

13. **Bulmer, J. N., Longfellow, M., and Ritson, A.**, Leukocytes and resident blood cells in endometrium, *Ann. N.Y. Acad. Sci.*, 622, 57, 1991.

14. **Christmas, S. E., Bulmer, J. N., Meager, A., and Johnson, P. M.**, Phenotypic and functional analysis of human CD3-decidual leucocyte clones, *Immunology*, 71, 182, 1990.

15. **Clark, D. A.**, Paraimmunology in the decidua, *Am. J. Reprod. Immunol.*, 24, 37, 1990.

16. **Clark, D. A., Falbo, M., Fowley, R. B. et al.**, Active suppression of host-vs-graft reaction in pregnant mice. IX. Soluble suppressor activity obtained from allopregnant mouse decidua that blocks the cytolytic effector response to IL-2 is related to transforming growth factor-β, *J. Immunol.*, 141, 3833, 1988.

17. **Clark, D. A., Flanders, K. C., Banwatt, D. et al.**, Murine pregnancy decidua produces a unique immunosuppressive molecule related to transforming growth factor β-2, *J. Immunol.*, 144, 3008, 1990.

18. **Dallenbach-Hellweg, G.**, The normal histology of the endometrium, in *Histopathology of the Endometrium*, 3rd ed., Springer-Verlag, Berlin, 1987, 25.

19. **Dietl, J., Horny, H. P., Ruck, P., Marzusch, K., Kaiserling, E., Griesser, H., and Kabelitz, D.**, Intradecidual T lymphocytes lack immunohistochemically detectable T-cell receptors, *Am. J. Reprod. Immunol.*, 24, 33, 1990.

20. **Dorman, P. J. and Searle, R. F.**, Alloantigen presenting capacity of human decidual tissue, *J. Reprod. Immunol.*, 13, 101, 1988.

21. **Earl, U., Lunny, D. P., and Bulmer, J. N.**, Leucocyte populations in ectopic tubal pregnancy, *J. Clin. Pathol.*, 40, 901, 1987.

22. **Earl, U., Estlin, C., and Bulmer, J. N.**, Fibronectin and laminin in the early human placenta, *Placenta*, 11, 223, 1990.

23. **Ferry, B. L., Starkey, P. M., Sargent, I. L. et al.**, Cell populations in the human early pregnancy decidua: natural killer activity and response to interleukin-2 of CD56-positive large granular lymphocytes, *Immunology*, 70, 446, 1990.

24. **Ferry, B. L., Sargent, I. L., Starkey, P. M., and Redman, C. W. G.,** Cytotoxic activity against trophoblast and choriocarcinoma cells of large granular lymphocytes from human early pregnancy decidua, *Cell. Immunol.,* 132, 140, 1991.

25. **Gambel, P., Rossant, J., Hunziker, R. D., and Wegmann, T. G.,** Origin of decidual cells in murine pregnancy and pseudopregnancy, *Transplantation,* 39, 443, 1985.

26. **Gendron, R. L. and Baines, M. G.,** Infiltrating decidual natural killer cells are associated with spontaneous abortion in mice, *Cell. Immunol.,* 133, 261, 1988.

27. **Golander, G., Zakuth, V., Shechter, Y., and Spirer, Z.,** Suppression of lymphocyte reactivity *in vitro* by a soluble factor secreted by explants of human decidua, *Eur. J. Immunol.,* 11, 849, 1981.

28. **Head, J. R.,** Can trophoblast be killed by cytotoxic cells? *In vitro* evidence and *in vivo* possibilities, *Am. J. Reprod. Immunol.,* 20, 100, 1989.

29. **Itohara, S., Farr, A. G., Lafaille, J. J., Bonneville, M., Takagaki, Y., Haas, W., and Tonegawa, S.,** Homing of a γδ thymocyte subset with homogeneous T-cell receptors to mucosal epithelia, *Nature,* 343, 754, 1990.

30. **Kabawat, S. E., Mostoufi-Zadeh, M., Berkowitz, R. S., Driscoll, S. G., and Bhan, A. K.,** Implantation site in molar pregnancy: a study of immunologically competent cells with monoclonal antibodies, *Am. J. Obstet. Gynecol.,* 152, 97, 1985.

31. **Khong, T. Y.,** Immunohistologic study of the leukocytic infiltrate in maternal uterine tissues in normal and pre-eclamptic pregnancies at term, *Am. J. Reprod. Immunol. Microbiol.,* 15, 1, 1987.

32. **King, A. and Loke, Y. W.,** Human trophoblast and JEG choriocarcinoma cells are sensitive to lysis by IL2-stimulated decidual NK cells, *Cell. Immunol.,* 129, 435, 1990.

33. **King, A., Birkby, C., and Loke, Y. W.,** Early human decidual cells exhibit NK activity against the K562 cell line but not against first trimester trophoblast, *Cell. Immunol.,* 118, 337, 1989.

34. **King, A., Kalra, P., and Loke, Y. W.,** Human trophoblast cell resistance to decidual NK lysis is due to lack of NK target structure, *Cell. Immunol.,* 127, 230, 1990.

35. **Lanier, L. L., Le, A. M., Civin, C. I., Loken, M. R., and Phillips, J. H.,** The relationship of CD16 (leu11) and leu19 (NKH1) antigen expression on human peripheral blood NK cells and cytotoxic T lymphocytes, *J. Immunol.,* 136, 4480, 1986.

36. **Longfellow, M. and Bulmer, J. N.,** Immunohistochemical and *in vitro* studies of MHC antigen expression by epithelial cells in human endometrium, submitted for publication.

37. **Manaseki, S. and Searle, R. F.,** NK Cell activity of first trimester human decidua, *Cell. Immunol.,* 121, 337, 1989.

38. **Matsui, S., Yoshimura, N., and Oka, T.,** Characterisation and analysis of soluble suppressor factor from early human decidual cells, *Transplantation,* 47, 678, 1989.

39. **Michel, M., Underwood, J., Clark, D. A., et al.,** Histologic and immunologic study of uterine biopsy tissue of women with incipient abortion, *Am. J. Obstet. Gynecol.,* 161, 409, 1989.

40. **Mues, B., Langer, D., Zwadlo, G., and Sorg, G.,** Phenotypic characterisation of macrophages in human term placenta, *Immunology,* 67, 303, 1989.

41. **Nagler, A., Lanier, L. L., Cwirla, S., and Phillips, J. H.,** Comparable studies of human FCRIII positive and negative natural killer cells, *J. Immunol.,* 143, 3183, 1989.

42. **Nebel, L., Fein, A., Rudak, E., Blank, M., Mushiach, S., Dor, J., Lerran, D., and Goldman, B.,** Structural aspects of embryo failure following *in vitro* fertilisation and embryo transfer; immune rejection or malimplantation, in *Reproductive Immunology 1986,* Clark, D. A. and Croy, B. A., Eds., Elsevier Science Publishers, Amsterdam, 1986, 227–235.

43. **Oksenberg, J. R., Mor-Yosef, S., Ezra, Y., and Brautbar, C.,** Antigen presenting cells in human decidual tissue. III. Role of accessory cells in the activation of suppressor cells, *Am. J. Reprod. Immunol. Microbiol.,* 16, 151, 1988.

44. **Pace, D., Morrison, L., and Bulmer, J. N.,** Proliferative activity in endometrial stromal granulocytes throughout the menstrual cycle and early pregnancy, *J. Clin. Pathol.,* 42, 35, 1989.

45. **Pace, D. P., Longfellow, M., and Bulmer, J. N.,** Intraepithelial lymphocytes in human endometrium, *J. Reprod. Fertil.,* 91, 165, 1991.

46. **Parhar, R. S., Yagel, S., and Lala, P. K.,** PGE$_2$-Mediated immunosuppression by first trimester human decidual cells blocks activation of maternal leukocytes in the decidua with potential anti-trophoblast activity, *Cell. Immunol.,* 120, 61, 1989.

47. **Peel, S.,** Granulated metrial gland cells, *Adv. Anat. Embryol. Cell Biol.,* Mongr. Ser. No. 115, 1989.

48. **Pijnenborg, R., Dixon, G., Robertson, W. B., and Brosens, I.,** Trophoblast invasion of human decidua from 8–18 weeks of pregnancy, *Placenta,* 1, 3, 1980.

49. **Redline, R. W. and Lu, C. Y.,** Localization of fetal major histocompatibility complex antigens and maternal leukocytes in murine placenta. Implications for maternal-fetal immunological relationship, *Lab. Invest.,* 61, 1989.

50. **Ritson, A. and Bulmer, J. N.,** Extraction of leucocytes from human decidua. A comparison of dispersal techniques, *J. Immunol. Meth.,* 104, 231, 1987.

51. **Ritson, A. and Bulmer, J. N.,** Endometrial granulocytes in human decidua react with a natural killer (NK) cell marker, NKH1, *Immunology,* 62, 329, 1987.

52. **Ritson, A. and Bulmer, J. N.,** Isolation and functional studies of granulated lymphocytes in first trimester human decidua, *Clin. Exp. Immunol.,* 77, 263, 1989.

53. **Robertson, W. B.,** Gestational endometrium, in *The Endometrium,* Butterworths, London, 1981, 73.

54. **Springer, T. A.,** Adhesion receptors of the immune system, *Nature,* 346, 425, 1990.

55. **Starkey, P. M., Sargent, I. L., and Redman, C. W. G.,** Cell populations in human early pregnancy decidua—characterization and isolation of large granular lymphocytes by flow cytometry, *Immunology,* 65, 129, 1988.

56. **Tabibzadeh, S.,** Evidence of T-cell activation and potential cytokine action in human endometrium, *J. Clin. Endocrinol. Metab.,* 71, 645, 1990.

57. **Wegmann, T. G.,** Maternal T cells promote placental trophoblast growth and prevent spontaneous abortion, *Immunol. Lett.,* 17, 297, 1988.
58. **Yeh, C.-J. G., Bulmer, J. N., Hsi, B. -L., Tian, W.-T., Rittershaus, C., and Ip, S.,** Monoclonal antibodies to T cell receptor γδ complex react with human endometrial glandular epithelium, *Placenta,* 11, 253, 1990.

Uterine Cells of Immunologic Relevance in Animal Systems

David A. Clark
Departments of Medicine/Obstetrics and Gynecology
McMaster University
Hamilton, Ontario, Canada

1. INTRODUCTION

Although the ethical restraints limiting availability of large quantities of animal uterine tissue for study are not so severe as in the human, immuno-histologic categorization equivalent to the elegant studies of Bulmer et al. in the human has not been done.[1] Antibodies for cell typing in sections in the sheep, goat, and horse have only recently become available[2] and in the mouse and rat, functional studies have been emphasized. In this treatise, the limited information that exists about uterine cells of immunologic relevance for different animal species at different stages of reproduction will be summarized.

2. NONPREGNANT ANIMALS

Unlike humans, who have a menstrual cycle and shed their uterine lining cells externally (with bleeding) at regular intervals, subprimates, such as the rodent, have an estrus cycle where excess uterine cells are resorbed internally. It is unfortunate that detailed phenotyping of uterine cells during the estrus cycle has not been done in the mouse, where the necessary antibodies already

8868-6/93/$0.00 + $.50
© 1993 by CRC Press, Inc.

exist, as this could indicate if there are unique cell types in the human potentially relevant to uterine bleeding.[3] In the murine uterus at estrus, a population of large-sized CD8[+] cells is found which can suppress proliferation of lymphocytes into allospecific cytotoxic T cells. The suppression is not antigen specific, and is activated by estrogen plus progesterone.[4] A similar population of large-sized, nonspecific suppressor cells that appear hormone dependent have been found in human luteal-phase endometrium.[5] The surface phenotype of these cells has not been determined. It should also be noted that in neither species does one know if the cells are located in uterine tissues or rather, are in the blood that circulates through uterine blood vessels.

The uterine cavity is potentially susceptible to assault by infectious agents, and is also exposed at intervals to male spermatozoa. In the mouse, bacteria are detectable with sperm in the uterine lumen.[6,7] Both bacteria and sperm that have not fertilized an egg appear to be rapidly cleared by phagocytic polymorphonuclear leukocytes.[6] A similar mechanism may operate in the vagina.[8] Exposure to sperm by the uterine route may lead to immune sensitization as measured by leukocyte adherence inhibition,[9] but this has proven controversial.[10] There may also be enlargement of the lymph nodes draining the uterus if washed spermatozoa are placed in the uterine lumen and in response to natural mating.[11,12] Evidence for sensitization as reflected in enhanced lymphoproliferative responses, T cell cytokine release, cytotoxic T cell generation, and antibody responses have not been published, but there has been evidence for negative types of immune responses, i.e., tolerance induction in the absence of a pregnancy.[13] Deliberate instillation of allogeneic adult cells into the uterine lumen may lead to sensitization as shown by Beer and Billingham,[11] and Lande[14] has shown uterine exposure to antigens can sensitize. This lack of sensitization in the case of sperm exposure may be due to sperm-associated immunosuppressive molecules.[15] Absence of lymphatic drainage is known to block immune reponses, even when antigen-presenting cells and lymphocytes may be present in the tissue.[16] The lymphatic drainage of the uterine lining appears minimal, particularly in the superficial regions near the luminal surface.[17] However, hormonal activation of the rodent uterus in early pregnancy appears to enhance lymphatic drainage,[18] so sensitization may be enhanced. Following mating, there is enhanced mRNA for certain cytokines such as colony-stimulating factor (CSF)-1, interleukin (IL)-3, granulocyte macrophage (GM)-CSF, IL-1, tumor necrosis factor (TNF)-α, IL-6 in mouse uterine lining cells which are infiltrated by lymphocytes, polymorphs, and macrophages after mating;[19,20] with the exception of IL-3 which is T cell specific, all of the cytokines may all arise from macrophages.

The uterus has been likened to other mucosa-lined organs such as the gut and respiratory tract that are exposed to the external environment. Secretory IgA plays a major role in protecting the latter from pathogens. IgA-producing B cells localize in the cervical area of the murine uterus and this localization is hormonally regulated.[21,22] There may also be some localization in the uterine lining of the mouse, but not rat[23,24] and secretory IgA as well as IgG and complement may be produced locally and gain access to the uterine lumen.[25] The production of secretory component may be estradiol stimulated.[26]

In mucosal epithelia, a population of intraepithelial lymphocytes (IEL) may be found. The majority contain cytoplasmic granules, and those with T cell receptors may bear the $\gamma\delta$ rather than the $\alpha\beta$ type that typifies most T cells in blood, lymph nodes, and spleen.[27] These cells are present in the human, rodent, sheep,[28] pig,[29] cow, and horse. The function of the uterine IEL is unknown. IEL from other mucosal organs of rodents have been found to show natural killer cell (NK) activity, sometimes of unique selectivity towards virus-infected cells,[30-32] suppressive activity, and to produce cytokines such as CSF.[33]

There appears to be some differential control of migration of eosinophiles into genital tissues. Estradiol stimulated eosinophil accumulation in the uterus of the rat whereas progesterone stimulated cervical infiltration.[34-36] CD4+ macrophages were also stimulated by estradiol.[35] In the sheep, however, withdrawal of estrogen and progesterone appeared to stimulate eosinophil and polymorphonuclear infiltration into the uterus.[29,37] Hormonally regulated migratory cell populations in the uterus may play important roles in eliminating infection in the response to male gametes, and in tissue remodeling.

3. PREGNANCY

Pregnancy begins with fertilization of one or more oocytes, and may be conveniently divided into a pre-implantation phase, an implantation and peri-implantation period, and a postimplantation phase when a distinct fetus and placenta can be identified. In species such as the rodent, the fetal trophoblast burrows into the uterine stroma and a decidual reaction develops, similar to the human. In species such as the pig and horse, the attachment is either epithelial or only a select population of trophoblast enters the stroma to form islands or cups (as seen in the horse).[38] A decidual reaction does not usually occur in this setting. A decidual reaction in the mouse or rat required only a mild traumatic stimulus in addition to estrogen and progesterone.[39] Production of the latter can be stimulated by an infertile mating, resulting in pseudopregnancy. If trauma is applied to the epithelium, extensive proliferation and decidualization results in a deciduoma. In the human, in contrast, decidual tissue will form in response to the hormonal milieu of a pregnancy; here the pregnancy may be remote and present ectopically in the fallopian tube.

3.1. Preimplantation/Preattachment Phase

Regrettably, I have been unable to locate any detailed characterization of the cell populations present in the uterine lining of animals during this phase of normal pregnancy. Infiltration by lymphocytes, macrophages, and release of cytokines has been mentioned.[19,20] The cell population in the mouse functionally characterized has been a CD8+ hormonally recruited or activated suppressor cell, as described above.[4] This cell population is probably thymus-derived, as mice that lack mature T and B cells due to the effect of the *scid/ scid* genotype are greatly deficient in suppressor cell activity at this phase in pregnancy and in response to administration of estrogen and progesterone.[40]

3.2. Attachment and Peri-implantation Phase

In the mouse, the blastocyst attaches to the antimesometrial side of the uterus and elicits a primary decidual reaction. Macrophages and lymphatics are excluded from this zone.[17,18,42] The hormonally induced CD8+ suppressor population persists but is masked in its activity by cells bearing receptors for the Fc end of IgG.[43] The nature and location of these two functionally antagonistic cell populations is unknown. Although a deficiency of CD8+ cells does not seem to lead to abortion in specific pathogen free (SPF) *scid/ scid* mice,[40] conventionally housed CBA/J mice injected with anti-CD8 have an increased loss rate,[43] and antibody that interferes with suppressor T cell function may likewise lead to pregnancy failure.[44-46] In the mouse, the peri-implantation phase lasts approximately 4 days. Within 2 days of implantation, granulated asialo-GM1+ cells become prominent in the uterine lining outside the primary decidual zone,[47,48] and the occasional activated lymphocyte cell may appear adjacent to the trophoblast.[48] NK activity is also present at this time[49] and as determined in the pig, may be recruited by the embryo itself.[50] The function of NK-like cells is uncertain, but they may be related to the CD56+ T/NK lineage cells found in the human and mature into large granulated cells called metrial gland (MG) cells.[51] Mast cells are also found in the uterus of certain species at the time of implantation, may play a role in the vascular changes at implantation, and are deficient in aged females.[52] No data on mast cells are available for the mouse.

3.3. Postimplantation Phase

In the mouse, the ectoplacental cone trophoblast grows across and obliterates the uterine lumen and attaches to mesometrial uterine lining, stimulating a basal decidual reaction wherein there is an ongoing maternal vascular proliferation.[42,48] A definitive placenta forms and is vascularized by these maternal vessels. The trophoblast cells at the placenta-decidua interface are initially trophoblast giant cells that were present in the periimplant phase, but these soon disappear allowing direct contact between spongiotrophoblast and decidua. Trophoblast invades into decidua and also invades and lines the maternal arterial feed within the placenta, but does not invade vessels in the decidua as in the human.[53]

A variety of maternal lymphomyeloid cells are present in the rodent decidua at this point in time and can be described in some detail.

3.3.1. Macrophages Are Present[53-56]

When removed from the uterus and studied *in vitro,* these cells can present antigen, can produce cytokines, and can release prostaglandin E$_2$ (PGE$_2$) in immunosuppressive concentrations.[55,57-61]*In situ,* macrophage function appears to be suppressed by a direct contact mechanism with stroma.[62] This suppression is reflected in a reduced ability to deal with intracellular pathogens such as *Listeria monocytogenes.*[63] Production of prostaglandins by macrophages and other cells may also be suppressed *in situ,* as reflected by reduced levels of histochemically detectable cyclooxygenase.[64,65] This makes biologic sense as prostaglandins appear to stimulate labor and in early pregnancy, may be abortogenic.[66,67] In the human, progesterone appears to trigger production of a protein that suppresses PG production, and it has been suggested that mechanisms may occur in the rodent.[67,68] Contrary to the report of Lala et al.,[69] indomethacin, an inhibitor of PGE$_2$ synthesis that blocks PGE$_2$-mediated suppression, does not appear to cause abortion in mice.[70-72] The production of suppressive concentrations of PGE$_2$ appears to be an *in vitro* artifact.

It is not known if macrophages can process or present antigen *in situ.* Antigen presentation may be due to dendritic-type cells.[18] Cytokines which may be produced by macrophages are many and include transforming growth factor (TGF)-β, TNF-α, and GM-CSF.[55] There is some evidence for *in situ* production of TGF-β1 in the periimplant phase of pregnancy,[73] and TNF-α appears to be produced early in the postimplant phase, but there is evidence that macrophages are not responsible for the latter,[54] perhaps due to the regulatory effects of stromal cells.[62] The role of these cytokines may lie in differentiation of trophoblast or other uterine cells bearing the appropriate receptors.

3.3.2. T Cells

Both CD8$^+$ and CD8$^-$ Lyt 1 cells are present, and the number is greater in allogeneic as compared to syngeneic pregnancy.[56] The accumulation peaks at about day 12 to 14 of mouse pregnancy. It is unknown if these cells are functional or bear T cell receptors.[74] Large CD8$^+$ suppressor cells have NOT been found at this timepoint in pregnancy[75,76] and similar large suppressor cells are also absent in the decidua of the human towards the end of the first trimester of pregnancy.[5] CD8$^+$ Cytotoxic cells such as alloantigen-specific cytotoxic lymphocytes (CTL) and nonspecific lymphokine-activated killer (LAK)-like cells have been isolated from the decidua and placental remnants of dying (aborting/resorbing) embryos.[77,78]

3.3.3. Novel Non-T Suppressor Cells

A small subpopulation of cells in murine decidua exert potent suppression *in vitro* by release of a factor related to TGF-β2.[75,79,80] Suppressive activity correlates with the presence of small granulated lymphocytes lacking T cell markers, asialo-GM1, MAC-1, but possessing Fc receptors.[76] Both suppressive activity and granulated cells predominant in the deeper regions of the decidua basalis.[76] A similar small lymphocytic population releasing a TGF-β-related suppressor factor has been found in human pregnancy decidua,[80,81] and there may be a factor-producing larger cell population in the mouse.[82] In both the mouse and human, the trophoblast appears to be able to activate the suppressor cells.[83,84] Small- and large-sized suppressor cells have also been found in the endometrium of the pregnant pig.[84] Suppression was present in pseudopregnant endometrium as well,[85] but it was not determined if these were the large-sized nonfactor-producing T-like suppressor cells that are hormonally recruited or activated.[4,5]

It has been suggested that the small-sized suppressor cells at the implantation site in the mouse arise from bone marrow, as the small cell component of bone marrow localizes selectively at implant sites[86] and cells in this fraction can be activated to suppress via release of a TGF-β.[87] Definite proof of the origin of implant-site non-T suppressor cells from bone marrow has yet to be obtained. TGF-β2-producing suppressor cells are present on the decidua of pregnant SCID mice, consistent with a non-T, non-B cell phenotype.[40]

3.3.4. Asialo-GM1⁺ Cells

Large granule-containing cells accumulate in the deep basal region of the decidua basalis and extend into the myometrium. This accumulation is called the metrial gland (MG).[88] The function of the large MG cells is uncertain. They are more numerous at allopregnant implant sites than syngeneic pregnancy sites.[89] Although difficult to isolate, explant culture techniques have allowed some *in vitro* studies to be done. Such MG cells can release various cytokines, including CSF-1, IL-1, and two unidentified factors: one stimulating growth of DA-1 cells and one cytotoxic to a macrophage cell line.[90] mRNA for leukemia inhibitory factor (LIF) was also detected. MG cells, even though they contain perforin,[91] do not kill YAC targets.[92,93] MG cells may arise by modification of NK cells;[47] the activity of which diminishes as large MG cells develop.[49,51] Mature MG cells appear more akin to lymphokine-activated killer cells (LAKs), as they can kill an NK-resistant, CTL-resistant, TNF-α insensitive, LAK-sensitive mouse trophoblast cell line *in vitro*[94] (and unpublished data) and may also lyse fresh trophoblast (which is similarly sensitive only to lysis by LAKs)[95] *in vitro.*[96] MG cells may be associated with dying trophoblast in the placental labyrinth *in situ,* but it is unknown if MG cells actually kill the trophoblast.[96,97] Supernatants conditioned by MG cells are toxic to early mouse embryo *in vitro.*[92] *In vivo* injection of asialo-GM1 antibody only partially depletes MG cells. Their morphology is altered, but there is no compromise of the pregnancy.[51] Bone marrow chimeras have been used to demonstrate that MG cells, like NK cells, are bone marrow derived.[97]

In certain strains of mice, such as the DBA/2-mated CBA/J, a high abortion rate can be reduced to normal by administration of antibody against asialo-GM1.[47] Although NK nonspecific, LAK, and alloantigen-specific CTL-type activity has been isolated from dying embryos, and asialo-GM1[+] cells may be involved in nonspecific cytotoxicity,[51,77,79,96] it is still uncertain that direct killing of targets, either trophoblast or vascular cells, is the cause of the embryo death and the mechanism of protection by antiasialo-GM1 antibody remains uncertain. TNF-α has also been implicated in abortion, and its administration enhances loss in the CBA-DBA/2 system[98] and anti-TNF-α antibody prevents it. Pentoxifylline which blocks TNF-α release also prevents abortion.[99] However, administration of antiasialo-GM1 antibody that stops abortion does *not* affect TNF-α levels,[81] there is no excessive *in situ* staining with anti-TNF-α associated with embryos doomed to abort as might have been expected from the distribution of asialo-GM1[+] cells[49] (M. Baines, personal communication), and the protection against abortion produced by anti-TNF-α antibody or by pentoxifylline may be direct.[81] Pentoxifylline can have a number of effects on the vascular system that might also be relevant.[100,101] Immunoglobulin itself in high doses can exert antiabortive effects in the mouse by mechanisms as yet unknown.[102]

3.3.5. Decidual Cells

Lala et al. have proposed that typical decidual cells from the mouse uterus elaborate immunosuppressive concentrations of PGE_2 that prevent lymphocyte/LAK activation and abortion.[60,61,69] Administration of indomethacin caused 100% abortion in some but not all lots of CD2 mice.[69] The possibility that high levels of PGE_2 production represent an *in vitro* artifact has been discussed above. An abortogenic effect of PGE_2 synthesis-blocking drugs such as acetyl salicylic acid (ASA) and indomethacin has not been confirmed by Gendron et al.,[103] Kamel and Wood,[70] Clark, and Chaouat.[72]

Using bone-marrow chimeric mice, Kearns and Lala[104] concluded that most typical decidual cells in the uterus arose from bone marrow rather than from stromal precursors in the uterus. This conclusion was refuted by Fowlis and Ansell[105] and by Gambel et al.[106,107] Only a subpopulation is bone-marrow derived.[106,107]

4. SUMMARY COMMENTS

There is much to be learned about uterine cell populations, their actions, interactions, and regulation in rodents. Much less is known about the uteri of domestic animals. Hopefully, investigation of the latter might provide some insight into how to increase productivity.

REFERENCES

1. **Bulmer, J. N.,** Decidual cellular responses, *Curr. Opinion Immunol.,* 1, 1141, 1989.
2. Proceedings of the First International Workshop on Leukocyte Antigens in Cattle, Sheep and Goats, Hanover, Germany, July 25, 1989, *Vet. Immunol. Immunopathol.,* 27, 1, 1991.
3. **Clark, D. A. and Daya, S.,** Macrophages and other migratory cells in endometrium: relevance to endometrial bleeding, in *Contraception and Mechanisms of Endometrial Bleeding,* D'Arcangues, C., Fraser, I., Newton, J., and Odlind, V., Eds., Cambridge University Press, Cambridge, 1990, 363.
4. **Brierley, J. and Clark, D. A.,** Characterization of hormone-dependent suppressor cells in the uterus of pregnant and pseudopregnant mice, *J. Reprod. Immunol.,* 10, 201, 1987.
5. **Daya, S., Clark, D. A., Devlin, C., and Jarrell, J.,** Preliminary characterization of two types of suppressor cells in the human uterus, *Fertil. Steril.,* 44, 778, 1985.
6. **Parr, E. L. and Parr, M. B.,** Secretory immunoglobulin binding to bacteria in the mouse uterus after mating, *J. Reprod. Immunol.,* 8, 71, 1985.
7. **Parr. E. L. and Parr, M. B.,** Deposition of C3 on bacteria in the mouse uterus after mating, *J. Reprod. Immunol.,* 12, 315, 1988.
8. **Phillips, D. M. and Mahler, S.,** Phagocytosis of spermatozoa by the rabbit vagina, *Anat. Rec.,* 189, 61, 1977.
9. **Dorsman, B. G., Tumboh-Oeri, A. G., and Roberts, T. K.,** Detection of cell-mediated immunity to spermatozoa in mice and man by the leucocyte adherence-inhibition test, *J. Reprod. Fertil.,* 53, 277, 1978.
10. **Faruki, S. and Hancock, R. J. T.,** Failure of spleen cell migration assays to detect cell-mediated immunity to spermatozoa after natural mating in female mice, *J. Reprod. Fertil.,* 69, 195, 1983.
11. **Beer, A. E. and Billingham, R. E.,** Host responses to intra-uterine tissue, cellular and fetal allografts, *J. Reprod. Fertil. Suppl.,* 21, 59, 1974.
12. **Shaya, E. I., McLean, J. M., and Gibbs, A. C.,** Accumulation and proliferation of lymphocytes in the lymph nodes of the female rat following first mating, *J. Anat.,* 132, 137, 1981.
13. **Prehn, R. T.,** Specific homograft tolerance induced by successive matings and implications concerning choriocarcinoma, *J. Natl. Cancer Inst.,* 25, 883, 1960.
14. **Lande, I. J. M.,** Systemic immunity developing from intrauterine antigen exposure in the non-pregnant rat, *J. Reprod. Immunol.,* 9, 57, 1986.
15. **Porat, O. and Clark, D. A.,** Analysis of immunosuppressive molecules associated with murine *in vitro* fertilized embryos, *Fertil. Steril.,* 54, 1154, 1990.
16. **Barker, C. F. and Billingham, R. E.,** Extension of skin homograft survival by prevention of graft-host skin contact, *Transplant. Proc.,* 5, 153, 1973.
17. **Head, J. R.,** Lymphoid components in the rodent uterus, in *Immunoregulation and Fetal Survival,* Gill, T. J., III and Wegmann, T. G., Eds., Oxford University Press, New York, 1987, 46.

18. **Head, J. R., Miller, S. T., and Kresge, C. K.,** Uterine lymphatic vessels and IA$^+$ cells: possible role in antigen processing,in *Reproductive Immunology 1986*, Clark, D. A. and Croy, B. A., Eds., Elsevier, Amsterdam, 1986, 201.

19. **Sanford, T. H., De, M., Andrews, G. A., and Wood, G. W.,** Cellular and molecular characterization of the post-mating uterine inflammatory response in the mouse, in *Cellular Signals Controlling Uterine Function*, Lavia, L. A., Ed., Plenum Press, New York, 1991, 172.

20. **Lobel, B. L., Levy, E., and Shelesnyak, M. C.,** Studies on the mechanism of nidation. XXXIV. Dynamics of cellular interactions during progestation and implantation in the rat. Part I, *Acta Endocrinol. Suppl.*, 123, 7, 1967.

21. **McDermott, M. R. and Bienenstock, J.,** Evidence for a common mucosal immunologic system. I. Migration of B immunoblasts into intestinal, respiratory, and genital tissues, *J. Immunol.*, 122, 1892, 1979.

22. **McDermott, M. R., Clark, D. A., and Bienenstock, J.,** Evidence for a common mucosal immunologic system. II. Influence of the estrous cycle on B immunoblast migration into genital and intestinal tissues, *J. Immunol.*, 124, 2536, 1980.

23. **Parr, M. B. and Parr, E. L.,** Immunohistochemical localization of immunoglobulins A, G and M in the mouse female genital tract, *J. Reprod. Fertil.*, 74, 361, 1985.

24. **Parr, M. B. and Parr, E. L.,** Immunohistochemical investigation of secretory component and immunoglobulin A in the genital tract of the female rat, *J. Reprod. Fertil.*, 85, 105, 1989.

25. **Bernard, O., Rachman, F., and Bennett, D.,** Immunoglobulins in the mouse uterus before implantation, *J. Reprod. Fertil.*, 63, 237, 1981.

26. **Wira, C. R., Bodwell, J. E., and Prabhala, R. H.,** *In vivo* response of secretory component in the rat uterus to antigen, IFN-γ, and estradiol, *J. Immunol.*, 146, 1893, 1991.

27. **Guy-Grand, D., Cerf-Bensussan, N., Malissen, B., Malassis-Seris, M., Briottet, C., and Vassalli, P.,** Two gut intraepithelial CD8$^+$ lymphocyte populations with different T cell receptors: a role for the gut epithelium in T cell differentiation, *J. Exp. Med.*, 173, 471, 1991.

28. **Staples, L. D., Heap, R. B., Wooding, F. B. P., and King, G. J.,** Migration of leucocytes into the uterus after acute removal of ovarian progesterone during early pregnancy in the sheep, *Placenta*, 4, 339, 1983.

29. **King, G. J.,** Reduction in uterine intra-epithelial lymphocytes during early gestation in pigs, *J. Reprod. Immunol.*, 14, 41, 1988.

30. **Tagliabue, A. A., Befus, A. D., Clark, D. A., and Bienenstock, J.,** Characteristics of natural killer cells in the murine intestinal epithelium and lamina propria, *J. Exp. Med.*, 155, 1785, 1982.

31. **Viney, J. L., Kilshaw, P. J., and MacDonald, T. T.,** Cytotoxic α/β^+ and γ/δ^+ T cells in murine intestinal epithelium, *Eur. J. Immunol.*, 20, 1623, 1990.

32. **Carman, P. S., Ernst, P., Rosenthal, K. L., Clark, D. A., Befus, A. D., and Bienenstock, J.,** Intraepithelial leukocytes contain a unique subpopulation of NK-like cytotoxic cells active in the defense of gut epithelium to enteric murine coronavirus, *J. Immunol.*, 136, 1548, 1986.

33. **Dillon, S. B., Dalton, B. J., and MacDonald, T. T.**, Lymphokine production by mitogen and antigen activated mouse intra-epithelial lymphocytes, *Cell. Immunol.*, 103, 326, 1986.

34. **Luque, E. H. and Montes, G. S.**, Progesterone promotes a massive infiltration of the rat uterine cervix by the eosinophilic polymorphonuclear leukocytes, *Anat. Rec.*, 223, 257, 1989.

35. **Zheng, Y., Sundstrom, A., Lyttle, C. R., and Teuscher, C.**, Differential expression of estrogen-regulated CD4 and Ia positive cells in the immature rat uterus, *J. Leuk. Biol.*, 46, 493, 1989.

36. **Lee, Y. H., Howe, R. S., Sha, S.-J., Teuscher, C., Sheehan, D. M., and Lyttle, C. R.**, Estrogen regulation of an eosinophilic chemotactic factor in the immature rat uterus, *Endocrinology*, 125, 3022, 1989.

37. **Murdoch, W. J.**, Treatment of sheep with prostaglandin F2α enhances production of a luteal chemoattractant for eosinophils, *Am. J. Reprod. Immunol. Microbiol.*, 15, 52, 1987.

38. **Allen, W. R., Kydd, J. H., and Antczak, D. F.**, Xenogeneic donkey-in-horse pregnancy created by embryo transfer: immunological aspects of a model of early abortion, in *The Immunology of the Fetus*, Chaouat, G., Ed., CRC Press, Boca Raton, FL, 1990, chap. 22.

39. **Kennedy, T. G., Squires, P. M., and Yee, G. M.**, Mediators involved in decidualization, in *Serono Symposia: Blastocyst Implantation*, Yoshinaga, K., Ed., Adams, Boston, 1989, 135.

40. **Clark, D. A., Banwatt, D. K., Manuel, J., Fulop, G., and Croy, B. A.**, Scid mice in reproductive biology, *Curr. Top. Microbiol. Immunol.*, 152, 227, 1989.

41. **Tachi, C. and Tachi, S.**, Macrophages and implantation, *Ann. N.Y. Acad. Sci.*, 476, 158, 1986.

42. **Lobel, B. L., Levy, E., and Shelesnyak, M. C.**, Studies on the mechanism of nidation. XXXIV. Dynamics of cellular interactions during progestation and implantation in the rat. Part III, *Acta Endocrinol. Suppl.*, 123, 77, 1967.

43. **Clark, D. A., Brierley, J., Banwatt, D., and Chaouat, G.**, Hormone-induced preimplantation Lyt 2⁺ murine uterine suppressor cells persist after implantation and may reduce the spontaneous abortion rate in CBA/J mice, *Cell. Immunol.*, 123, 334, 1989.

44. **Beaman, K. D. and Hoversland, R. C.**, Induction of abortion in mice with a monoclonal antibody specific for suppressor T-lymphocyte molecules, *J. Reprod. Fertil.*, 82, 691, 1988.

45. **Athanasas-Platsis, S., Quinn, K. A., Wong, T.-Y., Rolfe, B. E., Cavanagh, A. C., and Morton, H.**, Passive immunization of pregnant mice against early pregnancy factor causes loss of embryonic viability, *J. Reprod. Fertil.*, 87, 495, 1989.

46. **Hoversland, R. C. and Beaman, K. D.**, Embryo implantation associated with increase in T cell suppressor factor in the uterus and spleen of mice, *J. Reprod. Fertil.*, 88, 135, 1990.

47. **Gendron, R. L. and Baines, M. G.**, Infiltrating decidual natural killer cells are associated with spontaneous abortion in mice, *Cell. Immunol.*, 113, 261, 1988.

48. **Lobel, B. L., Levy, E., and Shelesnyak, M. C.,** Studies on the mechanism of nidation. XXXIV. Dynamics of cellular interactions during progestation and implantation in the rat. Part II, *Acta Endocrinol. Suppl.,* 123, 47, 1967.

49. **Gambel, P., Croy, B. A., Moore, W. D., Hunziker, R. D., Wegmann, T. G., and Rossant, J.,** Characterization of immune effector cells present in early murine decidua, *Cell. Immunol.,* 93, 303, 1985.

50. **Croy, B. A., Waterfield, A., Wood, W., and King, G. J.,** Normal murine and porcine embryos recruit NK cells to the uterus, *Cell. Immunol.,* 115, 471, 1988.

51. **Parr, E. L., Parr, M. B., Zheng, L. M., and Young, J. D.,** Mouse granulated metrial gland cells originate by local activation of uterine natural killer lymphocytes beginning at implantation and continuing through day 14 of pregnancy, *Biol. Reprod.,* 44, 834, 1991.

52. **Rahima, A. and Soderwall, A. L.,** Mast cells in uteri of pregnant young and senescent female golden hamsters, *Biol. Reprod.,* 17, 523, 1977.

53. **Redline, R. W. and Lu, C. Y.,** Localization of fetal major histocompatibility complex antigens and maternal leukocytes in murine placenta, *Lab. Invest.,* 61, 27, 1989.

54. **Hunt, J. S., Manning, L. S., Mitchell, D., Selanders, J. R., and Wood, G. W.,** Localization and characterization of macrophages in murine uterus, *J. Leuk. Biol.,* 38, 255, 1985.

55. **Hunt, J. S.,** Current topic: the role of macrophages in the uterine response to pregnancy, *Placenta,* 11, 467, 1990.

56. **Kearns, M. and Lala, P. K.,** Characterization of hematogenous cellular constituents of the murine decidua: a surface marker study, *J. Reprod. Immunol.,* 8, 213, 1985.

57. **Hunt, J. S., Manning, L. S., and Wood, G. W.,** Macrophages in murine uterus are immunosuppressive, *Cell. Immunol.,* 85, 499, 1984.

58. **Matthews, C. J. and Searle, R. F.,** The role of prostaglandins in the immunosuppressive effects of supernatants from adherent cells of murine decidual tissue, *J. Reprod. Immunol.,* 12, 109, 1987.

59. **Wood, G. W., Kamel, S., and Smith, K.,** Immunoregulation and prostaglandin production by mechanically-derived and enzyme-derived murine decidual cells, *J. Reprod. Immunol.,* 13, 235, 1988.

60. **Lala, P. K., Kearns, M., Paraher, R. S., Scodras, J., and Johnson, S.,** Immunological role of the cellular constituents of the decidua in the maintenance of semiallogeneic pregnancy, *Ann. N.Y. Acad. Sci.,* 476, 183, 1986.

61. **Scodras, J. M., Parhar, R. S., Kennedy, T. G., and Lala, P. K.,** Prostaglandin-mediated inactivation of natural killer cells in the murine decidua, *Cell. Immunol.,* 127, 352, 1990.

62. **Redline, R. W., McKay, D. B., Vazquez, M. A., Papaioannou, V. E., and Lu, C. Y.,** Macrophage functions are regulated by the substratum of murine decidual stromal cells, *J. Clin. Invest.,* 85, 1951, 1990.

63. **Redline, R. W. and Lu, C. Y.,** Specific defects in the anti-listerial immune response in discrete regions of the murine uterus and placenta account for susceptibility to infection, *J. Immunol.,* 140, 3947, 1988.

64. **Parr, M. B., Parr, E. L., Munaretto, K., Clark, M. R., and Dey, S. K.,** Immunohistochemical localization of prostaglandin synthase in the rat uterus and embryo during the peri-implantation period, *Biol. Reprod.,* 38, 333, 1988.

65. **Rees, M., Parry, D. M., Anderson, A. B., and Turnbull, A. C.**, Immunohistochemical localisation of cyclooxygenase in the human uterus, *Prostaglandins*, 23, 207, 1982.
66. **Wilson, L., Jr. and Freinkel, N.**, Alterations in uterine and placental prostaglandin F and E with gestational age in the rat, *Prostaglandins*, 24, 567, 1982.
67. **Wiqvist, N., Lundstrom, V., and Green, K.**, Premature labor and indomethacin, *Prostaglandins*, 10, 515, 1975.
68. **Smith, S. K. and Kelly, R. W.**, The release of PGF2α and PGE2 from separated cells of human endometrium and decidua, *Prost. Leuk. Ess. Fatty Acids*, 33, 91, 1988.
69. **Lala, P. K., Scodras, J. M., Graham, C. H., Lysiak, J. J., and Parhar, R. S.**, Activation of maternal killer cells in the pregnant uterus with chronic indomethacin therapy, IL-2 therapy, or a combination therapy is associated with embryonic demise, *Cell. Immunol.*, 127, 368, 1990.
70. **Kamel, S. and Wood, G. W.**, Failure of *in vitro*-expanded hyperimmune cytotoxic T lymphocytes to affect survival of mouse embryos *in vivo*, *J. Reprod. Immunol.*, 19, 69, 1991.
71. **Chaouat, G., Menu, E., and Wegmann, T. G.**, Role of lymphokines of the CSF family and of TBF, gamma interferon, and IL-2 in placental growth and fetal survival studied in 2 murine models of spontaneous resorptions, in *Materno-Fetal Relationship: Molecular and Cellular Biology*, Chaouat, G., Ed., Proc. INSERM Colloque, John Libbey, Paris, 1991, 91.
72. **Clark, D. A.**, Controversies in reproductive immunology, *Crit. Rev. Immunol.*, 11, 215, 1991.
73. **Tamada, H., McMaster, M. T., Flanders, K. C., Andrews, G. K., and Dey, S. K.**, Cell type-specific expression of TGF-β1 in the mouse uterus during the periimplantation period, *Mol. Endocrinol.*, 4, 965, 1990.
74. **Clark, D. A.**, Paraimmunology in the decidua, *Am. J. Reprod. Immunol.*, 24, 37, 1990.
75. **Slapsys, R. M. and Clark, D. A.**, Active suppression of host versus graft reaction in pregnant mice. V. Kinetics, specificity, and *in vivo* activity of non-T suppressor cells localized to the genital tract of mice during first pregnancy, *Am. J. Reprod. Immunol.*, 3, 65, 1982.
76. **Slapsys, R. M., Richards, C. D., and Clark, D. A.**, Active suppression of host-versus-graft reaction in pregnant mice. VIII. The uterine decidua-associated suppressor cell is distinct from decidual NK cells, *Cell. Immunol.*, 99, 140, 1985.
77. **Chaouat, G., Clark, D. A., and Wegmann, T. G.**, Genetic aspects of the CBA × DBA/2 and B10 × B10.A models of murine pregnancy failure and its prevention by lymphocyte immunisation, in *Early Pregnancy Loss: Mechanisms and Treatment*, Beard, R. W. and Sharp, F., Eds., Peacock Press, Ashton-under-Lyne, 1988, 89.
78. **Croy, B. A., Rossant, J., and Clark, D. A.**, Effects of alterations in the immunocompetent status of *Mus musculus* females on the survival of transferred *Mus caroli* embryos, *J. Reprod. Fertil.*, 74, 479, 1985.

79. **Clark, D. A., Flanders, K. C., Banwatt, D., Millar-Book, W., Manuel, J., Stedronska-Clark, J., and Rowley, B.**, Murine pregnancy decidua produces a unique immunosuppressive molecule related to TGF-β2, *J. Immunol.*, 144, 3008, 1990.

80. **Clark, D. A., Lea, R. G., Denburg, J., Banwatt, D., Manuel, J., Namji, N., Underwood, J., Michel, M., Mowbray, J., Daya, S., and Chaouat, G.**, TGF-β related suppressor factor in mammalian pregnancy decidua: homologies between the mouse and human in successful pregnancy and in recurrent unexplained abortion, in *Materno-Fetal Relationship: Molecular and Cellular Biology,* Chaouat, G., Ed., INSERM Colloque, John Libbey, Paris, 1991, 171.

81. **Clark, D. A., Lea, R. G., Podor, T., Daya, S., Banwatt, D., and Harley, C.**, Cytokines determining the success or failure of pregnancy, *Ann. N.Y. Acad. Sci.*, 626, 524, 1991.

82. **Clark, D. A., Damji, N., Chaput, A., Daya, S., Rosenthal, K. L., and Brierley, J.**, Decidua-associated suppressor cells and suppressor factors regulating interleukin-2: their role in the survival of the "fetal allograft", in *Proceedings of VI International Congress in Immunology,* Cinader, B. and Miller, R. G., Eds., Academic Press, New York, 1986, 1089.

83. **Slapsys, R. M., Younglai, E., and Clark, D. A.**, A novel suppressor cell is recruited to decidua by fetal trophoblast-type cells, *Regul. Immunol.*, 1, 182, 1988.

84. **Daya, S., Johnson, P. M., and Clark, D. A.**, Trophoblast induction of suppressor type cell activity in human endometrial tissue, *Am. J. Reprod. Immunol.*, 19, 65, 1989.

85. **Croy, B. A., Wood, W., and King, G. J.**, Evaluation of intrauterine immune suppression during pregnancy in a species with epitheliochorial placentation, *J. Immunol.*, 139, 1088, 1987.

86. **Krcek, J. and Clark, D. A.**, Localization of a small sized bone marrow subpopulation at the implantation site in the murine fetus, *Am. J. Reprod. Immunol.*, 7, 95, 1985.

87. **Moore, S. C. and Sorderberg, L. S. F.**, Mouse bone marrow natural suppressor cells: induction and activity, *FASEB J.*, 4, 435, 1990.

88. **Peel, S.**, Granulated metrial gland cells, *Adv. Anat. Embryol. Cell Biol.*, 115, 1, 1989.

89. **Jbara, K. and Stewart, I.**, Granulated metrial gland cells in the uterus and labyrinthine placenta of inbred and outbred pregnancies in mice, *J. Anat.*, 135, 311, 1985.

90. **Croy, B. A., Guilbert, L., Browne, M., Gough, N., Stinchcomb, D., Reed, N., and Wegmann, T. G.**, Characterization of cytokine production by the metrial gland and granulated metrial gland cells, *J. Reprod. Immunol.*, 19, 149, 1991.

91. **Parr, E. L., Parr, M. B., and Young, J. D.**, Localization of a pore-forming protein (perforin) in granulated metrial gland cells, *Biol. Reprod.*, 37, 1327, 1987.

92. **Parr, E. L., Szary, A., and Parr, M. B.**, Measurement of natural killer activity and target cell binding by mouse metrial gland cells isolated by enzymic or mechanical methods, *J. Reprod. Fertil.*, 88, 283, 1990.

93. **Croy, B. A. and Kassouf, S. A.,** Evaluation of the murine metrial gland for immunological function, *J. Reprod. Immunol.,* 15, 51, 1989.

94. **McDougall, J. R., Croy, B. A., Chapeau, C., and Clark, D. A.,** Demonstration of a splenic cytotoxic effector cell in mice of genotype *scid/scid.bg/ bg, Cell. Immunol.,* 130, 106, 1990.

95. **Drake, B. L. and Head, J. R.,** Murine trophoblast can be killed by lymphokine-activated killer cells, *J. Immunol.,* 143, 9, 1989.

96. **Stewart, I. and Mukhtar, D. Y.,** The killing of mouse trophoblast cells by granulated metrial gland cell *in vitro, Placenta,* 9, 417, 1988.

97. **Peel, S. and Stewart, I.,** Rat granulated metrial gland cells differentiate in pregnant chimeric mice and may be cytotoxic for mouse trophoblast, *Cell Differ. Dev.,* 28, 55, 1989.

98. **Chaouat, G., Menu, E., Clark, D. A., Minkowsky, M., Dy, M., and Wegmann, T. G.,** Control of fetal survival in CBA × DBA/2 mice by lymphokine therapy, *J. Reprod. Fertil.,* 89, 447, 1990.

99. **Gendron, R. L., Nestel, F. P., Lapp, W. S., and Baines, M. G.,** Lipopolysaccharide induced early pregnancy failure in mice is associated with decidual natural killer-like cells, uterine production of tumor necrosis factor and is preventable by pentoxifylline, *J. Reprod. Fertil.,* 90, 395, 1990.

100. **Crowell, R. E., Chick, T. W., and Reed, W. P.,** Pentoxifylline relaxes isolated pulmonary after preconstriction with norepinephrine, *Respiration,* 57, 45, 1990.

101. **Boogaerts, M. A., Malbrain, S., Meeus, P., van Hove, L., and Verhoef, G. E.,** *In vitro* modulation of normal and diseased human neutrophil function by pentoxifylline, *Blut,* 61, 60, 1990.

102. **Heine, O., Mueller-Eckhardt, G., Stitz, L., and Pabst, W.,** Influence of treatment with mouse immunoglobulin on the rate of viable neonates in the CBA/J × DBA/2J model, *Res. Exp. Med.,* 192, 49, 1992.

103. **Gendron, R. L., Farooki, R., and Baines, M. G.,** Resorption of CBA/J and DBA/2 mouse conceptuses in CBA/J uteri correlates with failure of the fetoplacental unit to suppress natural killer cell activity, *J. Reprod. Fertil.,* 89, 277, 1990.

104. **Kearns, M. and Lala, P. K.,** Radioautographic analysis of surface markers on decidual cells shared by cells of the lymphomyeloid tissues, *Am. J. Reprod. Immunol. Microbiol.,* 9, 39, 1985.

105. **Fowlis, D. J. and Ansell, J. D.,** Evidence that decidual cells are not derived from bone marrow, *Transplantation,* 39, 445, 1985.

106. **Gambel, P., Rossant, J., Hunziker, R. D., and Wegmann, T. G.,** Origin of decidual cells in murine pregnancy and pseudo-pregnancy, *Transplantation,* 39, 443, 1985.

107. **Gambel, P., Rossant, J., Hunziker, R. D., and Wegmann, T. G.,** Decidual cells in murine pregnancy and pseudo-pregnancy: origin and natural killer activity, *Transplant. Proc.,* 17, 905, 1985.

Decidua-Associated Immunoregulatory Factors

R. F. Searle
Department of Immunology
The Medical School
University of Newcastle upon Tyne
Newcastle upon Tyne, England

1. INTRODUCTION

While maternal immune recognition of the semiallogeneic intrauterine conceptus as indicated by limited maternal antifetal humoral and cell-mediated immune responses during pregnancy is an infrequent event which is not obligatory for pregnancy success, it has been suggested that active regulation of maternal effector immune pathways is required to operate locally at the level of the fetal placental unit to ensure fetal survival.[11,29] Maternal immune responses leading to spontaneous resorption or miscarriage with fetal demise during murine and human pregnancy is apparently associated with the presence of natural killer (NK)-like cells, cytotoxic T lymphocytes (CTL), as well as the absence of a distinct decidua-associated cell population with soluble suppressor activity.[12,14,21] The proposal that active immunoregulatory processes represent a primary mechanism essential for successful pregnancy outcome, however, has been questioned.[5]

To date there is a large body of evidence that a range of soluble products of the two components of the placenta, namely fetal trophoblast and maternal decidual tissue, display immunoregulatory properties and therefore have the capacity to regulate maternal immunity *in vivo*. Whether these placental-associated regulatory factors represent a secondary rather than a primary mechanism in the maternal-fetal immunointeraction is unknown and provides a focus for future studies. In this chapter, the extent of decidua-associated immunoregulation is outlined.

2. IMMUNOREGULATORY ACTIVITY OF MURINE DECIDUAL TISSUE

Support for the proposal that the decidua has an important *in vivo* immunoregulatory role in the maternal-fetal relationship has been strengthened by the findings from several laboratories that murine decidual tissue produces soluble factors which regulate a variety of immune responses *in vitro*.

Globerson and co-workers[23] first reported that crude extracts of decidual tissue obtained from pseudopregnant rats suppressed the *in vitro* T cell-dependent antibody response to α-2, 4-dinitrophenyl-polylysine. Although the nature of the immunoregulatory agent in the decidual preparation was not characterized further, this study demonstrated unequivocally the potential of decidua to regulate immune responses. Subsequently, Kirkwood and Bell[28] reported that supernatants from a culture system in which murine uterine cells undergo artificially induced decidual cell differentiation *in vitro* display immunoregulatory activity. Supernatants from decidual cell cultures derived from syngeneically and allogeneically mated mice resulted in significant inhibition of the mixed lymphocyte reaction (MLR) and phytohemagglutinin (PHA)-induced lymphoproliferation with the inhibitory activity being produced during the period of decidual cell differentiation and later during involution of the cultures. The production of inhibitory factor by both syngeneic and allogeneic decidual cell cultures, however, suggested that this production is a basic property of decidua rather than an immunologically related response. The finding that supernatants added 24 h after the start of the MLR inhibited the MLR to the same extent as addition at 0 h indicated that the immunoregulatory soluble factor in the culture supernatants probably acted at the proliferative phase of the MLR rather than during the immune recognition phase. By contrast, no inhibitory activity was detected in supernatants from cultures of embryonic tissues. In a preliminary attempt to define further the nature of the decidual immunoregulatory factor, culture supernatant inhibitory activity was demonstrated to be associated with both high- (>1500) and low- (<1500) molecular-weight fractions.

Although the precise identity of the immunoregulatory factors, their mechanism of immunosuppression, and the uterine cell population undergoing decidual cell differentiation *in vitro* responsible for soluble factor production were not resolved, the study served to focus attention on the capacity of murine decidual tissue in normal pregnancy to produce a range of soluble immunosuppressor factors with the capacity to regulate the maternal immune response *in vivo*.

Similarly, supernatants from short-term cultures of syngeneic murine decidual tissue obtained from the uteri of pregnant mice inhibited a third-party MLR.[1] The immunoregulatory factor which acted during the proliferative phase of the MLR lacked immunological specificity. The degree of inhibitory activity was markedly affected by the seeding density of the two morphologically distinct adherent decidual cell populations of the cultures, the period of culture, and the stage of pregnancy from which the decidua was obtained for culture, inhibitory activity being maximal on day 8 post coitus (pc). By contrast, supernatants from cultures of nonpregnant uteri did not produce any significant inhibitory effect on the MLR.

Subsequent studies have focused on the physiochemical nature of the soluble factors produced during short-term *in vitro* culture. A comparison of the electrophoretic and gel filtration profiles of supernatants from cultures of decidual tissue from uteri of pregnant mice on day 8 pc and from pseudopregnant mice showed that the range of immunoregulatory factors synthesized by decidua from pregnant uteri with a fetus and by artificially induced deciduoma without a fetal contribution were identical.[20] Several, rather than a single, nonspecific inhibitory factors appeared to be involved. Fractionation revealed that MLR inhibitory activity was associated with three different molecular size fractions, namely <1.5 kDa, 60 kDa, and 1000 kDa, but only the low- (<1.5 kDa) molecular-weight fraction was capable of inhibiting both MLR and spontaneous neonatal thymocyte proliferation.[2] The kinetics of production of the inhibitory factors are different with the maximum production of the MLR-inhibitory high-molecular-weight fraction by decidua obtained from day 8 of pregnancy, whereas the low-molecular-weight fraction is produced throughout early pregnancy. Furthermore, the 60-kDa and 1000-kDa fractions also inhibited cytotoxic T cell (CTL) generation, but had no effect on preexisting CTL lytic activity.[20] In addition, crude supernatants impaired the anti-Srbc antibody response while the 60-kDa fraction proved to be strongly stimulatory for the T-dependent plaque-forming antibody response. These findings indicated that the immunoregulatory activity of crude culture supernatants of decidual tissue appeared to be derived from several soluble factors with different properties rather than due to a single factor with a particular biological activity.

3. PROSTAGLANDIN E$_2$-MEDIATED IMMUNOSUPPRESSOR ACTIVITY OF MURINE DECIDUA

Other workers reported that the nonspecific immunosuppressive property of culture supernatants of murine decidual tissue from day 8 pc reflected a major contribution of a low-molecular-weight soluble factor.[37] The immunosuppressive activity of culture supernatants in a panel of *in vitro* assays of T cell lymphoproliferation, including MLR, thymocyte proliferation assay, CTL generation, and mitogen- and antigen-induced proliferation assays, was completely abrogated after dialysis with a low-molecular-weight cut-off. Furthermore, supernatants from indomethacin-treated cultures to prevent prostaglandin synthesis, unlike the paired untreated cultures, showed a significant loss of suppressive activity. The substantial production of immunoregulatory prostaglandins by decidual tissue *in vitro* introduced the possibility of an immunoregulatory role of decidua-derived prostaglandins at the maternal-fetal interface during pregnancy.

Similarly, studies in which supernatants were generated from short-term cultures of uterine cell suspensions obtained later from days 14 to 19 of allopregnancy have reported immunoregulatory prostaglandin production by late decidual tissue. Different soluble suppressor factors, however, were generated depending on whether murine decidual cells were mechanically or enzymatically dispersed.[55,60] Although the degree of nonspecific suppression of MLRs produced by culture supernatants of enzymatically or mechanically dispersed uterine cells was quantitatively similar, major qualitative differences existed in the suppression mediated by the two methodologic approaches. Suppressor activity was completely lost with indomethacin-treated cultures of enzyme-prepared cells, while the level of suppression by cultured, mechanically prepared cells was not affected.[55,60] Enzymatically dispersed cells produced very high levels of the prostaglandin PGE_2 compared to the insignificant PGE_2 levels by mechanically dispersed cells. The prostaglandin contribution to supernatant suppressor activity of cultured, enzymatically dispersed cells was further indicated by the complete loss of suppression after charcoal adsorption which selectively removes lipids, while there was no apparent effect after protein depletion.

Further evidence for a possible immunoregulatory role of decidua-derived prostaglandins in materno-fetal cellular immunointeractions came from studies *in vitro* which have demonstrated an inactivation of NK cell activity in murine decidua.[46] Typical decidual cells, decidual macrophages as well as decidual cell culture supernatants, inhibited NK cell activity in an MHC-unrestricted manner. Indomethacin or anti-PGE_2 antibody treatment abrogated this suppression and revived NK cell activation. These findings suggested that PGE_2 produced by decidual macrophages and by typical decidual cells, as identified by their uninucleate morphology and cell surface phenotype, is responsible for the suppression of NK cell activity in murine decidua. Moreover, the levels of suppressor activity by decidua correlated with the increased levels of PGE_2 production in late gestation decidua. When pregnant mice were treated with chronic indomethacin therapy via drinking water to block prostaglandin synthesis *in vivo,* embryo resorption (89 to 100%) resulted and this abortifacient effect could be prevented by anti-asialo GM1 (a NK cell and activated macrophage marker) antibody treatment. Mononuclear cells isolated from the uteri of the aborting mice showed killer activity.

Moreover these findings suggested that PGE_2-mediated immunoregulation of NK cells within decidua may be obligatory for fetal survival *in vivo*.[31]

Although PGE_2 makes a major contribution to decidua-associated suppressor factor-mediated suppression, there is unequivocal evidence that more than one soluble factor is generated by enzymatically dispersed uterine cells. Supernatants from indomethacin-treated cultures suppressed the MLR when added late in culture, which suggests that other soluble factors, in addition to PGE_2, block T cell proliferation. The nature of the other soluble factor is unknown, except that it is not a protein and might be a nonprostaglandin lipid. It is the production of these other nonprostaglandin soluble factors which is held to account for the incomplete loss of suppression in some indomethacin-treated decidual cell cultures.[55] In contrast, mechanically dispersed decidual cells produced only insignificant amounts of PGE_2 and generated indomethacin-insensitive nonprostaglandin soluble suppressor factors.

The cellular source of the prostaglandins and other soluble suppressor factors in culture supernatants is unknown. Decidual tissue in pregnant and in pseudopregnant mice is a mixture of several distinct cell types. Short-term cultures of murine decidual tissue from early in pregnancy contain two distinct adherent cell populations which have been identified as F4/80 antigen-positive macrophages and stroma-derived decidual cells.[36,47] Macrophages which are present in large numbers in the pregnant uterus produce prostaglandins PGE_2 and $PGF_{2\alpha}$, prostacyclin, and thromboxane, but only PGE_2 has extensively documented immunoregulatory effects on T cell function. Typical decidual cells have also been reported to release PGE_2 *in vitro*. Although decidual macrophage (at least 95% pure) cultures from late pregnancy[55] produce more PGE_2 than macrophage-depleted decidual cell cultures (which contained less than 1% contaminating macrophages), there is evidence that these latter morphologically heterogeneous decidual cell cultures also produce PGE_2 and are highly immunosuppressive of MLRs, indomethacin treatment relieving macrophage-depleted uterine cell-mediated MLR suppression. PGE_2 regulates T cell lymphoproliferative responses by inhibiting the production of interleukin (IL)-2 and the expression of transferrin and IL-2 receptors, but does not inhibit responses to IL-2 once IL-2R are expressed. Decidua-derived PGE_2 could therefore protect the fetus from a variety of maternal effector mechanisms by regulating T cell-dependent lymphoproliferative responses and CTL generation. Additional immunoregulatory effects of PGE_2 include the inhibition of NK cell lytic activity and the downregulation of MHC class II expression.

The overall significance of a decidua-derived PGE_2-mediated local regulation of maternal immunity, however, remains unclear, since the basal levels of PG release by murine decidual tissue *in vivo* is unknown. It is essential to establish whether in the mouse PGE_2 production by the various distinct decidual cell populations also occurs *in vivo* or only when cultured after enzymic dispersal *in vitro*. However, the failure of indomethacin to block completely suppression indicates that decidual macrophages and other decidual cell populations produce additional soluble suppressor factors. The precise mechanism of action of these high-molecular-weight soluble factors remains unknown. The culture supernatants are unlikely to contain the immunosuppressor factor, transforming growth factor (TGF)-β_2-related factor, which is produced exclusively by granular small lymphocytic non-T suppressor cells within decidua which are nonadherent *in vitro*. It is important for further studies to define the relative amounts of immunoregulatory PGE_2 and the other high-molecular-weight soluble factors produced by murine decidual tissue *in vivo*. The studies to date indicate that the range of soluble suppressive molecules produced by murine decidual cells *in vitro* is critically influenced both by the methodological approaches used to disperse the decidua for culture and by the appropriate stage in gestation. It is clear, however, that these factors are not specifically induced following antigenic exposure of the fetal-placental unit and act *in vitro* without MHC specificity or restriction to block nonspecifically the immune response.

4. TGF-β_2-MEDIATED IMMUNOSUPPRESSOR ACTIVITY OF MURINE DECIDUA

Clark and co-workers[13,15,16,49] have described a trophoblast-dependent decidua-associated suppressor cell population which produces a soluble suppressor factor *in vitro*. Suppressor cell activity is obtained from allopregnant decidua on days 9.5 to 16.5 of pregnancy by mechanical dispersal followed by velocity sedimentation. It was noted that enzymic dispersal eliminated suppressor activity. The predominant suppressor cell population *in vitro* is a small granulated FcR-bearing cell with a modal sedimentation velocity of 3.0 ± 0.5 mm/h and a null phenotype (Thy 1^-, Ly 1^-2^-, asialo-GM1$^-$, and Mac 1^-) but their precise *in situ* localization is unclear. These cells nonspecifically inhibited the generation of CTL *in vitro* and *in vivo*, did not affect the activity of performed CTLs, but were deficient in decidua destined to abort in the CBA/DBA J mice. A lesser degree of inhibitory activity was noted with a large-size decidua-associated suppressor cell population isolated by velocity sedimentation at 8 to 10 mm/h. As with the cell-associated suppressor activity crude supernatants from cultures of Thy 1.2 plus complement-treated resistant decidua-derived cells displayed similar nonspecific and non-MHC-restricted suppressor activity *in vitro* for CTL and lymphokine-activated killer (LAK) cell generation as well as NK cell activation. This nonspecific soluble suppressor activity was initially reported to be associated with a single peak of activity of approximately 100 kDa on Sephacryl 200 chromatography and thus appeared to be due to a single factor and not to various molecular species from decidua. The soluble factor inhibited the proliferation of IL-2-dependent cell lines as well as IL-2-dependent generation of cytotoxic effector cells *in vitro* and acted to block the action of IL-2 but did not block the binding of IL-2 to the IL-2R. This activity blocked the proliferative response to IL-2 by cells with IL-2R and may thereby effectively regulate immune responses *in vivo*.

Subsequent studies have characterized further the soluble suppressor factor associated with this distinct decidual cell population. The suppressive activity was unchanged or only slightly affected by indomethacin treatment, anti-PGE$_2$ antibody, dextran-activated charcoal and lipid extraction to remove steroids and prostaglandins, but was abrogated by hydroxylapatite and Con A-agarose. The suppressive activity of supernatants was completely abolished by anti-TGF-β antibody treatment. Furthermore, high-performance liquid chromatography under acidic conditions revealed a dominant peak of suppressor activity at 13 kDa with some residual activity at 65 kDa and at 1000 kDa but the activity which had been seen under neutral conditions at 80 to 100 kDa and 300 kDa disappeared. Moreover, suppression by the 13-kDa peak was completely reversed by treatment with anti-TGF-β antibody. Members of the TGF-β family, however, are known to be homodimers with a molecular size of 25 kDa. This suggests that the decidua-associated small cell soluble suppressor activity was primarily mediated by a 13-kDa decidua-associated factor which represents a distinct regulatory molecule related to TGF-β that associates with protein and glycoprotein carrier molecules. It is unclear whether either the 65-kDa and 1000-kDa molecules are related in any manner to the 13-kDa activity. The suppressive activity of both the crude and purified decidual soluble suppressor factor was neutralized by antibodies to TGF-β$_2$ but not to TGF-β$_1$. A subsequent study with nonreducing polyacrylamide gel electrophoresis and Western blotting of the purified suppressive factor showed that the TGF-β$_2$-reactive molecules in highly purified decidual supernatants was approximately in the 20- to 23-kDa range rather than 13 kDa. This is slightly smaller than TGF-β$_2$ and suggests that the soluble decidual immunosuppressor factor is a distinct molecule which is closely related to TGF-β$_2$ but is indistinguishable from TGF-β$_2$ by specific antibodies. The precise relationship of the 23-kDa decidua-associated suppressor factor with TGF-β$_2$ will only be established by molecular cloning and sequencing analysis.

As in the case of decidual PGE$_2$ production, it remains to be determined whether the production of the TGF-β$_2$-related factor by murine decidua occurs *in vivo* or rather is elaborated only *in vitro*. Messenger RNA for TGF-β$_2$, however, has been demonstrated in decidua and *in situ* hybridization has revealed a small population of positive cells in decidua basalis. This suggests that production of this decidua-associated regulatory agent probably takes place *in vivo*.

5. OTHER MURINE DECIDUAL PROTEINS WITH POTENTIAL IMMUNOREGULATORY ACTIVITY

Pregnancy-associated serum protein with α_1-electrophoretic mobility (α_1-PAP) which is present in murine pregnancy sera and the sera of some strains of virgin females, but is absent from males,[57] is immunohistochemically localized to mononuclear leukocytes in the intestinal mucosa and associated lymphoid tissue, liver hepatocytes, placental trophoblast, and to α_1-PAP$^+$ cells in the decidua during pregnancy.[58] The identity of the α_1-PAP-positive decidual cell population, however, is unknown, but it has been suggested they may represent decidual macrophages. Macrophages in other locations appear to be closely involved with the production of this protein. Although its functional role is unclear, rat pregnancy-associated globulin (PAG), a purported analog to α_1-PAP, is immunosuppressive *in vitro* and suppresses delayed-type hypersensitivity reactions in both mice and rats *in vitro*. Whether α_1-PAP is synthesized by the murine decidua is unclear, as is its immuno-suppressive properties *in vitro*. It is a matter for speculation whether decidual α_1-PAP production will prove to be involved in regulation of local immune responses during pregnancy.

6. IMMUNOREGULATORY ACTIVITY OF HUMAN DECIDUA

Several workers have demonstrated the capacity of human decidual tissue to suppress lymphocyte alloreactivity *in vitro*. This immunoregulatory activity of human decidua, as in the case of mouse, is mediated by a range of soluble suppressor factors.

6.1. Immunoregulatory Properties of Soluble Factors Synthesized by Human Decidua

As in the case of the mouse, culture supernatants from explants of early human decidua inhibited the MLR and mitogen-induced lymphoprolifera-tion.[24] The identity of the soluble suppressor factor, however, was not characterized, although the contribution of immunoregulatory prostaglandins was apparently excluded. Dialysis to remove low-molecular-weight factors did not affect the level of immunoinhibitory activity and the PGE$_2$ concentration present in the culture supernatants was reported to be not sufficient to be suppressive *in vitro*.

Other workers subsequently confirmed that culture supernatants from early human decidua contain a soluble suppressor factor and further inves-tigated the mechanism of immunosuppressive activity.[34] In these studies an adherent decidual cell fraction was obtained by enzymic and mechanically dispersed human decidua between 8 to 10 weeks of pregnancy and then enriched with a discontinuous density gradient. The decidual cultures contained in excess of 90% round cytoplasmic-rich typical decidual cells, lacked stromal fibroblasts, macrophages, and leukocytes by morphological criteria, and did not express the macrophage antigen MY4. Crude culture supernatants inhibited both T and B cell *in vitro* assays such as PHA-induced lymphoproliferation, the MLR, allogeneic cytotoxic T cell generation, and immunoglobulin production, and appeared to act at the level of lymphokine production and lymphocyte activation since the levels of IL-2 and interferon IFN-γ production as well as IL-2R expression were decreased. Gel filtration of the supernatants revealed a single peak of suppressive activity with a molecular weight between 43 and 67 kDa while any contribution of regulatory prostaglandins was excluded by dialysis.

The suppressor factor has now been further purified by serial biochemical procedures and immunochemically characterized.[35] The purified soluble factor is a protein, is not a glycoprotein, and inhibits T cell function in an identical manner as the crude culture supernatants. This protein inhibited IL-2, IFN-γ and B cell-stimulating factor-2 (BSF-2) production and decreased IL-2R and transferrin receptor expression on PHA-stimulated blasts at 5 μg/ml. Isoelectric focusing displayed four bands, the protein isoelectric point was approximately 7.5 in one band and between 6.85 and 7.35 in the other three. This protein appears to be decidual cell specific and is not produced by other cell types derived from other fractions of early human decidua nor by endometrial cells from nonpregnant women. This fraction may contain several distinct molecular species and requires further purification.

Whether the partially purified protein is identical to the immunosuppressor factor obtained from a cell line transformed from human decidual cells is not known,[54] nor is its relationship to the high-molecular-weight immunosuppressor factors in culture supernatants of murine decidual tissue. Although this protein is apparently human decidual cell specific and displays immunosuppressive properties *in vitro,* the *in vivo* role of the soluble factor awaits clarification. The future development of purified soluble suppressor protein-specific monoclonal antibodies would permit not only its immunohistological localization but also analysis of the kinetics of the protein's synthesis, secretion, and serum levels during pregnancy.

6.2. Immunoregulatory Factor Synthesized by a Cell Line Derived from Human Decidual Cells

Culture supernatants from the cell line, TTK-1, established from human early decidual tissue contain a soluble immunosuppressor factor.[54] The crude supernatant inhibited both the one-way and two-way MLR to a greater extent than culture supernatants of other transformed cell lines. The supernatant had a dose-dependent suppressive activity in the MLR which was inhibited when supernatants were added 5 days after the start of the MLR culture. In addition, the TTK-1 supernatant suppressed the proliferation of an IL-2-dependent T cell line but failed to inhibit that of IL-2-independent T cell lines. These findings suggest that the mechanism of TTK-1 supernatant-mediated immunosuppression is by inhibition of the action of IL-2 in the proliferative phase of the immune response. Biochemical characterization and partial purification of the TTK-1 supernatant revealed that the molecular weight of the soluble suppressor factor(s) in the MLR and proliferation of IL-2-dependent T cell line was between 43 and 67 kDa. This immunosuppressive fraction, however, was reported to contain several components by gel electrophoresis. Further purification of the suppressor factors will clarify the precise mechanism of immunosuppression.

An important point to be resolved is whether the 43- to 67-kDa immunoregulatory factor(s) produced by the transformed decidual cell line is identical to that synthesized by normal early human decidua. This will ultimately necessitate comparison of the amino acid sequences of the two factors. Although the transformed TTK-1 cell line morphologically resembles decidual cells at the fine structural level, the decidua-derived cell line has lost some of the surface markers associated with normal decidua and, in addition, fails to produce detectable levels of the decidua-associated hormone, prolactin.

6.3. Prostaglandin E_2-Mediated Immunosuppressor Function of Early Human Decidua

Addition of a heterogeneous population of decidua-derived cells from early in gestation, 6.5 to 9.5 weeks menstrual age, as well as the enriched typical decidual cell fraction (identified as 96% pure on the basis of morphological and other surface and cytoplasmic phenotype properties) to the MLR suppressed lymphoproliferation and CTL generation.[42] The level of MHC-unrestricted suppression was greater than that with either the mixed decidual fraction which contained numerous decidual macrophages or later gestational age first-trimester decidua. This early decidua-associated suppression, however, was either substantially or completely relieved by indomethacin- or anti-PGE_2 antibody-treated decidual cultures. Moreover, the degree of suppression correlated positively with PGE_2 concentrations *in vitro*. These findings suggested that the suppression of alloreactivity was mediated predominantly by the *in vitro* synthesis of prostaglandins secreted by typical decidual cells and by decidual macrophages in first-trimester decidua. The inverse relationship between the degree of suppression and gestational age of the decidua, moreover, appeared to correlate with the decline in incidence of typical decidual cells from later gestational age decidua. This strengthened the view that the typical nonphagocytic, uninucleate, Dec-1 antigen-positive typical decidual cell represents a major suppressor cell population within early human decidua in addition to suppression mediated by decidual macrophages.

The *in vitro* PGE_2-mediated suppression of lymphocyte activation and proliferation by early typical decidual cells is mediated by the downregulation of IL-2R development on lymphocytes and the inhibition of IL-2 production in the mixed lymphocyte culture (MLC).[30] These effects blocked T cell proliferation but PGE_2 did not interfere with either the interaction of IL-2 and IL-2R nor the lytic activity of preformed CTLs. In addition to this afferent blockade of T cell activation, decidua-associated PGE_2 completely inhibited IL-2R expression on, as well as IL-2 production by, the maternal leukocytic population in dispersed decidual tissue cultures.[43] IL-2R expression and IL-2R production were stimulated in indomethacin- or anti-PGE_2 antibody-treated decidual cultures and this was further enhanced by exogenous rIL-2, findings which suggest that PGE_2 produced by first-trimester decidua may block the activation of the maternal decidual leukocytic population *in situ*.

It should be noted that there was a much-reduced residual level of immunosuppression by decidual cells in the presence of indomethacin which may indicate an additional nonprostaglandin-mediated suppression. Alternatively, it may have been due to preformed PGE_2, since there was near complete abrogation of this inhibition in the presence of anti-PGE_2 antibody.

The actual levels of prostaglandin release by human decidua *in vivo* during pregnancy are not known. *In vitro* glandular preparations of early human decidua produce markedly less immunoregulatory PGE_2 than glandular cells of the nonpregnant proliferative endometrium,[50] the *in vitro* synthesis of prostaglandins being inhibited by progesterone after ovulation. In addition, it has been reported that the trauma of collecting decidual tissue may result in the artificial and rapid release of PGE_2. It is therefore important to establish whether human decidua produces PGE_2 *in situ* or rather only when decidua is cultured *in vitro*.

6.4. Trophoblast-Induced Decidua-Associated Soluble Immunosuppressor Factors

Workers have described three distinct populations of decidua-associated suppressor cells, two of which produce soluble immunosuppressor factors.[17-19] The surface phenotype, cytoplasmic and other morphological properties of these decidua-associated suppressor cells and their *in situ* localization, however, have not been fully investigated, except for their size and sedimentation velocity. Mitogen-induced maternal lymphoproliferation is nonspecifically suppressed predominantly by a population of small suppressor cells obtained from first-trimester decidua after mechanical dispersal and isolation by velocity sedimentation. These cells had a modal sedimentation velocity of 4.16 $\pm$ 0.08 mm/h. Occasionally a small amount of suppressive activity is seen in association with a large cell population with a sedimentation velocity of

7 mm/h, a cell type which is characteristic of luteal-phase endometrium and which does not produce soluble suppressor factors. The overall levels of suppressive activity were considered to be higher in later- (weeks 13 to 16) stage first-trimester decidua than in decidua at 10 to 11 weeks of pregnancy. Crude supernatants from these later first-trimester decidua-associated cell cultures differentially inhibited the proliferation of IL-2-dependent cell lines while non-IL-2-dependent cells were unaffected. No suppressive activity was noted when culture supernatants were added 18 h after the start of assay. Suppressive activity was mainly associated with two soluble factors of molecular size 21 kDa and 43 kDa, while a reduced level of suppression was detected with a 60-kDa factor. The suppression by the soluble suppressor factors produced by the decidua-associated small cell population is mediated by the block to IL-2 action and acts at the level either of the cell or IL-2 before IL-2 and IL-2R interaction, thereby preventing lymphoproliferation. The finding that decidua-associated suppressor activity correlated with successful pregnancy[14] and was absent in women with a missed abortion at 10 to 11 weeks of pregnancy[17] suggested that the production of IL-2 blocking factors may immunoregulate maternal effector alloreactivity *in vivo*. Whether the range of soluble factors represent distinct suppressor molecules or polymers or breakdown products is unknown, as is their relationship to other human decidual secretory products. Furthermore, it remains to be determined whether the suppressive activity is mediated by a TGF-β_2-like molecule as is the case of the murine decidua-associated small cell suppressor factor. The finding that these soluble suppressor factors are elaborated when small cells from luteal-phase endometrium are incubated with trophoblast suggests that the small suppressor cell population in pregnant decidua is trophoblast dependent as in the case of the mouse.

Other studies have demonstrated a third distinct decidua-associated suppressor cell population in the uterine decidua obtained only from women early in first trimester with a tubal ectopic pregnancy; i.e., where the fetal placental unit is located outside the uterus. The large decidua-associated suppressor cell population with a mean sedimentation velocity of 6.7 ± 0.12 mm/h, as well as crude culture supernatants, inhibited mitogen-induced lymphoproliferation. This suppressor cell population in uterine decidua remote from the ectopic pregnancy not only differed in size from the small decidua-associated suppressor cell associated with intrauterine pregnancy but also released soluble factors unlike the large suppressor cells associated with luteal-phase endometrium. These soluble suppressor factors, moreover, differed in molecular size from those associated with normal pregnancy decidua, suppressive activity being associated with two major fractions corresponding to molecular sizes of 135 and 100 kDa. Furthermore, when endometrial luteal-phase large cells were cultured in medium conditioned by ectopic pregnancy trophoblast, soluble suppressor activity was induced, which suggests that, as in the case of the small decidua-associated suppressor cells in intrauterine pregnancy, the large cell population associated with ectopic pregnancy is trophoblast dependent.

The absence of the large trophoblast-dependent suppressor cell population with soluble suppressor factor activity from intrauterine pregnant decidua may reflect the possibility that the large cell population in luteal-phase endometrium are activated by trophoblast-derived factors during early pregnancy and are then replaced by the decidua-associated small cell population with soluble suppressor activity.

7. DEFINED IMMUNOREGULATORY SECRETORY PROTEINS OF THE DECIDUA

The endometrium during pregnancy is known to synthesize and secrete a number of proteins many of which are required for the maintenance of embryonic growth and viability. Although their precise role *in vivo* requires clarification, some of these secretory proteins produced apparently uniquely by decidua have immunoregulatory properties *in vitro*.

7.1. Endometrial Protein 15

One of the major secretory endometrial proteins is a glycosylated β-lactoglobulin homolog, endometrial protein 15, which was originally isolated from extracts of term human placenta[9] and termed placental protein 14 (PP14). Subsequent immunochemical and biochemical studies have shown this protein to possess identical characteristics to a number of other proteins independently described by several workers. These include pregnancy-associated endometrial α_2-globulin (α_2-PEG), progesterone-dependent endometrial protein (PEP), chorionic α_2-microglobulin, placenta-specific α_2-microglobulin, and human alpha uterine protein.[3,26,53] The complete amino acid sequence homology of PP14 with β-lactoglobulins, however, indicates that this protein belongs to the β-lactoglobulin secretory protein family.[27] Endometrial protein 15 serum levels during pregnancy peak between weeks 6 to 12 of pregnancy and decline thereafter.[25] The levels of this protein in the maternal circulation during the first trimester concur with *in vitro* studies of its synthesis *de novo* and secretion rates which show that this protein represents a major soluble protein produced by decidua in early pregnancy and is not absorbed serum protein. It forms quantitatively 10% of the total soluble protein extracted from decidua. In amniotic fluid the protein levels are two to three orders of magnitude higher than in serum and are derived from the endometrial glands. Immunohistological studies have localized this protein primarily to the secretory glandular epithelium in the nondecidualized decidua spongiosa region of the pregnant endometrium during the early trimester while glands in the decidua compacta are either nonsecretory or contain less immunoreactive protein.[59] Although this protein is also synthesized by secretory endometrial glands during the mid to late luteal phase of the menstrual cycle, it is not uniquely synthesized by endometrial glands since human male seminal plasma contains high protein levels where it forms 2.5% of the total protein. Although the *in vivo* role of this protein is unclear,[4] there is no evidence that, in man, it is involved in the binding and transport of a vitamin or small-molecular-weight hydrophobic ligand as would be expected from its membership of the β-lactoglobulin protein family. The protein is reported to display marked immunosuppressive properties *in vitro*.

Crude human decidual extracts as well as the purified endometrial protein 15 inhibited the MLR and PHA-induced lymphoproliferation, the suppression being dose dependent and relating to the PP14 content.[10,44] Treatment of the decidual extracts and the purified protein preparations with a monoclonal anti-PP14 immunoadsorbent confirmed the specificity of this immunosuppressive activity, the reduction in suppressive activity being related to the reduction in PP14 content of the decidual extracts and not to the total protein content of the extracts. Moreover, the use of immunoadsorption ruled out the possibility that the inhibitory activity of any decidual proteins might reflect the contribution of contaminating impurities in the protein preparations. Recent attention has focused on the molecular and cellular mechanism by which the protein exerts its immunosuppressive effects. Crude decidual extracts inhibited interleukin-2 (IL-2) production and soluble IL-2 receptor (IL-2R) release from PHA-stimulated lymphocytes.[45] Specific reduction of the PP14 content of the decidual extracts by monoclonal anti-PP14 immunoadsorbent markedly reduced the inhibitory activity. This suggests that the purified decidual protein may act at the IL-2/IL-2R level of the immune response.

Whether the *in vitro* activities of this protein have physiological importance *in vivo* remains to be elucidated. It is noteworthy that the protein levels at which immunosuppressive activity occurred *in vitro* are similar to the endometrial protein 15 levels in uterine luminal fluid and cervical secretions, which suggests that this secretory protein could act *in vivo* as a local immunoregulatory factor of cell-mediated immunity.

7.2. Pregnancy-Associated Plasma Protein A

Pregnancy-associated plasma protein -A (PAPP-A) was first detected in the plasma of pregnant women.[32] Subsequent purification and biochemical characterization demonstrated that PAPP-A is a macromolecular glycoprotein of dimeric structure.[52] During pregnancy, PAPP-A levels increase in the maternal circulation to reach peak levels at parturition.[51] Although this protein was first demonstrated to be produced by placental trophoblast,[22,56] direct measurement and immunohistological studies have shown PAPP-A to be localized to and synthesized by the decidua and endometrial glands of pregnant uteri. PAPP-A is synthesized and released *in vitro* by early and term decidual explants as well as by trophoblast. The decidual tissue also released human placental lactogen and prolactin. The *de novo* production of this protein *in vitro* by decidua is significantly increased by a factor present only in pooled pregnancy-associated serum. Interestingly, the decreased production of the protein by term trophoblast would suggest that decidua-derived PAPP-A can account for the increased levels of PAPP-A in the maternal circulation in late pregnancy. PAPP-A, however, is neither pregnancy nor decidua specific but is present in seminal plasma, in preovulatory ovarian follicular fluid, and in nonpregnant endometrial glandular and stromal cells. It is a progesterone-dependent protein.[8]

Although the physiological role of the protein is unknown, PAPP-A has been claimed to display immunosuppressive properties *in vitro,* inhibiting PHA-induced lymphocyte proliferation.[6] Subsequent studies have proved to be contradictory. This immunoregulatory effect has not been confirmed for lectin-induced lymphocyte proliferation nor for the MLR.[33,48] PAPP-A, however, displays a marked inhibitory effect on complement-induced hemolysis.[7] Heparin-free PAPP-A purified from heparinized plasma specifically inhibits the third component of human complement (C3) by binding to this complement subcomponent. The effect of PAPP-A on the other complement subunits is not known. The inhibitory effect of PAPP-A on C3 is obtained with physiological levels of PAPP-A which occur in the plasma of normal pregnant women. Whether this protein operates *in vivo* to reduce complement-mediated lysis and phagocytosis *in vivo* is unknown, but the earlier suggestion that PAPP-A is an immunosuppressive agent on lymphocyte function appears to be discredited.

8. DECIDUAL ANTIGEN-PRESENTING CELL-DEPENDENT IMMUNOREGULATION

In addition to decidua-associated immunoregulation mediated by soluble suppressor factors, Oksenberg and co-workers[41] have reported decidual antigen-presenting cell (APC)-dependent immunoregulation. A distinct decidual cell population isolated from first-trimester decidua by mechanical dispersal, density centrifugation, and adherence to plastic coated with gelatin and autologous plasma displayed the capacity to present soluble and particulate antigens to maternal T cells *in vitro* in an MHC class II-restricted manner and induced lymphoproliferation. The fibronectin-adherent decidual antigen-presenting cell population lacked PAN-T cell surface markers and expressed MHC class II antigen and fibronectin receptors. The greater majority of the heterogeneous APC population were 63D3 antigen-positive macrophages.[40] When decidual APC were challenged with mechanically dispersed fetal cells *in vitro* and then cocultured with autologous maternal peripheral blood fibronectin nonadherent cells, a radiosensitive suppressor cell population was induced in the fibronectin nonadherent maternal lymphocytes in an MHC class II-restricted manner. These regulatory cells nonspecifically suppressed

MLC, CTL generation, mitogen-induced lymphoproliferation, as well as B cell antibody-forming cells in an MHC class II nonrestricted manner, but did not inhibit preformed CTL lytic activity. The suppressor cell population was only induced by decidual APC challenged with viable fetal cells but not with fetal cell supernatants, homogenates, and fetal cell membranes, nor with allogeneic adult cells nor other soluble antigens. Suppressor activity was not stimulated by either naive decidual APC or adult peripheral blood APC after challenge with fetal antigens. These suppressor cells, however, were dependent for their *in vitro* induction upon a nylon wool adherent MHC class II and Ig-positive B cell population within the peripheral blood fibronectin nonadherent cells. The phenotype of the regulatory nonadherent cell is MHC class II antigen and Ig-negative but Leu 1 (Pan-T) and Leu 2 (CD8) T cell positive. These findings indicate that decidual APC are capable of inducing an antigen nonspecific cytotoxic/suppressor T cell which operates in a non-MHC-restricted manner. The capacity of decidual APC *in vitro* to induce selectively functional suppressor T cells suggests that cells within the decidua may have the capacity to immunorecognize fetal antigens *in vivo* and thereby regulate maternal immune responses. The precise nature of the fetal antigenic challenge which stimulates decidual APC for regulatory cell induction *in vitro* is unknown. Whether this *in vitro* finding of decidual APC-dependent regulatory cell induction operates *in vivo* remains to be determined. Although the existence of antigen-specific CD8-positive suppressor T cells is controversial, the existence of a functional T cell subset to immunoregulate the immune response is well documented.[38,39] The finding of decidual APC-dependent immunoregulation by CD8$^+$ T cell which is nonantigen specific and MHC class II unrestricted requires independent confirmation.

The relative importance of decidual APC-dependent immunoregulation and decidua-associated suppressor factor-mediated immunoregulation for the maternal-fetal immunorelationship remains to be determined.

9. CONCLUDING REMARKS

A number of suppressor factors are elaborated by decidua during rodent and human pregnancy. Notably PGE$_2$, TGF-β_2-related factor as well as a number of higher-molecular-weight secretory products have nonspecific immunoregulatory activity *in vitro*. The higher-molecular-size suppressor factors require further characterization and their precise molecular and cellular mechanism of action to be defined. Some of the higher-molecular-size products may prove to be merely carrier molecules for the active immunosuppressor agent(s). The relative importance of the various decidua-associated suppressor factors highlighted by *in vitro* approaches to the maternal-fetal relationship is the subject for speculation and will provide the focus for further study. In all cases molecular cloning will determine whether their production occurs *in vivo* or, rather, suppressor activity is elaborated only *in vitro*. Whether these decidua-associated immunoregulatory factors have a crucial immunoregulatory role *in vivo* remains a major unanswered issue. In addition to their immunosuppressive properties and proposed *in vivo* role in immunoregulating maternal effector cells at the level of the fetoplacental unit, the decidual-associated soluble factors may be pivotally involved in controlled fetoplacental growth and development. Complex interactive events probably exist between these soluble factors and the various growth factors and cytokines which have been demonstrated to operate locally throughout pregnancy.

REFERENCES

1. **Badet, M.-T., Bell, S. C., and Billington, W. D.,** Immunoregulatory activity of supernatants from short-term cultures of mouse decidual tissue, *J. Reprod. Fertil.,* 68, 351–358, 1983.
2. **Badet, M.-T., Bell, S. C., and Billington, W. D.,** Partial characterization of immunosuppressive factors from short-term cultures of murine decidual tissue, *Ann. Immunol. (Inst. Pasteur),* 134C, 321–329, 1983.
3. **Bell, S. C. and Bohn, H.,** Immunochemical and biochemical relationship between human pregnancy-associated secreted endometrial α_1- and α_2-globulins (α_1- and α_2-PEG) and the soluble placental proteins 12 and 14 (PP12 and PP14), *Placenta,* 7, 283–294, 1986.
4. **Bell, S. C. and Drife, O. J.,** Secretory proteins of the endometrium: potential markers for endometrial dysfunction, *Baillière's Clin. Obstet. Gynaecol.,* 3, 271–391, 1989.
5. **Billington, W. D.,** Maternal-fetal interactions in normal human pregnancy, *Baillière's Clin. Immunol. Allergy,* 2, 527–549, 1988.
6. **Bischof, P., Lauber, K., de Wurstemberger, B., and Girard, J. P.,** Inhibition of lymphocyte transformation by pregnancy-associated plasma protein-A (PAPP-A), *J. Clin. Lab. Immunol.,* 7, 61–65, 1982.
7. **Bischof, P., Geinoz, A., Herrman, W. L., and Sizonenko, P. C.,** Pregnancy-associated plasma protein-A (PAPP-A) specifically inhibits the third component of human complement (C3), *Placenta,* 5, 1–8, 1984.
8. **Bischof, P. and Tseng, L.,** *In vitro* release of pregnancy-associated plasma protein-A (PAPP-A) by human endometrial cells, *Am. J. Reprod. Immunol. Microbiol.,* 10, 139–142, 1986.
9. **Bohn, H., Kraus, W., and Winckler, W.,** New soluble placental tissue proteins: their isolation, characterization, localization and quantification, *Placenta,* 4 (Suppl.), 67–81, 1982.
10. **Bolton, A. E., Pockley, A. G., Clough, K. J., Mowles, E. A., Stoker, R. J., Westwood, O. M. R., and Chapman, M. G.,** The identification of placental protein 14 (PP14) as an immunosuppressant factor involved in human reproduction, *Lancet,* i, 593–595, 1987.

11. **Chaouat, G., Kolb, J. P., and Wegmann, T. G.,** The murine placenta as an immunological barrier between the mother and the fetus, *Immunol. Rev.,* 75, 31–54, 1983.

12. **Clark, D. A., Slapsys, R. M., Croy, B. A., and Rossant, J.,** Suppressor cell activity in uterine decidua correlates with success or failure of murine pregnancies, *J. Immunol.,* 131, 540–542, 1983.

13. **Clark, D. A., Chaput, A., Walker, C., and Rosenthal, K. L.,** Active suppression of host-vs-graft reaction in pregnant mice. VI. Soluble suppressor activity obtained from decidua of allopregnant mice blocks the response to IL-2, *J. Immunol.,* 134, 1659-1664, 1985.

14. **Clark, D. A., Mowbray, J., Underwood, J., and Lidell, H.,** Histopathologic alterations in the decidua in human spontaneous abortion: loss of cells with large cytoplasmic granules, *Am. J. Reprod. Immunol. Microbiol.,* 13, 19–22, 1987.

15. **Clark, D. A., Falbo, M., Rowley, R. B., Banwatt, D., and Stedronska-Clark, J.,** Active suppression of host-versus-graft reaction in pregnant mice. IX. Soluble suppressor activity obtained from allopregnant mouse decidua that blocks the cytolytic effector response to IL-2 is related to transforming growth factor β, *J. Immunol.,* 141, 3833–3840, 1988.

16. **Clark, D. A., Flanders, K. C., Banwatt, D., Millar-Book, W., Manuel, J., Stedronska-Clark, J., and Rowley, B.,** Murine pregnancy decidua produces a unique immunosuppressive molecule related to transforming growth factor β-$_2$, *J. Immunol.,* 44, 3008–3014, 1990.

17. **Daya, S., Clark, D. A., Devlin, C., and Jarrell, J.,** Preliminary characterization of two types of suppressor cells in the human uterus, *Fertil. Steril.,* 44, 778–785, 1985.

18. **Daya, S., Rosenthal, K. L., and Clark, D. A.,** Immunosuppressor factor(s) produced by decidua-associated suppressor cells: a proposed mechanism for fetal allograft survival, *Am. J. Obstet. Gynaecol.,* 156, 344–350, 1981.

19. **Daya, S., Johnson, P. M., and Clark, D. A.,** Trophoblast induction of suppressor-type cell activity in human endometrial tissue, *Am. J. Reprod. Immunol.,* 19, 65–72, 1989.

20. **Dearden-Badet, M.-T.,** Comparative study of biological properties of proteins synthesised *in vitro* by murine decidua and deciduoma, *Am. J. Reprod. Immunol. Microbiol.,* 10, 20–25, 1986.

21. **de Fougerolles, A. R. and Baines, M. G.,** Modulation of natural killer cell activity in pregnant mice alters the spontaneous abortion rate, *J. Reprod. Immunol.,* 11, 147–154, 1987.

22. **Dobashi, K., Ajika, K., Ohkawa, T., Okano, H., Okinaga, S., and Arai, K.,** Immunohistochemical localization of pregnancy-associated plasma protein A (PAPP-A) in placentae from normal and pre-eclamptic pregnancies, *Placenta,* 5, 205–212, 1984.

23. **Globerson, A., Bauminger, S., Abel, S., and Peleg, S.,** Decidual extracts suppress antibody response *in vitro, Eur. J. Immunol.,* 7, 120–122, 1977.

24. **Golander, G., Zakuth, V., Shechter, Y., and Spirer, Z.,** Suppression of lymphocyte reactivity *in vitro* by a soluble factor secreted by explants of human decidua, *Eur. J. Immunol.,* 11, 849–851, 1981.

25. **Julkunen, M., Rutanen, E.-M., Koskimies, A. I., Ranta, T., Bohn, H., and Seppälä, M.,** Distribution of placnetal protein 14 in tissue and body fluids during pregnancy, *Br. J. Obstet. Gynaecol.,* 92, 1145–1151, 1985.

26. **Julkunen, M., Raiker, R. S., Joshi, S. G., Bohn, H., and Seppälä, M.,** Placental protein 14 and progestagen-dependent endometrial protein are immunologically indistinguishable, *Hum. Reprod.,* 1, 7–8, 1986.

27. **Julkunen, M., Seppälä, M., and Jänne, O. A.,** Complete amino acid sequence of human placental protein 14: a progesterone-regulated uterine protein homologous to beta-lactoglobulins, *Proc. Natl. Acad. Sci. U.S.A.,* 85, 8845–8849, 1988.

28. **Kirkwood, K. J. and Bell, S. C.,** Inhibitory activity of supernatants from murine decidual cell cultures on the mixed lymphocyte reaction, *J. Reprod. Immunol.,* 3, 243–252, 1981.

29. **Lala, P. K., Chatterjee-Hasrouni, S., Kearns, M., Montgomery, B., and Colavincenzo, V.,** Immunobiology of the feto-maternal interface, *Immunol. Rev.,* 75, 87–116, 1983.

30. **Lala, P. K., Kennedy, T. G., and Parhar, R. S.,** Suppression of lymphocyte alloreactivity by early gestational human decidua. II. Characterisation of the suppressor mechanism, *Cell. Immunol.,* 116, 411–422, 1988.

31. **Lala, P. K., Scodras, J. M., Graham, C. H., Lysiak, J. J., and Parhar, R. S.,** Inactivation of maternal killer cells in the pregnant uterus with chronic indomethacin therapy, IL-2 therapy or a combination of therapy is associated with embryonic demise, *Cell. Immunol.,* 127, 368–381, 1990.

32. **Lin, T. M., Halbert, S. P., Kiefer, D., and Spellacy, W. N.,** Three pregnancy-associated human plasma proteins: purification, monospecific antisera and immunological identification, *Int. Arch. Allergy,* 47, 35–53, 1984.

33. **McIntyre, J. A., Hsi, B., Faulk, W. P., Klopper, A., and Thomson, R.,** Immunological studies of the human placenta. Functional and morphological analysis of pregnancy-associated plasma protein-A (PAPP-A), *Immunology,* 44, 577–584, 1981.

34. **Matsui, S., Yoshimura, N., and Oka, T.,** Characterization and analysis of soluble suppressor factor from early human decidual cells, *Transplantation,* 47, 678–683, 1989.

35. **Matsui, S., Yoshimura, N., and Oka, T.,** Immunochemical characterization of the suppressor factor from early human decidua, *Transplantation,* 48, 651–654, 1989.

36. **Matthews, C. J., Adams, A. M., and Searle, R. F.,** Detection of macrophages and the characterization of Fc receptor bearing cells in the mouse decidua, placenta and yolk sac using the macrophage-specific monoclonal antibody F4/80, *J. Reprod. Immunol.,* 7, 315–323, 1985.

37. **Matthews, C. J. and Searle, R. F.,** The role of prostaglandins in the immunosuppressive effects of supernatants from adherent cells of murine decidual tissue, *J. Reprod. Immunol.,* 12, 109–124, 1987.

38. **Mitchison, N. A.,** Suppression, *Immunol. Today,* 12, 392–393, 1989.

39. **Moller, G.,** Do suppressor cells exist?, *Scand. J. Immunol.,* 27, 247–250, 1988.

40. **Oksenberg, J. R., Mor-Yosef, S., Persitz, E., Schenker, Y., Mozes, E., and Brautbar, C.,** Antigen-presenting cells in human decidual tissue, *Am. J. Reprod. Immunol. Microbiol.,* 11, 82–88, 1986.

41. **Oksenberg, J. R., Mor-Yosef, S., Ezra, Y., and Brautbar, C.,** Antigen-presenting cells in human decidual tissue. III. Role of accessory cells in the activation of suppressor cells, *Am. J. Reprod. Immunol. Microbiol.,* 16, 151–158, 1988.

42. **Parhar, R. S., Kennedy, T. G., and Lala, P. K.,** Suppression of lymphocyte alloreactivity by early gestational human decidua (I) characterization of suppressor cells and suppressor molecules, *Cell. Immunol.,* 116, 392–410, 1988.

43. **Parhar, R. S., Yagel, S., and Lala, P. K.,** PGE$_2$-mediated immunosuppression by first trimester human decidual cells blocks activation of maternal leukocytes in decidua with potential anti-trophoblast activity, *Cell. Immunol.,* 120, 61–74, 1989.

44. **Pockley, A. G., Mowles, E. A., Stoker, R. J., Westwood, O. M. R., Chapman, M. G., and Bolton, A. E.,** Suppression of *in vitro* lymphocyte reactivity to phytohemagglutinin by placental protein 14, *J. Reprod. Immunol.,* 13, 31–40, 1988.

45. **Pockley, A. G. and Bolton, A. E.,** Placental protein 14 (PP14) inhibits the synthesis of interleukin-2 and the release of soluble interleukin-2 receptors from phytohaemagglutinin-stimulated lymphocytes, *Clin. Exp. Immunol.,* 77, 252–256, 1989.

46. **Scodras, J. M., Parhar, R. S., Kennedy, T. G., and Lala, P. K.,** Prostaglandin-mediated inactivation of natural killer cells in the murine decidua, *Cell. Immunol.,* 127, 352–367, 1990.

47. **Searle, R. F., Bell, S. C., and Billington, W. D.,** Ia antigen-bearing decidual cells and macrophages in cultures of mouse decidual tissue, *Placenta,* 4, 139–148, 1983.

48. **Sinosich, M. J., Porter, R., Sloss, P., Bonifacio, M. D., and Saunders, D. M.,** Pregnancy-associated plasma protein-A in human ovarian follicular fluid, *J. Clin. Endocrinol. Metab.,* 58, 500–504, 1984.

49. **Slapsys, R. M. and Clark, D. A.,** Active suppression of host-versus-graft reaction in pregnant mice. V. Kinetics, specificity and *in vivo* activity of non-T suppressor cells localized to the genital tract of mice during first pregnancy, *Am. J. Reprod. Immunol. Microbiol.,* 3, 65–71, 1983.

50. **Smith, S. K. and Kelly, R. W.,** The release of PGF$_{2\alpha}$ and PGE$_2$ from separated cells of human endometrium and decidua, *Prostaglandins Leukotrienes Essential Fatty Acids,* 33, 91–96, 1988.

51. **Smith, R., Bischof, P., Hughes, G., and Klopper, A.,** Studies on pregnancy associated plasma protein-A in the third trimester of pregnancy, *Br. J. Obstet. Gynaecol.,* 86, 882–887, 1979.

52. **Sutcliffe, R. G., Kukulska-Langlands, B. M., Coggins, J. R., Hunter, J. B., and Gore, C. H.,** Studies on human pregnancy-associated plasma protein A. Purification by affinity chromatography and structural comparison with α_2-macroglobulin, *Biochem. J.,* 191, 799–809, 1980.

53. **Sutcliffe, R. G., Joshi, S. G., Paterson, W. F., and Bank, J. F.,** Serological identity between human alpha uterine protein and human progestagen-dependent endometrial protein, *J. Reprod. Fertil.,* 65, 207–209, 1982.

54. **Tatsumi, K., Mori, T., Mori, E., Kanzaki, H., and Mori, T.,** Immunoregulatory factor released from a cell line derived from human decidual tissue, *Am. J. Reprod. Immunol. Microbiol.,* 13, 87–92, 1987.

55. **Tawfik, O. W., Hunt, J. S., and Wood, G. W.,** Implication of prostaglandin E$_2$ in soluble factor-mediated immune suppression by murine decidual cells, *Am. J. Reprod. Immunol. Microbiol.,* 12, 111–117, 1986.
56. **Wahlström, T., Teisner, B., and Folkersen, J.,** Tissue localization of pregnancy-associated plasma protein A (PAPP-A) in normal placenta, *Placenta,* 2, 253–258, 1981.
57. **Waites, G. T. and Bell, S. C.,** Identification of a murine pregnancy-associated serum protein (α_1-PAP) as a female-specific acute phase reactant, *J. Reprod. Fertil.,* 70, 581–589, 1984.
58. **Waites, G. T., Udagawa, Y., Armstrong, S. S., Sewell, H. F., Bell, S. C., and Thomson, A. W.,** Immunohistochemical localization of murine α_1-pregnancy-associated protein (α_1-PAP) in pregnant mice: relationship between serum α_1-PAP levels and incidence of positive cells, *J. Reprod. Immunol.,* 8, 173–185, 1985.
59. **Waites, G. T. and Bell, S. C.,** Immunohistological localization of human pregnancy-associated endometrial α-globulin (α_2-PEG), a glycosylated β-lactoglobulin homologue, in the decidua and placenta during pregnancy, *J. Reprod. Fertil.,* 87, 291–300, 1989.
60. **Wood, G. W., Kamel, S., and Smith, K.,** Immunoregulation and prostaglandin production by mechanically-derived and enzyme-derived murine decidual cells, *J. Reprod. Immunol.,* 13, 235–248, 1988.

Early Embryonic Development and the Immune System

Hideharu Kanzaki and Takahide Mori
Department of Gynecology and Obstetrics
Faculty of Medicine
Kyoto University
Kyoto, Japan

1. INTRODUCTION

During early embryogenesis, the embryo is a floating mass of cells in the maternal fallopian tube and uterus, and can grow and differentiate without exogenous growth factors. A growing body of evidences suggests that the preimplantation embryo produces a variety of growth factors and biologically active molecules. Most of these factors are considered to work in an autocrine manner, but some of them can modulate the microenvironment in the fallopian tube and uterus. On the other hand, many humoral factors released from the fallopian tube and uterine endometrium have been known to affect the development of the embryo, and it has been suggested that preimplantation embryos may be affected under some pathological conditions characterized by an unusual immune response. For example, mouse blastocyst growth *in*

0-8493-8868-6/93/$0.00 + $.50

vitro was reported to be suppressed by the addition of sera from women with unexplained habitual abortions and infertility.[5,25]

Although the immunological functions of the uterine endometrium during the peri-implantation period are largely unknown, it has become apparent that the uterine endometrium, a target tissue of ovarian steroid hormones, is a unique tissue that not only produces biologically active substances such as cytokines, but can also respond to them. In this chapter, we discuss the immune factors which influence early embryonic development and endometrial function during the peri-implantation period.

2. FACTORS INFLUENCING EARLY EMBRYONIC DEVELOPMENT

The significance of antisperm antibodies in both male and female infertility has been recognized, and many experimental studies have demonstrated that the antisperm antibodies affect not only sperm motility in the female genital tract, but can also prevent the fertilization process itself. However, *in vitro* fertilization (IVF) technology has made it possible to achieve pregnancies in women with antisperm antibodies by using *in vitro* fertilization without the presence of autologous serum containing the antisperm antibodies.

The effect of antisperm antibodies on early embryonic development after fertilization is unclear. Based on isoimmunization with experimental animals, Menge et al.[19] suggested that the antisperm immune response exerted an embryotoxic effect in the oviduct, and that this effect persisted throughout the implantation period. It was also suggested that the embryos might be affected by sperm cell surface antigens incorporated into the embryos by embryonic cross-reaction antigens developed after fertilization, or by an indirect effect of the antisperm antibodies.[20] However, in humans, an anti-implantation or embryotoxic effect caused by antisperm antibodies is unlikely, because in most IVF-ET (embryo transfer) programs, there seems to be no difference in the pregnancy and abortion rates between women with antisperm antibodies and those with other causes of infertility.

A causal relationship between uterine leukocytosis and infertility has long been suggested. Parr and Shirley[28] reported that mouse embryo development from the two-cell stage to blastocysts was inhibited by leukocytes, and Smith et al.[35] found that rat morulae were killed by leukocyte extract *in vitro*. Several other studies[1,10] also showed similar toxic effects for leukocyte extracts or products on preimplantation embryos. Recently, Hill et al.[12] cultured CD1 mouse embryos from the two-cell stage for 4 d with leukocyte culture supernatants and various cytokines, including interleukin (IL)-1, IL-2 interferon (IFN), colony-stimulating factor (CSF), B cell growth factor (BCGF), and tumor necrosis factor (TNF). They found that supernatants from mitogen-stimulated (phytohemagglutinin [PHA], concanavalin [Con]A, and lipopolysaccharides [LPS]) and alloantigen-stimulated lymphocytes markedly arrested the growth of embryos. Among the cytokines tested, IL-2, CSF, BCGF, and IFN-γ significantly inhibited embryo development over a wide range of concentrations; IL-1 and TNF showed an inhibition only at very high concentrations (IL-1: 1×10^3 U/ml; TNF: 1×10^6 U/ml). However, Sueldo et al.[36] have reported the inhibitory effect of IL-1 on F_1-hybrid mice (C3H × C57 Black) embryo development at low (5 U/ml) concentrations. Based on these findings, it is tempting to speculate that some mechanisms which activate the maternal immune response may increase the cytokine levels which inhibit the growth of embryos and results in immunological infertility or abortion.

However, Schneider et al.[32] observed no inhibitory effect of these cytokines in a mouse embryo culture system, and our experiments with F_1-hybrid mice (C57 Black × C3H) showed enhanced embryo growth in conditioned media obtained from activated lymphocytes.[11] We cultured two-cell mouse embryos to the blastocyst stage with or without the supernatants of activated human lymphocytes (Con A and alloantigen stimulation), and found that those supernatants facilitated embryo development to the hatching blastocyst stage (control cultures: 54.8%; cultures with Con A supernatants: 86.5%; cultures with MCL supernatants: 96.2%). Our results agree with the previous *in vivo* study of Chaouat et al.,[4] in which vaccination with paternal antigens led to increased fetal protection in the mouse abortion model. Activation of the maternal immune response resulting in a local increase of cytokines was suggested to enhance fetal placental growth (placental immunotrophism).[40]

At present, controversial results have been reported as to the effects of cytokines on embryonic development. Embryos may require stage-specific growth factors at each developmental step, and a given factor may have different effects at different stages of embryogenesis. The complicated relationship between cytokines and embryonic development will be elucidated with the future establishment of an appropriate *in vitro* culture system for mammalian embryos.

3. EMBRYONIC SIGNALS TO THE MATERNAL IMMUNE SYSTEM

Preimplantation embryos are known to release a number of hormones and proteins, but their importance is mostly unknown. A key enzyme of steroid biosynthesis, hydroxysteroid dehydrogenase, has been detected in rat and mouse blastocysts,[41] and it has been reported that mouse blastocysts can metabolize progesterone *in vitro*.[42]

Rappolee et al.[27] reported the existence of mRNA for transforming growth factor (TGF)-α, TGF-β1, platelet-derived growth factor (PDGF)-A, Kaposi's sarcoma-type fibroblast growth factor (kFGF), and insulin-like growth factor (IGF)-II in mouse preimplantation embryos. Since the amount of these hormones and growth factors endogenous to embryos is very small, these substances have been suggested to work in an autocrine manner. However, their local effects on maternal endometrial cells and immune cells at the implantation site cannot be ignored. O'Neill[26] reported that mouse embryos can produce platelet-activating factor (PAF), a biologically active phospholipid which modulates vascular permeability and initiates many events associated with inflammation. Subsequently, PAF from human embryos was reported,[7] and it has been suggested that embryo-derived PAF plays an important role in the process of implantation.

To explain the survival of alloantigenic embryos in the uterus, a protective mechanism of pregnancy-induced immunosuppression was proposed, and a number of factors have been suggested as candidates at the fetomaternal interface. A low-molecular-weight, immunosuppressive protein termed early pregnancy factor (EPF), initially detected by the Rosette inhibition test,[21] was found in the maternal serum within hours of fertilization. EPF was shown to be produced by the ovary and oviduct upon stimulation with an unknown humoral factor(s) released from the fertilized ovum,[22] and it is believed to mediate immunosuppression in cases of maternal immunological rejection. However, the nature of EPF, as well as the embryo-derived EPF-inducing factor(s), remains to be clarified.

Rabbit or mouse blastocysts were reported to release some factor(s) which could inhibit lymphoproliferation induced by mitogens and alloantigens *in vitro*.[9,29] Mayumi et al.[18] reported that mouse blastocyst-conditioned media contained some heat labile factor(s) which could induce suppressor T lymphocytes in mixed lymphocyte culture (MLC). In humans, Daya and Clark[8] observed significant suppressive activity of ConA-stimulated lymphoproliferation brought about by the spent culture media from early embryos obtained from an IVF-ET program. They reported that the presence of this suppressive factor(s) was correlated significantly with successful implantations (clinical pregnancy establishment) after ET. Armstrong et al.[2] were not able to find such correlation, whereas Segars et al.[33] reported a significant suppressive effect caused by human embryo culture media, especially by blastocyst culture media; they found that pregnancy was achieved in 66% of the patients in whom the culture media demonstrated a significant suppressive effect. The correlation between the immunosuppressive activity by early embryo culture media (0 to 24 hours) and a successful pregnancy outcome in human IVF-ET was also reported by Sheth et al.,[34] and they found a slight increase of IL-1α levels in the media which exhibited a significant immunosuppression, and suggested that the synthesis of suppressive factor(s) by embryo might be stimulated by IL-1.

Imakawa and Roberts[13] reported the molecular structure and gene of a biologically active substance named trophoblast protein-1 (TP-1), and found that TP-1 from both ovines (oTP-1) and bovines (bTP-1) were closely related to IFN-α. Both oTP-1 and bTP-1 showed antiviral activity *in vitro*, and have many physiological effects that mimic recombinant IFN-α. oTP-1 affected early and late events in the *in vitro* proliferative response of mitogen- and IL-2-stimulated lymphocytes.[23] Therefore, this protein may have a pivotal role in controlling the maternal immune response to embryonic alloantigens in these species.

Considering the above fact, it is clear that some of the substances released from periimplantation embryos could modulate the function of the maternal immune system. Further investigations to characterize these substances, especially in humans, will provide an answer to the question of implantation failure and immunological abortion.

4. ENDOMETRIAL FUNCTION AND THE IMMUNE SYSTEM

Although the proliferation/differentiation of endometrial cells is mainly controlled by ovarian steroid hormones, some other substances, such as histamines, prostaglandins, leukotrienes, and platelet-activating factor (PAF), have been reported to modulate endometrial stromal cell transformation (decidualization). These substances are the mediators of the inflammatory process, modulate local immune responses, and are released not only from the periimplantation embryos but also from uterine endometrial tissues. A number of estrogen- and progesterone-dependent proteins have been reported in the endometrium, but very little is known of their biological or immunological activities. The human endometrium is known to release some unknown progesterone-dependent suppressive factor(s) that attenuates mitogen- and alloantigen-stimulated lymphoproliferation.[39] A well-characterized protein in the human endometrium, β-lactoglobulin homolog (βLG/PP14), is produced by endometrial glandular epithelial cells[15] and has been suggested to have immunosuppressive activity.[3] The plasma level of PP14 was elevated after ovulation and reached its highest value in the late secretory phase during the normal menstruation cycle.[14] In our experiments, PP14 exhibited a significant suppressive effect on natural killer cell activity, supporting a role in protecting embryos from maternal killer cells during the periimplantation period.[24]

The endometrium is composed of a variety of cells, including glandular epithelial cells, fibroblast-like stromal cells, leukocytes, tissue macrophages, and vascular endothelial cells. Recently, the functional significance of endometrial stromal cells has become apparent. Estrogen failed to enhance the proliferation of primary cultures of purified endometrial epithelial cells, but the proliferation was enhanced when stromal cells were cocultured.[6,30] Tabibzadeh et al.[37] reported the *in vitro* production of IFN-β_2/IL-6 by human endometrial stromal cells in response to the inflammation-associated cytokines, IL-1 TNF, and IFN-γ. However, LPS and serum had no effect on IFN-β_2/IL-6 production. They also observed that estrogen suppressed IFN-β_2/IL-6 secretion from stimulated endometrial stromal cells, suggesting a physiologic link between the endocrine and immune systems in the uterus.

The effect of IL-1 on endometrial function was demonstrated by the fact that IL-1 stimulated prostaglandin E2 (PGE2) production in human endometrial tissue.[38] Because PGE2 is a potent immunosuppressant, this report and that of Kauma et al.,[17] which showed increased IL-1 levels in the endometrium after pregnancy, suggest an immunoregulatory role for IL-1 in the human endometrium. On the other hand, we found that IL-1 could inhibit progesterone-induced decidualization of human endometrial stromal cells *in vitro,* assessed by morphological changes and prolactin production.[16] Human endometrial stromal cells separated from the proliferative endometrium were transformed to decidual cells and produced prolactin in the presence of 10^{-6} *M* progesterone during an *in vitro* culture of 2 weeks. The addition of rIL-1 (2 U/ml) into the culture medium completely inhibited this *in vitro* decidualization, with no cytotoxic effects as judged by cell numbers and [^{3}H]-thymidine incorporation into the cultured cells. At present the role(s) of IL-1 in the endometrium is not fully understood, but it is reasonable to speculate that infertility caused by endometrial inflammation or foreign bodies (e.g., intrauterine devise; IUD) may be caused by an increase in IL-1 released from activated uterine macrophages.

The intimate relationship between the immune and endocrine systems in the endometrium was further suggested by a report that mRNA encoding macrophage colony-stimulating factor (M-CSF, CSF-1) was present mainly in the glandular epithelial cells of the endometrium during mouse pregnancy. Its role as a growth factor for placental development was also suggested in mice.[31] In our culture system of human endometrial cells, M-CSF was detected in the supernatants of both epithelial and stromal cell cultures. This assay was performed using enzyme-linked immunosorbent assay (ELISA) based on a dual antibody immunometric sandwich principle using horse and rabbit polyvalent antibodies against human urinary CSF (CSF-HU) (manuscript in preparation). The addition of estrogen to the culture had no effect on M-CSF production by epithelial and stromal cells, but progesterone stimulated M-CSF production in stromal cells, but not in epithelial cells, in a dose-dependent manner. The colony-stimulating activity of the culture supernatants was confirmed by a monolayer agar culture system containing mouse unfractionated bone marrow cells. Thus, it was demonstrated that biologically active M-CSF was produced by the nonpregnant human endometrium under the control of progesterone. M-CSF in human endometrium may play a role(s) in the differentiation and maturation of tissue macrophages and endometrial cells, and in embryonic (placental) development during the periimplantation period.

5. CONCLUSIONS

There is considerable evidence to suggest that the maternal immune system responds to fetal alloantigens, including the major histocompatibility complex (MHC), during pregnancy. However, the immune response is usually not unfavorable for fetal development. At present it is unclear when the maternal immune system first recognizes embryonic antigens. Nevertheless, many factors that can modify immunological function have been shown to be released from both pre-implantation embryos and the uterine endometrium, and an intimate relationship between the immune and endocrine systems has been revealed in the uterus. Studies on these immune factors in relation to the embryo and endometrium should yield an understanding of the immunology of implantation, and may lead to increased pregnancy rates in human IVF-ET through an improvement in embryo culture *in vitro* and implantation after ET.

REFERENCES

1. **Anderson, D. J. and Alexander, N. J.,** Induction of uterine leukocytosis and its effect on pregnancy in rats, *Biol. Reprod.,* 21, 1143, 1979.
2. **Armstrong, D. T., Chaouat, G., Guichard, A., Cedard, L., Andreu, G., and Denver, L.,** Lack of correlation of immunosuppressive activity secreted by human *in vitro* fertilization (IVF) ova with successful pregnancy, *J. In Vitro Fertil. Embryo Transfer,* 6, 15, 1989.
3. **Bolton, A. E., Clough, K. J., Stoker, R. J., Pockley, A. G., Mowles, E. A., Westwood, O. M. R., and Chapman, M. G.,** Identification of placental protein 14 as an immunosuppressive factor in human reproduction, *Lancet,* i, 593, 1987.
4. **Chaouat, G., Kolb, J. P., Kiger, N., Stanislawski, M., and Wegmann, T. G.,** Immunologic consequences of vaccination against abortion in mice, *J. Immunol.,* 134, 1594, 1985.
5. **Chavez, D. J. and McIntyre, J. A.,** Sera from women with histories of repeated fetal wastage causes abnormalities in mouse periimplantation blastocysts, *J. Reprod. Immunol.,* 6, 273, 1984.
6. **Chen, L., Linder, H. R., and Lancet, M.,** Mitogenic action of oestrogen-17β on human myometrium and endometrial cells in long term tissue cultures, *J. Endocrinol.,* 59, 87, 1973.
7. **Collier, M., O'Neill, C., Ammit, A. J., and Saunders, D. M.,** Biochemical and pharmacological characterization of human embryo-derived platelet activating factor, *Hum. Reprod.,* 3, 993, 1987.
8. **Daya, S. and Clark, D. A.,** Production of immunosuppressor factor(s) by preimplantation human embryo, *Am. J. Reprod. Immunol. Microbiol.,* 11, 98, 1986.
9. **Dey, S. K., Stechschulte, D. J., and Abdou, N. I.,** Modulation of the *in vitro* lymphocyte response by rabbit blastocysts, *J. Reprod. Immunol.,* 3, 141, 1981.
10. **El Sahwi, S. and Moyer, D. L.,** *In vitro* study of the embryotoxic activity of leukocytes, *Contraception,* 16, 453, 1977.

11. **Fukuda, A., Mori, Ts., Mori, E., Tatsumi, K., Kanzaki, H., and Mori, Ta.,** Effects of the supernatants of mixed lymphocyte cultures and decidual cell line cultures on mouse embryo development *in vitro, J. In Vitro Fertil. Embryo Transfer,* 6, 59, 1989.

12. **Hill, J. A., Haimovici, F., and Anderson, D. J.,** Production of activated lymphocytes and macrophages inhibit mouse embryo development *in vitro, J. Immunol.,* 139, 2250, 1987.

13. **Imakawa, K. and Roberts, M.,** Interferons and maternal recognition of pregnancy, in *Development of Preimplantation Embryos and Their Environment,* Yoshinaga, K. and Mori, T., Eds., Alan R. Liss, New York, 1989, 347–358.

14. **Julkunen, M., Apter, D., Seppala, M., Stenman, U. H., and Bohn, H.,** Serum levels of placental protein 14 reflect ovulation in nonconceptional menstrual cycles, *Fertil. Steril.,* 45, 47, 1986.

15. **Julkunen, M., Seppala, M., and Janne, O. A.,** Molecular cloning of complementary DNAs for two human endometrial proteins and cellular localization of their messenger RNAs, in *Frontiers in Human Reproduction,* Seppala, M. and Hamberger, L., Eds., The N.Y. Academy of Sciences, New York, 1991, 284–294.

16. **Kariya, M., Kanzaki, H., Takakura, K., Imai, K., Okamoto, N., Emi, N., Kariya, Y., and Mori, T.,** Interleukin-1 inhibits *in vitro* decidualization of human endometrial stromal cells, *J. Clin. Endocrinol. Metab.,* 73, 1170, 1991.

17. **Kauma, S., Matt, D., Strom, S., Eierman, D., and Turner, T.,** Interleukin-1β, human leukocyte antigen HLA-DRα, and transforming growth factor-β expression in endometrium, placenta, and placental membranes, *Am. J. Obstet. Gynecol.,* 163, 1430, 1990.

18. **Mayumi, T., Bithoh, S., Anan, S., Hama, T., Fujimoto, S., and Yamamoto, H.,** Suppressor T lymphocyte induction by a factor released from cultured blastocysts, *J. Immunol.,* 134, 404, 1985.

19. **Menge, A. C., Burkons, D. M., and Friedlander, G. E.,** Occurrence of embryo mortality in rabbit isoimmunization against semen, *Int. J. Fertil.,* 17, 93, 1972.

20. **Menge, A. C. and Naz, R. K.,** Immunologic reactions involving sperm and preimplantation embryos, *Am. J. Reprod. Immunol.,* 18, 17, 1988.

21. **Morton, H., Hegh, V., and Clunie, G. J. A.,** Studies of the rosette inhibition test in pregnant mice: evidence of immunosuppression?, *Proc. R. Soc. London Ser. B,* 193, 413, 1976.

22. **Morton, H., Wolfe, B. E., McNiell, L., Clarke, F. M., and Clunie, G. J. A.,** Early pregnancy factor: tissues involved in its production in the mouse, *J. Reprod. Immunol.,* 2, 73, 1980.

23. **Newton, G. R., Vallet, J. L., Hansen, P. J., and Bazer, F. W.,** Inhibition of lymphocyte proliferation by ovine trophoblast protein-1 and a high molecular weight glycoprotein produced by the peri-implantation sheep conceptus, *Am. J. Reprod. Immunol.,* 19, 99, 1989.

24. **Okamoto, N., Uchida, A., Kanzaki, H., Takakura, K., Kariya, Y., Kanzaki, H., Riittinen, L., Koistinen, R., Seppala, M., and Mori, T.,** Suppression by human placental protein 14 of natural killer cell activity and T cell proliferative response, *Am. J. Reprod. Immunol.,* 26, 137, 1991.

25. **Oksenberg, J. R. and Brautbar, C.**, *In vitro* suppression of murine blastocysts growth by sera from women with reproductive disorders, *Am. J. Reprod. Immunol.*, 11, 118, 1986.
26. **O'Neill, D.**, Thrombocytopenia is an initial maternal response to fertilization in mice, *J. Reprod. Fertil.*, 73, 559–566, 1985.
27. **Rappolee, D. A., Sturn, K. S., Schultz, G. A., Pedersen, R. A., and Werb, Z.**, The expression of growth factor ligands and receptors in preimplantation mouse embryos, in *Early Embryo Development and Paracrine Relationship*, Heyner, S. and Wiley, L. M., Eds., Alan R. Liss, New York, 1989, 11–25.
28. **Parr, E. L. and Shirley, R. L.**, Embryotoxicity of leukocyte extracts and its relationship to intrauterine contraception in humans, *Fertil. Steril.*, 27, 1067, 1976.
29. **Pavia, C. S. and Stites, D. P.**, Trophoblast regulation of maternal-placental lymphocyte interactions, *Cell. Immunol.*, 58, 202, 1981.
30. **Pavlik, E. J. and Katzenellenbogen, B. S.**, Human endometrial cells in primary tissue culture: estrogen interactions and modulation of cell proliferation, *J. Clin. Endocrinol. Metab.*, 47, 333, 1978.
31. **Pollard, J. W., Bartocci, A., Arceci, R. J., Orlofsky, A., Lander, M. B., and Stanley, E. R.**, Apparent role of the macrophage growth factor, CSF-1, in placental development, *Nature (London)*, 330, 484, 1987.
32. **Schneider, E. G., Armant, D. R., Kupper, T. S., and Polan, M. R.**, Absence of a direct effect of recombinant interleukins and cultured peritoneal macrophages on early embryonic development in mouse, *Biol. Reprod.*, 40, 825, 1989.
33. **Segars, J. H., Rogers, B. J., Niblack, G. D., Wentz, A. C., and Osteen, K. G.**, The human blastocyst produces a soluble factor(s) that interferes with lymphocyte proliferation, *Fertil. Steril.*, 52, 381, 1989.
34. **Sheth, K. V., Parhar, R. S., Roca, G. L., Hamilton, C. J. C. M., Al-Sedairy, S. T., and Jabbar, F. A.**, Prediction of successful embryo implantation by measuring interleukin-1-alpha and immunosuppressive factor(s) in preimplantation embryo culture fluid, *Fertil. Steril.*, 55, 952, 1991.
35. **Smith, D. M., El Sahwi, S., Wilson, N., and Moyer, D. L.**, Effect of polymorphonuclear leukocytes on the development of mouse embryos cultured from the two-cell stage to blastocysts, *Biol. Reprod.*, 4, 74, 1971.
36. **Sueldo, C. E., Kelly, E., Montro, L., Subias, E., Baccaro, M., Swanson, J. A., Steinleitner, A., and Lambert, H.**, Effect of interleukin-1 on gamete interaction and mouse embryo development, *J. Reprod. Med.*, 35, 868, 1990.
37. **Tabibzadeh, S. S., Santhananm, U., Sehgel, P. B., and May, L. T.**, Cytokine-induced proliferation of IFN-β_2/IL-6 by freshly explanted human endometrial stromal cells. Modulation by estradiol-17β, *J. Immunol.*, 142, 3134, 1989.
38. **Tabibzadeh, S. S., Kaffka, K. L., Satyaswaroop, P. G., and Kilian, P. L.**, Interleukin-1 (IL-1) regulation of human endometrial function: presence of IL-1 receptor correlates with IL-1-stimulated prostaglandin E_2 production, *J. Clin. Endocrinol. Metab.*, 70, 1000, 1990.
39. **Wang, H. S., Kanzaki, H., Tokushige, M., Sato, S., Yoshida, M., and Mori, T.**, Effect of ovarian steroids on the secretion of immunosuppressive factor(s) from human endometrium, *Am. J. Obstet. Gynecol.*, 158, 629, 1988.

40. **Wegmann, T. G.,** Maternal T cells promote placental growth and prevent spontaneous abortion, *Immunol. Lett.,* 17, 297, 1988.
41. **Wu, J.-T. and Lin, G. M.,** The presence of 17β-hydroxysteroid dehydrogenase activity in preimplantation rat and mouse blastocyst, *J. Exp. Zool.,* 220, 121–124, 1982.
42. **Wu, J.-T.,** Metabolism of progesterone by preimplantation mouse blastocyst in culture, *Biol. Reprod.,* 36, 549–556, 1987.

Chapter

9

Late Trophoblast Immunoregulatory Factors

Fumitaka Saji
Department of Obstetrics and Gynecology
Osaka University Medical School
Osaka, Japan

1. INTRODUCTION

From an immunological viewpoint, the fetus with its paternally inherited alloantigens may be considered a successful allograft residing in the maternal host.[40,61] The ability of an allogeneic fetus to survive without suffering rejection by the mother, despite its potential to stimulate a maternal antifetal immune response, has given rise to a number of postulates to explain this phenomenon. The suggested mechanisms of survival of the allogeneic conceptus include (1) local and systemic suppression of the immune response by maternal lymphocytes;[18,68,70] (2) weak immunogenicity of the trophoblast, possibly due to the lack of class II major histocompatibility complex (MHC) antigen expression, restricted class I MHC antigens, and/or unique class I antigen expression;[30,39,51,54,100] and (3) the production of anti-idiotypic antibody to maternal cells coded to respond to paternal alloantigens.[4] In addition, (4) the production of blocking antibodies or antigen-antibody complexes; (5) adsorption of cytotoxic antibodies or antigen-antibody complexes by Fcγ receptor-bearing cells in the placenta;[50,102] and (6) the blockade of afferent lymphatics by the decidua[14] have been suggested; as well as (7) local immunoregulation by cells at the fetomaternal interface, including trophoblast cells, decidual cells, and endometrial leukocytes via cell products; (8) impaired susceptibility of the trophoblast to natural killer (NK) cells and lymphokine-activated killer (LAK) cells;[81,106] and (9) the physiological barrier that the placenta itself provides to the passage of both maternal and fetal cells. Although some of these hypotheses still remain controversial and may represent secondary or back-up systems contributing to the survival of the fetoplacental allograft, the above-mentioned mechanisms would appear to be reasonably able to prevent immunological rejection during pregnancy. Among these various mechanisms, the key role appears to be played by trophoblast (placenta)-secreted factors by the trophoblast itself acting at the fetomaternal interface.[82] The trophoblast originates as a single layer of trophectoderm constituting the wall of the unimplanted blastocyst, and progresses rapidly through various stages of proliferation and differentiation to form a number of different types of trophoblast cells incorporated into the structually complex definitive hemochorial placenta.

A number of trophoblast-associated factors have been proposed as immunoregulatory agents involved in the survival of the allogeneic fetoplacental unit. These factors are possibly involved in inhibiting the effects of allogeneic cytotoxic T cells upon the alloantigen-bearing trophoblast, as well as in generating the split tolerance/facilitation reaction. Thus, it seems that these factors can be classified into two main categories, immunosuppressive factors and immunostimulatory factors.

2. IMMUNOSUPPRESSIVE MECHANISMS OF TROPHOBLAST-DERIVED FACTORS

Degenne et al.[25] studied the immunosuppressive effects of human syncytiotrophoblast extracts obtained from placental villi by mechanical homogenization on the proliferative response of lymphocytes to different lectins (phytohemagglutinin [PHA] and concanavalin [Con] A) and allogeneic cells in one-way mixed lymphocyte cultures. The trophoblast extract reduced the spontaneous proliferation of a human erythroleukemic cell line (K562) and a human B lymphoma line (LHN13) that were maintained in culture prior to testing, and this inhibition was due to a cytostatic effect. A similar cytostatic effect was observed when a soluble factor secreted from cultured human placental trophoblasts was studied.[23,80] Trophoblast cells prepared by collagenase digestion followed by differential centrifugation were cultured briefly, and the culture supernatant was examined for its effect on *in vitro* lymphocyte functions. The supernatant suppressed the reaction of peripheral blood lymphocytes from healthy donors to PHA and pokeweed mitogen (PWM), and also suppressed their activity in the mixed lymphocyte reaction. These findings were later confirmed by Sanyal et al.[83] In addition to inhibiting blast transformation by allogeneic lymphocytes, the culture supernatant of normal placental trophoblast cells generated an *in vitro* population of suppressor lymphocytes which are generally considered to be responsible for immunologic tolerance. The supernatant also reduced NK cell activity against K562 target cells. It was found that the generation of cytotoxic T-lymphocytes was markedly depressed, but inhibition of the effector phase of lymphocyte-mediated cytotoxicity was less clear. The supernatant impaired the cell-mediated lympholysis of PHA-stimulated allogeneic target lymphocytes at the effector level,[23] but it showed no inhibition of the effector phase of lymphocyte-mediated cytotoxicity against the RPMI 8866 and Daudi tumor cell lines.[80]

The situation for rodent trophoblast cells is very similar to that in humans. Modification of the alloimmune response at both the humoral and cellular levels by placental extracts syngeneic to the recipient was observed in the mouse.[27,35] Placental extracts prepared by either mechanical homogenization or sodium deoxycholate solubilization delayed the rejection of *in vivo* tumor allografts. Serological analysis revealed that the placental extract did not modify overall hemagglutinating antibody production, but simultaneously caused both a decrease in the production of cytotoxic complement-fixing antibodies (IgG2) and an increase of specific anaphylactic mast cell degranulating antibodies (IgG1). Placental extracts promoted class deviations of the alloantibody response, such as enhancing the production of antibodies and suppressor cells favoring allograft survival.

Immunosuppressive molecules observed in both culture supernatants and extracts of normal trophoblastic cells were also found not only in the vesicle fluid and tissue extracts of hydatidiform mole,[22] but also in the culture supernatants of choriocarcinoma cell lines.[58-60,101] Samples obtained by direct aspiration of hydatidiform mole vesicles or homogenization of molar tissues produced a significant suppression of mitogen-induced lymphocyte proliferation. The major suppressive effect was found in the <50-kDa fractions resolved by molecular weight chromatography of molar extracts.[22] On the other hand, cultured JEG-3 human choriocarcinoma cells secrete a protein complex of about 150 to 200 kDa that inhibits tetanus toxoid- and PHA-induced lymphocyte transformation.[101] This JEG-3 cell factor appears to be identical to the normal trophoblast-derived immunoregulatory factor on the basis of its various *in vitro* effects on lymphocyte responses.[59] The site of action of this factor in the T cell signal transduction pathway was investigated using a phorbol ester and a calcium ionophore, reagents which strongly stimulate interleukin (IL)-2-mediated T cell responses,[58-60] and the factor was found to completely suppress the human T cell responses activated by the phorbol ester and calcium ionophore. It failed to inhibit CD25 expression and IL-2 production by T cell blasts in the T cell activation phase ($G_0 \rightarrow G_1$ phase of the cell cycle), but completely blocked the recombinant IL-2-induced proliferation of T cell blasts in the T cell proliferative phase ($G_1 \rightarrow S$ phase). Thus, this factor acted on the cytoplasmic signal transduction pathways

TABLE 1.
Trophoblast-Associated Factors with Nonspecific
Immunosuppressive Activity

Category	Factor
Steroid hormones	Cortisol
	Progestin
	Estrogen
Protein hormones	Chorionic gonadotrophin (hCG)
	Chorionic somatomammotrophin (hCS, hPL)
Proteins and glycoproteins	Pregnancy-associated α_2-glycoproteins (α_2-PAG, PAG, PZP, SP-3, PAM)
	Pregnancy-specific β_1-glycoproteins (PSβ_1G, SP1, PAPP-C, TBG)
	Pregnancy-associated plasma protein A (PAPP-A)
	Placental protein 14 (PP14)
	Transforming growth factor β(TGF-β)

without interfering with the IL-2 molecules themselves or their interaction with the IL-2 receptor. This factor also suppressed the IL-2-independent proliferative response of T cells to the phorbol ester. Recent studies examining the effect of the factor on LAK cell generation induced by recombinant IL-2 have shown that it inhibits LAK cell proliferation.[60] These findings taken together suggest that the choriocarcinoma-derived factor only suppresses the proliferative function of immunocompetent cells and does not inhibit either activation or differentiation events.

3. TROPHOBLAST FACTORS WITH NONSPECIFIC IMMUNOSUPPRESSIVE ACTIVITY

A number of pregnancy-associated serum factors have been proposed as immunosuppressive agents contributing to fetal survival during pregnancy. Many of these factors are synthesized by the placenta, especially the trophoblast, and have been championed in recent years (reviewed in References 9, 17, and 34). These factors can be classified under three main headings: (1) steroid hormones; (2) protein hormones; and (3) proteins and glycoproteins (Table 1). The majority of them are detectable in the maternal serum at levels lower than those which affect the various *in vitro* assays used to assess their immunosuppressive function. However, it seems reasonable to assume that higher concentrations may be achieved in the uterine environment.

3.1. Steroid Hormones

Steroid hormone concentrations increase during pregnancy, and these hormones exert a profound influence on immunologic reactivity. Estrogens as well as progestins have been reported to suppress both *in vitro* and *in vivo* immune reactions.[20,62,103] In pregnant women and in women taking oral contraceptives, a significant decrease of PHA-induced lymphoblast transformation and *in vitro* cytotoxicity has been observed.[12,24,36] Furthermore, progesterone combined with prostaglandin E (which increases in the gestational endometrium and decidua) has a synergistic effect on the mitogenic response of human peripheral lymphocytes.[33] Progesterone inhibits thymidine incorporation by PHA-stimulated lymphocytes, with the peak suppression occurring when it is added together with PHA at the initiation of culture and a gradual decline in suppression being produced by delaying the time of addition. From these findings, it appears that progesterone may be effective in inhibiting the initial activation processes of T cell mitogenesis.

The immunosuppressive properties of steroid hormones are now well known, but there are indications that the serum and placental levels of available steroids are too low to have a significant direct effect on lymphocytes.[72,84,96] For this reason, it is reasonable to assume that higher steroid hormone levels may be achieved in the uterine environment and at the fetomaternal interface than in the peripheral blood, and that such hormones may then regulate the immune response. Elevated steroid hormone levels in the vicinity of the placenta could, hence, participate in facilitating fetal survival as nonspecific local immunosuppressive factors. Another possibility is that steroids may affect the immune response indirectly, by inducing several proteins/glycoproteins having immunosuppressive properties and/or by inducing the thymic production of immunoregulatory factors or cells.[89] Their mode of action is not yet totally determined. Persellin and Rhodes[74] detected the inhibition of HLA-DR receptors at the level of the Fc fragment of monocytes by a pregnancy-associated protein which can be induced in women by the administration of estrogens/progestins. The functional role of steroid receptors on thymic cells has also been assessed by examining the effects of steroids on the secretion of immunoregulatory factors by cultured thymic epithelial cells.[92,93] Rat epithelial cells were cultured for up to 40 days in the presence of steroids and the culture supernatants were examined for their capacity to regulate PHA-induced thymocyte proliferation. Supernatants from estradiol- and corticosterone-treated cultures actually caused mitogenic stimulation to fall below control levels during much of the culture period. Subsequent studies have shown that the phenomenon occurs at the circulating hormone levels found during pregnancy.

3.2. Protein Hormones

Human chorionic gonadotropin (hCG), a glycoprotein of about 46 kDa, is produced by placental syncytiotrophoblasts during pregnancy. Biochemical studies of its α- and β-subunits suggest that hCG is related to several pituitary glycoprotein hormones, follicle stimulating hormone (FSH), luteinizing hormone (LH), and thyroid stimulating hormone (TSH). The β-subunits of these glycoprotein hormones are both immunologically and biologically specific for each individual hormone, although the biological activity of hCG is not clearly understood. Several reports have suggested that hCG profoundly inhibits the lymphocyte responses to PHA and allogeneic cells.[1,21,37,47] The hCG preparations studied were not cytotoxic to lymphocytes, and the suppressive effect was reversed by washing the cells after incubation with hCG. Experimental animal studies have shown that daily hCG injections prolonged skin graft survival[73] and decreased the incidence of graft-vs.-host disease.[86] However, these studies employed relatively impure commercial hCG preparations and highly purified hCG has since been found to be almost devoid of such activity. A comparison of purified hCG with the crude hCG obtained from different suppliers showed that the purified preparation produced no suppression of lymphocyte responses.[15]

The hormonal and immunosuppressive properties of hCG can be separated by chromatography,[55,64,65] indicating that the active factor is a substance other than hCG, which is probably a contaminant in the urine obtained from pregnant women. Bulk commercial preparations of hCG normally utilize urine obtained from women in the first trimester of pregnancy as a starting material and are purified by selective precipitation followed by ion exchange and gel chromatography. The crude commercial hCG preparations yielded by such purification procedures appear to contain a considerable amount of material of unknown composition that is also concentrated from the urine during processing. An immunosuppressive glycoprotein termed uromodulin, which is noncytotoxic and blocks the early events of T cell proliferation *in vitro,* has been purified from the urine of pregnant women.[66] A subsequent study showed that uromodulin could possibly be the IL-1 receptor, since it is a high-affinity ligand of IL-1 and is able to regulate IL-1 activity *in vitro.*[67]

Similarly to hCG, early studies on human placental lactogen (hPL) implied that this glycoprotein hormone possessed an immunosuppressive activity.[16,21,44] However, Morse[63] found that after extensive purification hPL could only suppress PHA-induced lymphocyte proliferation and the mixed lymphocyte reaction (MLR) at higher concentrations than those used in previoius studies. The physiological levels noted in pregnant serum and the placenta are inadequate to depress the immune response, suggesting that a contaminant might have been responsible for the inhibitory effects shown by the protein in other studies.

3.3. Proteins and Glycoproteins

A number of placental proteins and glycoproteins have been described in recent reports, but little is known yet about their biological roles. Some of these proteins have been reported to possess immunosuppressive properties (Table 1).

Pregnancy-associated α_2-glycoprotein (α_2-PAG) is a glycoprotein with a molecular size of 360 to 380 kDa which has a potent immunosuppressive effect when added to the MLR and also suppresses mitogen-induced lymphocyte proliferation.[87,88] Alpha$_2$-PAG preferentially inhibits T cell-mediated responses at a concentration below that normally found during pregnancy.[90] Since the serum α_2-PAG level increases with estrogen treatment,[91] estrogen-modulated immune reactions might be mediated by this glycoprotein.

Pregnancy-specific β_1-glycoprotein (PSβ_1G) is synthesized by the syncytiotrophoblast and reaches a maximum concentration in late pregnancy. Although this 90-kDa molecule suppresses the response of lymphocytes to PHA *in vitro,* maternal serum does not contain enough of this protein to have an *in vivo* suppressive effect,[44] suggesting that PSβ_1G may modulate immune reactivity locally in the periplacental environment.

Pregnancy-associated plasma protein A (PAPP-A) is a 750-kDa macroglobulin that is synthesized by the placental trophoblast and reaches its highest serum level in late pregnancy. Similarly to other pregnancy-associated α-glycoproteins, PAPP-A has the capacity to suppress the mitogenic response of lymphocytes.[49]

Among the placental proteins, placental protein 14 (PP14) is known to exhibit immunosuppressive activity *in vitro*. PP14 was originally isolated from the term placenta[10] and has been shown to have immunological and structural similarities to the other pregnancy-associated proteins.[6] Purified PP14 exhibits an immunosuppressive effect on allogeneically and mitogenically stimulated peripheral blood lymphocytes,[11,77] and also inhibits the secretion of IL-1 and the production of IL-2 by PHA-stimulated peripheral blood lymphocytes.[75,76] However, PP14 does not appear to inhibit the interaction of IL-2 with its receptor once the receptor has been expressed,[75] and the immunosuppressive activity of this protein could perhaps be mediated by the suppression of IL-1 secretion.[76]

Transforming growth factor-β (TGF-β) is a multifunctional polypeptide with a molecular size of 25 kDa that is composed of two disulfide-linked 12.5-kDa subunits.[56] It is produced by neoplastic and hematopoietic cells as well as by cells associated with the reproductive organs. Placenta, decidua, and ovarian granulosa cells have all been reported to produce TGF-β.[19,32,48] TGF-β blocks the ability of IL-1 to stimulate lymphocyte proliferation, while both TGF-β_1 and its homolog, TGF-β_2, suppress IL-1-dependent murine thymocyte proliferation. TGF-β also inhibits human peripheral blood T lymphocyte mitogenesis. The inhibition of cell division appears to occur after lymphocyte activation, since neither IL-2 receptor gene expression nor translation is suppressed. Furthermore, TGF-β does not block the synthesis of IL-2.[97] These findings are very similar to the data obtained on the mode of action of the immunosuppressive factor derived from cultured trophoblasts.[58,59]

TABLE 2.
Trophoblast-Associated Cytokines with Immunostimulatory Activity

Category	Cytokine
Interleukins	Interleukin-1 (IL-1)
	Interleukin-6 (IL-6)
Colony-stimulating factors (CSF)	Granulocyte macrophage-CSF (GM-CSF)
	Macrophage-CSF (M-CSF, CSF-1)
Other cytokines	Tumor necrosis factor (TNF)
	Interferon (IFN)

4. TROPHOBLAST FACTORS WITH IMMUNOSTIMULATORY ACTIVITY

In addition to immunosuppressive factors, placental cells produce various cytokines with immunostimulatory activity that promote the growth of placental tissues. Some of these cytokines are released from trophoblast cells, and may alter cellular growth differentiation, and/or function in an autocrine or paracrine manner.[57,78,80,99] So far IL-1, IL-6, two colony-stimulating factors (GM-CSF, M-CSF), tumor necrosis factor (TNF), and interferon (IFN) have been shown to be trophoblast-associated cytokines (Table 2).

Interleukin-1 is a 17-kDa glycoprotein that has a wide range of biological functions, such as regulation of the immune response[26,71] and stimulation of the release of hormones, both *in vivo*[46] and *in vitro*.[8] IL-6 is a 26-kDa glycoprotein, which is another representative cytokine with multiple biological activities.[38] These cytokines share a number of biological functions because IL-1 acts by inducing the secretion of IL-6 in various cellular systems, including fibroblasts,[105] endothelial cells,[85] and endometrial stromal cells.[95] In the human placenta, both of these cytokines are produced by trophoblasts and regulate hCG release from trophoblast cells.[45,69] Placental IL-1[31] has been shown to stimulate trophoblast cell lines to secrete hCG,[104] and the precise molecular regulatory mechanism of the endocrine hormone release mediated by IL-1 was very recently determined.[57] Trophoblasts purified by Percoll density gradient centrifugation released hCG from 120 min after stimulation with recombinant (r)IL-1α in an rIL-1α concentration-dependent manner. The IL-1α-stimulated trophoblasts released a molecule with IL-6 activity, and rIL-1-mediated hCG release from trophoblasts was reduced to the basal level by pretreatment of trophoblasts with an anti-IL-6-receptor monoclonal antibody, indicating that this hCG release was totally dependent on IL-6 and IL-6-receptor-mediated signal transduction. Furthermore, rIL-6 was found to stimulate hCG release by trophoblasts to a level similar to that produced by a gonadotropin releasing hormone (GnRH) analog.[69] The analog, however, released hCG by an IL-6-independent mechanism because a monoclonal antibody specific to the IL-6-receptor failed to block the analog-mediated response, but completely blocked IL-6-mediated hCG release. These findings suggested the existence of two distinct regulatory pathways for hCG release.

Tumor necrosis factor-α (TNF-α) is a glycoprotein with a molecular weight of 17 kDa that was originally called cachectin. It has multiple biological activities, including a direct cytotoxic effect on tumor cells, the stimulation of immunocompetent cells, the induction of cellular proliferation and differentiation, and an antiviral activity.[52] The presence of a receptor for TNF-α on villous trophoblasts[29] and the production of TNF-α during parturition[43] have both been reported. The interrelationships between IL-1, IL-6, TNF-α, and hCG have also been studied, since trophoblasts produce all these cytokines and the placental hormone. It was found that TNF-α and its receptor system were also involved in hCG release from trophoblasts by stimulating IL-6 release and activating the IL-6-receptor system. Simultaneous stimulation of trophoblasts with TNF-α and IL-1 resulted in a synergistic enhancement of IL-6 release and subsequent enhancement of hCG release.[53] Thus, trophoblast-derived TNF-α and IL-1 appear to synergistically regulate the level of IL-6 secretion by these cells, which in turn determines the level of hCG release that occurs following activation of the IL-6-receptor system.

Besides IL-1 and IL-6, various other growth factors and cytokines can be found in the placenta, especially in trophoblast cells. Duc-Goiran et al.[28] reported the expression of interferon (IFN)-α-like mRNA in placental tissues collected during the third trimester. By Northern blot analysis with RNA probes, IFN-α-like transcripts correlated with the presence of the functionally active protein purified by immunoaffinity chromatography. Considering the fact that the placenta contains IFN-α-specific receptors,[13] IFN-α-like molecules may function as physiological regulators of placental cellular processes and could actively participate in downregulating the tissue proliferation previously promoted by various growth factors. IFN-α could also participate in the protection of the fetus against rejection by maternal cytolytic cells, probably by its reported capacity to induce anticytolytic resistance in target cells.[7] Furthermore, IFN-α-like proteins were shown to be present in ovine trophoblasts and could also play a role in the nidation of the activated oocyte.[41,42]

It has been shown that IL-3 and granulocyte macrophage colony-stimulating factor (GM-CSF), as well as colony-stimulating factor-1 (CSF-1), all lymphokines of T lymphocyte origin, enhance the phagocytosis and proliferation of a mouse placental cell line.[3,98,99] CSF-1 was originally identified as a hematopoietic growth factor required for the proliferation, differentiation, and survival of mononuclear cells. Uterine CSF-1 levels in pregnant mice increase 1000-fold during gestation,[5] and the mRNA of the CSF-1 receptor, which is thought to be the protooncogene product of c-fms, has been detected in the mouse placenta. The expression and cellular sites of synthesis of CSF-1 and the CSF-1 receptor mRNA were also identified in the reproductive tract of pregnant mice,[2] implying a role for CSF-1 in the regulation of placental growth and differentiation.

Recently, the expression of the gene for macrophage colony-stimulating factor (M-CSF), a human counterpart of mouse CSF-1, and its receptor in the placenta and decidua throughout pregnancy was examined by Northern blot hybridization using specific probes. M-CSF and *c-fms* mRNAs were detected by Northern blotting in early-stage placentas and their levels subsequently increased during pregnancy. These mRNAs were not detected in the nonpregnant endometrium but were strongly induced in the maternal decidua with the same mRNA size as found in the placenta.[84] Northern blot analysis of the endometrium of a pseudopregnant uterus revealed that the expression of M-CSF and *c-fms* mRNA is regulated by the synergistic action of female sex steroid hormones.[4] The closely parallel increase of M-CSF mRNA in the placenta and endometrium during pregnancy strongly suggests that the dramatic changes occurring in placental development and/or uterine hypertrophy are associated with the increase of M-CSF mRNA in the pregnant uterus. It has also been reported that the concentration of CSF-1, a murine homolog of M-CSF, was significantly elevated in nonuterine tissues and serum during gestation,[5] and that CSF-1 could have an immunostimulatory effect on murine fetally derived placental cells[3] that resulted in the promotion of placental development and function.[78]

The expression of *c-fms* protooncogene transcripts, a M-CSF receptor mRNA, parallels M-CSF mRNA expression in the placenta and uterine endometrium during pregnancy and is further evidence to support the hypothesis that M-CSF may cause the local proliferation and differentiation of cells at the feto-maternal interface. The abundance of both M-CSF and *c-fms* mRNA in the human placenta and decidua indicates that M-CSF is deeply involved, in an autocrine and/or paracrine manner, in the physiological changes of these tissues. These observations, together with the previous report on the accumulation of CSF-1 in amniotic fluid during gestation, are consistent with the localized production and consumption of M-CSF by the materno-fetal interface.[79]

REFERENCES

1. **Adcock, E. W., Teasdale, F., August, C. S., Cox, S., Meschia, G., Battaglia, F. C., and Naughton, M. A.,** Human chorionic gonadotrophin: its possible role in maternal lymphocyte suppression, *Science,* 181, 845, 1983.

2. **Arceci, R. J., Shanahan, F., Stanley, E. R., and Pollard, J.,** Temporal expression and location of colony-stimulating factor 1 (CSF-1) and its receptor in the female reproductive tract are consistent with CSF-1-regulated placental development, *Proc. Natl. Acad. Sci. U.S.A.,* 86, 8818, 1989.

3. **Athanassakis, I., Bleackley, R. C., Paekau, V., Guilbert, L., Barr, P. J., and Weggman, T. G.,** The immunostimulatory effect of T cells and T cell lymphokines on murine fetally derived placental cells, *J. Immunol.,* 138, 37, 1987.

4. **Azuma, C., Saji, F., Kimura, T., Tokugawa, Y., Takemura, M., Samejima, Y., and Tanizawa, O.,** Steroid hormones induce macrophage colony-stimulating factor (MCSF) and MCSF receptor mRNAs in the human endometrium, *J. Mol. Endocrinol.,* 5, 103, 1990.

5. **Bartocci, A., Pollard, J. W., and Stanley, E. R.,** Regulation of colony-stimulating factor-1 during pregnancy, *J. Exp. Med.,* 164, 956, 1986.

6. **Bell, S. and Bohn, H.,** Immunochemical and biochemical relationships between human pregnancy-associated secreted endometrial alpha$_1$-alpha$_2$-globulins (alpha$_1$-alpha$_2$-PEG) and the soluble placental proteins 12 and 14 (PP12 and PP14), *Placenta,* 7, 283, 1986.

7. **Bergeret, M., Fouchard, M., Gregoire, A., Chany, C., and Zagury, D.,** Interferon effect on cytolytic T lymphocytes in a single cycle assay, *Immunology,* 48, 101, 1983.

8. **Bernton, E. W., Beach, J. E., Holaday, J. W., Smallridge, R. C., and Fein, H. G.,** Release of multiple hormones by a direct action of interleukin-1 on pituitary cells, *Science,* 238, 519, 1987.

9. **Billington, W. D. and Bell, S. C.,** Immunoregulatory factors in pregnancy: essential or irrelevant in the maintenance of the fetoplacental allograft?, in *Immunology of Human Placental Proteins,* Klopper, A., Ed., Praeger Publishers, London, 1982, 13–23.

10. **Bohn, H., Kraus, W., and Winckler, W.,** New soluble placental tissue proteins. Their isolation, characterization, localisation and quantification, *Placenta,* 4 (Suppl.), 67, 1982.

11. **Bolton, A. E., Pockley, A. G., Clough, K. J., Mowles, E. A., Stoker, R. J., Westwood, O. M. R., and Chapman, M. G.,** Identification of placental protein 14 as an immunosuppressive factor in human reproduction, *Lancet,* i, 593, 1987.

12. **Bousquet, J. and Fizet, D.,** Evidence of immunosuppressor factor in the serum of women taking oral contraceptives, *Gynecol. Obstet. Invest.,* 18, 178, 1984.

13. **Branca, A. A.,** High-affinity receptors for human interferon in bovine lung and human placenta, *J. Interferon Res.,* 6, 305, 1986.

14. **Bulmer, J. N.,** Decidual cellular responses, *Curr. Opinion Immunol.,* 1, 1141, 1989.

15. **Caldwell, J. L., Stites, D. P., and Fudenburg, H. H.,** Human chorionic gonadotropin: effects of crude and purified preparations on lymphocyte responses to phytohemagglutinin and allogeneic stimulation, *J. Immunol.,* 115, 1249, 1975.

16. **Cerni, C., Tatra, G., and Bohn, H.,** Immunosuppression by human placental lactogen (HPL) and the pregnancy-specific α_1 glycoprotei (PS-1), *Arch. Gynecol.,* 223, 1, 1977.

17. **Chaouat, G.**, Placental immunoregulatory factors, *J. Reprod. Immunol.*, 10, 179, 1987.

18. **Clark, D. A., Slapsys, R. M., Croy, B. A., and Rossant, J.**, Local active suppression by suppressor cells in the decidua: a review, *Am. J. Reprod. Immunol.*, 5, 78, 1984.

19. **Clark, D. A., Flanders, K. C., Banwatt, D., Millar-Book, W., Manuel, J., Stedronska-Clark, J., and Rowley, B.**, Murine pregnancy decidua produces a unique immunosuppressive molecule related to transforming growth factor β-2, *J. Immunol.*, 144, 3008, 1990.

20. **Clemens, L. E., Siiteri, P. K., and Stites, D. P.**, Mechanism of immunosuppression of progesterone on maternal lymphocyte activation during pregnancy, *J. Immunol.*, 122, 1978, 1979.

21. **Contractor, S. F. and Davies, H.**, Effect of human chorionic somatomammotrophin and human chorionic gonadotrophin on phytohemagglutinin-induced lymphocyte transformation, *Nature*, 243, 284, 1973.

22. **Cowan, B. D., Bennet, W. A., Brackin, M. N., and McGehee, R. P.**, Suppression of lymphocyte proliferation *in vitro* by macromolecules in the vesicle fluid and tissue extracts of hydatidiform mole, *J. Reprod. Immunol.*, 15, 39, 1989.

23. **Culouscou, J. M., Remacle-Bonnet, M. M., Pommier, G., Rance, R. J., and Depieds, R. C.**, Immunosuppressive properties of human placenta: study of supernatants from short-term syncytiotrophoblast cultures, *J. Reprod. Immunol.*, 9, 33, 1986.

24. **Davis, J. C. and Hapkin, L. S.**, Depressed lymphocyte transformation in women taking oral contraceptives, *Lancet*, i, 217, 1974.

25. **Degenne, D., Canepa, S., Horowitz, R., Khalfoun, B., Gutman, N., and Bardos, P.**, Effect of human syncytiotrophoblast extract on *in vitro* proliferative responses, *Am. J. Reprod. Immunol. Microbiol.*, 8, 20, 1985.

26. **Dinarello, C. A.**, Interleukin-1 and the pathogenesis of the acute-phase response, *New Engl. J. Med.*, 311, 1413, 1984.

27. **Duc, H. T., Masse, A., Bobe, P., Kinsky, R. G., and Voisin, G. A.**, Deviation of humoral and cellular alloimmune reactions by placental extracts, *J. Reprod. Immunol.*, 7, 27, 1985.

28. **Duc-Goiran, P., Chany, C., and Doly, J.**, Unusually large interferon-α-like mRNAs and high expression of interleukin-6 in human fetal annexes, *J. Biol. Chem.*, 264, 16507, 1989.

29. **Eades, D. K., Cornelius, P., and Pekela, P. H.**, Characterization of the tumor necrosis factor receptor in human placenta, *Placenta*, 9, 247, 1988.

30. **Ellis, S. A., Sargent, I. L., Redman, C. W., and McMichael, A. J.**, Evidence for a novel HLA antigen found on human extravillous trophoblast and a choriocarcinoma cell line, *Immunology*, 59, 595, 1986.

31. **Flynn, A., Finke, J. H., and Hiliker, M. L.**, Placental mononuclear phagocytes as a source of interleukin-1, *Science*, 218, 475, 1982.

32. **Frolik, C. A., Dart, L. L., Meyers, C. A., Smith, D. M., and Sporn, M. B.**, Purification and initial characterization of a type β transforming growth factor from human placenta, *Proc. Natl. Acad. Sci. U.S.A.*, 80, 3676, 1983.

33. **Fujisaki, S., Kawano, K., Haruyama, Y., and Mori, N.**, Synergistic effect of progesterone on prostaglandin E modulation of the mitogenic response of human peripheral lymphocytes, *J. Reprod. Immunol.*, 7, 15, 1985.

34. **Gill, T. J. and Repetti, C. F.**, Immunologic and genetic factors influencing reproduction, *Am. J. Pathol.*, 95, 465, 1979.

35. **Gupta, G. S., Kinsky, R. G., Duc, H. T., and Voisin, G. A.**, Effects of placental extracts on the immune response to histocompatibility antigens: class deviation of alloantibody response and allograft enhancement, *Am. J. Reprod. Immunol.*, 6, 117, 1984.

36. **Hagen, C. and Hipkin, L. S.**, Depressed lymphocyte response to PHA in women taking oral contraceptives, *Lancet*, i, 1185, 1972.

37. **Han, T.**, Inhibitory effect of human chorionic gonadotrophin on lymphocyte blastogenic response to mitogen, antigen and allogeneic cells, *Clin. Exp. Immunol.*, 18, 529, 1974.

38. **Hirano, T. and Kishimoto, T.**, Peptide growth factors and their receptor, in *Handbook of Experimental Pharmacology*, Sporn, M. M. and Roberts, A. B., Eds., Springer-Verlag, New York, 1990, 633–665.

39. **Hunt, J. S., Andrews, G. K., and Wood, G. W.**, Normal trophoblasts resist induction of class I HLA, *J. Immunol.*, 138, 2481, 1987.

40. **Hunziker, R. D. and Wegmann, T. G.**, Placental immunoregulation, *Crit. Rev. Immunol.*, 6, 245, 1986.

41. **Imakawa, K., Anthony, R. V., Kazemi, M., Marotti, K. R., Polites, H. G., and Roberts, R. M.**, Interferon-like sequence of ovine trophoblast protein secreted by embryonic trophectoderm, *Nature*, 330, 377, 1987.

42. **Imakawa, K. and Roberts, R. M.**, Interferons and maternal recognition of pregnancy, in *Development of Preimplantation Embryos and Their Environment*, Yoshinaga, K. and Mori, T., Eds., Allan R. Liss, New York, 1989, 347–358.

43. **Jaattela, M., Kuusela, P., and Saksela, E.**, Demonstration of tumor necrosis factor in human amniotic fluids and supernatants of placenta and decidual tissues, *Lab. Invest.*, 58, 48, 1988.

44. **Johannsen, R., Haupt, H., Bohn, H., Heid, K., Seiler, F. R., and Schwick, H. G.**, Inhibition of the mixed lymphocyte culture (MLC) by proteins: mechanism and specificity of the reaction, *A. Immunitat. A. Immunobiol.*, 152, 280, 1976.

45. **Kameda, T., Matsuzaki, N., Sawai, K., Okada, T., Saji, F., Matsuda, T., Hirano, T., Kishimoto, T., and Tanizawa, O.**, Production of interleukin-6 by normal human trophoblast, *Placenta*, 11, 205, 1990.

46. **Katsuura, G., Gottshall, P. E., Dahl, R. R., and Arimura, A.**, Adrenocorticotropin release induced by intracerebroventricular injection of recombinant human interleukin-1 in rats: possible involvement of prostaglandin, *Endocrinology*, 122, 1773, 1988.

47. **Kaye, M. D. and Jones, W. R.**, Effect of human chorionic gonadotropin on *in vitro* lymphocyte transformation, *Am. J. Obstet. Gynecol.*, 109, 1029, 1971.

48. **Kim, I. and Schomberg, D. W.**, The production of transforming growth factor-β activity by rat granulosa cell cultures, *Endocrinology*, 124, 1345, 1989.

49. **Klopper, A., Smith, R., and Davidson, I.**, The measurement of trophoblastic proteins as a test of placental function, in *Placental Protein*, Klopper, A. and Chard, T., Eds., Springer-Verlag, Heidelberg, 1979, 23–42.

50. **Koyama, M., Saji, F., Azuma, C., Negoro, T., Nakamuro, K., and Tanizawa, O.**, Immunologic properties of immunoglobulin eluted from human placenta, *Int. J. Feto-Maternal Med.*, 3, 187, 1990.

51. **Lala, P. K., Chatterjee-Hasrouni, S., Kearns, M., Montgomery, B., and Colavincenzo, V.**, Immunology of feto-maternal interface, *Immunol. Rev.*, 75, 87, 1983.

52. **Le, J. and Vilcek, J.**, Biology of disease. Tumor necrosis factor and interleukin-1: cytokines with multiple overlapping biological activities, *Lab. Invest.*, 56, 234, 1987.

53. **Li, Y., Matsuzaki, N., Masuhiro, K., Kameda, T., Taniguchi, T., Saji, F., Yone, K., and Tanizawa, O.**, Trophoblast-derived tumor necrosis factor-α induces release of human chorionic gonadotropin using IL-6 and IL-6-receptor dependent system in the normal human trophoblast, *J. Clin. Endocrinol. Metab.*, 74, 184, 1992.

54. **Loke, Y. W.**, Trophoblast antigen expression, *Curr. Opinion Immunol.*, 1, 1131, 1989.

55. **Maes, R. F. and Claverie, N.**, The effect of preparations of human chorionic gonadotropin on lymphocyte stimulation and immune response, *Immunology*, 33, 351, 1977.

56. **Massague, J.**, The TGF-β family of growth and differentiation, *Cell*, 49, 437, 1987.

57. **Masuhiro, K., Matsuzaki, N., Nishino, E., Taniguchi, T., Kameda, T., Li, Y., Saji, F., and Tanizawa, O.**, Trophoblast-derived interleukin-1 stimulates the release of human chorionic gonadotropin by activating IL-6 and IL-6-receptor systems in first trimester human trophoblast, *J. Clin. Endocrinol. Metab.*, in press.

58. **Matsuzaki, N., Okada, T., Kameda, T., Negoro, T., Saji, F., and Tanizawa, O.**, Analysis of the site of action induced by the choriocarcinoma-derived immunoregulatory factor on IL-2-mediated T cell responses, *J. Reprod. Immunol.*, 15, 181, 1989.

59. **Matsuzaki, N., Okada, T., Negoro, T., Saji, F., and Tanizawa, O.**, Trophoblast derived immunoregulatory factor: demonstration of the biological function and the physicochemical characteristics of the factor from choriocarcinoma cell lines, *Am. J. Reprod. Immunol.*, 19, 121, 1989.

60. **Matsuzaki, N., Saji, F., Okada, T., Sawai, K., Kameda, T., and Tanizawa, O.**, Analysis of immunoregulatory activity of a choriocarcinoma-derived factor: specific suppression of proliferative process of cell-mediated immune responses including LAK cell generation, *J. Reprod. Immunol.*, 19, 101, 1991.

61. **Medawar, P. B.**, Some immunological and endocrinological problems raised by evolution of viviparity in vertebrates, *Symp. Soc. Biol.*, 7, 320, 1953.

62. **Mori, T. and Kobayashi, H.**, Inhibitory effect of progesterone and 20α-hydroxypregn-4-en-3-one on the phytohemagglutinin induced transformation of human lymphocytes, *Am. J. Obstet. Gynecol.*, 127, 151, 1977.

63. **Morse, J. H.**, The effect of human chorionic gonadotrophin and placental lactogen on lymphocyte transformation *in vitro*, *Scand. J. Immunol.*, 5, 779, 1976.

64. **Morse, J. H., Stearns, G., Arden, J., Agosto, G. M., and Canfield, R. E.**, The effect of crude and purified human gonadotropin on *in vitro* stimulated human lymphocyte cultures, *Cell. Immunol.*, 25, 178, 1976.

65. **Morse, J. H., Erlich, P. H., and Canfield, R. E.**, Extracts of pregnancy urine contain a mitogen for human peripheral blood lymphocytes (PBL), *J. Immunol.*, 128, 2187, 1982.

66. **Muchmore, A. V. and Decker, J. M.**, Uromodulin: a unique 85-kilodalton immunosuppressive glycoprotein isolated from urine of pregnant women, *Science*, 229, 479, 1985.

67. **Muchmore, A. V.**, Uromodulin: an immunoregulatory glycoprotein isolated from pregnancy urine that binds to and regulates the activity of interleukin 1, *Am. J. Reprod. Immunol. Microbiol.*, 11, 89, 1986.

68. **Nagarkatti, P. S. and Clark, D. A.**, *In vitro* activity and *in vivo* correlates of alloantigens-specific murine suppressor T cells induced by allogeneic pregnancy, *J. Immunol.*, 131, 638, 1983.

69. **Nishino, E., Matsuzaki, N., Masuhiro, K., Kameda, T., Taniguchi, T., Takagi, T., Saji, F., and Tanizawa, O.**, Trophoblast-derived IL-6 regulates human chorionic gonadotropin secretion through IL-6 receptor on human trophoblasts, *J. Clin. Endocrinol. Metab.*, 71, 436, 1990.

70. **Olding, L. B. and Oldstone, M. B. A.**, Thymus-derived peripheral lymphocytes from human newborns inhibit division of their mothers' lymphocytes, *J. Immunol.*, 116, 682, 1976.

71. **Oppenheim, J. J., Kovacs, E. J., Matsushima, K., and Durum, S. K.**, There is more than one interleukin 1, *Immunol. Today*, 7, 45, 1986.

72. **Pavia, C., Siiteri, P. K., Perlman, J. D., and Stites, D. P.**, Suppression of murine allogeneic cell interactions by sex hormones, *J. Reprod. Immunol.*, 1, 33, 1979.

73. **Pearse, W. H. and Kaiman, H.**, Human chorionic gonadotropin and skin graft survival, *Am. J. Obstet. Gynecol.*, 98, 573, 1967.

74. **Persellin, R. H. and Rhodes, J.**, Inhibition of human monocyte FC receptor and HLA-DR antigen, *Clin. Exp. Immunol.*, 46, 350, 1981.

75. **Pockley, A. G. and Bolton, A. E.**, Effect of decidual placental protein 14 on interleukin-2-lymphocyte interactions, *Biochem. Soc. Trans.*, 16, 793, 1988.

76. **Pockley, A. G. and Bolton, A. E.**, The effect of human placental protein 14 (PP14) on the production of interleukin-1 from mitogenically stimulated mononuclear cell cultures, *Immunology*, 69, 277, 1990.

77. **Pockley, A. G., Mowles, E. A., Stoker, R. J., Westwood, O. M. R., Chapman, M. G., and Bolton, A. E.**, The suppression of *in vitro* lymphocyte reactivity to phytohemagglutinin (PHA) by placental protein 14 (PP14), *J. Reprod. Immunol.*, 13, 31, 1988.

78. **Pollard, J. W., Bartocci, A., Arecci, R., Orlofsky, A., Ladner, M. B., and Stanley, E. R.**, Apparent role of the macrophage growth factor, CSF-1, in placental development, *Nature*, 330, 484, 1987.

79. **Ringler, G. E., Coutifaris, C., Strauss, J. F., III, Allen, J. I., and Geier, M.**, Accumulation of colony-stimulating factor 1 in amniotic fluid during human pregnancy, *Am. J. Obstet. Gynecol.*, 160, 655, 1989.

80. **Saji, F., Koyama, M., Kameda, T., Negoro, T., Nakamuro, K., and Tanizawa, O.**, Effect of a soluble factor secreted from cultured human trophoblast cells on *in vitro* lymphocyte reactions, *Am. J. Reprod. Immunol. Microbiol.*, 13, 121, 1987.

81. **Saji, F., Kameda, T., Koyama, M., Matsuzaki, N., Negoro, T., and Tanizawa, O.,** Impaired susceptibility of human trophoblast to MHC nonrestricted killer cells: implication in the maternal-fetal relationship, *Am. J. Reprod. Immunol.,* 19, 108, 1989.

82. **Saji, F., Negoro, T., Matsuzaki, N., Koyama, M., Kameda, T., and Tanizawa, O.,** An immunoregulatory role of human trophoblasts, in *Development of Preimplantation Embryos and Their Environment,* Yoshinaga, K. and Mori, T., Eds., Alan R. Liss, New York, 1989, 435–446.

83. **Sanyal, M. K., Brami, C. J., Bischof, P., Simmons, E., Barnea, E. R., Dwyer, J. M., and Neftolin, F.,** Immunoregulatory activity in supernatants from cultures of normal human trophoblast cells of the first trimester, *Am. J. Obstet. Gynecol.,* 161, 446, 1989.

84. **Schiff, R. I., Mercier, D., and Buckley, R. H.,** Inability of gestational hormones to account for inhibitory effects of pregnancy plasmas on lymphocyte responses *in vitro, Cell. Immunol.,* 20, 69, 1975.

85. **Sironi, M., Breviario, F., Proserpio, P., Biondi, A., Vecchi, A., Damme, J. V., Dejano, E., and Mantovani, A.,** IL-1 stimulated IL-6 production in endothelial cells, *J. Immunol.,* 142, 549, 1989.

86. **Slater, L. M., Bostick, W., and Fletcher, L.,** Decreased mortality of murine graft-versus-host disease by human chorionic gonadotropin, *Transplantation,* 23, 103, 1977.

87. **Stimson, W. H.,** Transplantation—nature's success, *Lancet,* i, 684, 1972.

88. **Stimson, W. H.,** Studies on the immunosuppressive properties of a pregnancy-associated α-macroglobulin, *Clin. Exp. Immunol.,* 25, 199, 1976.

89. **Stimson, W. H. and Hunter, I. C.,** An investigation into the immunosuppressive properties of oestrogen, *J. Endocrinol.,* 28, 445, 1976.

90. **Stimson, W. H.,** Identification of pregnancy-associated α-macroglobulin on the surface of peripheral blood leukocyte populations, *Clin. Exp. Immunol.,* 28, 445, 1977.

91. **Stimson, W. H.,** Pregnancy-associated α_2-glycoprotein. Pregnancy-specific β_1-glycoprotein and pregnancy-associated plasma protein A and B, *Bibl. Reprod.,* 31, 225, 1978.

92. **Stimson, W. H., Crilly, P. J., and McCruden, A. B.,** Effect of sex steroids on the synthesis of immunoregulatory factors by thymic epithelial cell cultures, *IRCS Med. Sci.,* 8, 263, 1980.

93. **Stimson, W. H. and Crilly, P. J.,** Effects of steroids on the secretion of immunoregulatory factors by thymic epithelial cell cultures, *Immunology,* 44, 401, 1981.

94. **Suciu-Foca, N., Reed, E., Rohowsky, C., Kung, P., and King, D. W.,** Anti-idiotypic antibodies to anti-HLA receptors induced by pregnancy, *Proc. Natl. Acad. Sci. U.S.A.,* 80, 830, 1983.

95. **Tabibzadeh, S. S., Santhanam, U., Seghal, P. B., and May, L. T.,** Cytokine-induced production of IFN-β_2/IL-6 freshly explanted human endometrial stromal cells. Modulation by estradiol 17-β, *J. Immunol.,* 142, 3134, 1989.

96. **Tomoda, Y., Fuma, M., Miwa, T., Saka, N., and Ishizuka, N.,** Cell-mediated immunity in pregnant women, *Gynecol. Invest.,* 7, 280, 1976.

97. **Wahl, S. M., Hunt, D. A., Wong, H. L., Dougherty, S., McCartney-Francis, N., Wahl, L. M., Ellingsworth, L., Schmidt, J. A., Hall, G., Roberts, A. B., and Sporn, M. B.,** Transforming growth factor-β is a potent immunosuppressive agent that inhibits IL-1-dependent lymphocyte proliferation, *J. Immunol.,* 140, 3026, 1988.
98. **Weggman, T. G.,** Placental immunotrophism: maternal T cells enhance placental growth and function, *Am. J. Reprod. Immunol. Microbiol.,* 15, 67, 1987.
99. **Weggman, T. G.,** Maternal T cells promote placental trophoblast growth and prevent spontaneous abortion, *Immunol. Lett.,* 17, 297, 1988.
100. **Wei, X. and Orr, H. T.,** Differential expression of HLA-E, HLA-F, and HLA-G transcripts in human tissue, *Hum. Immunol.,* 29, 131, 1990.
101. **Wolf, R. L., Ilekis, J., and Benveniste, R.,** Characterization of an immune suppressor from transformed human trophoblastic JEG-3 cells, *Cell. Immunol.,* 78, 356, 1983.
102. **Wood, G. W. and King, C. R.,** Trapping antigen-antibody complexes within the human placenta, *Cell. Immunol.,* 69, 347, 1982.
103. **Wyle, F. A. and Kent, J. R.,** Immunosuppression by sex steroid hormones, *Clin. Exp. Immunol.,* 27, 407, 1977.
104. **Yagel, S., Lala, P. K., Powell, W. A., and Casper, R. F.,** Interleukin-1 stimulates human chorionic gonadotropin secretion by first trimester human trophoblast, *J. Clin. Endocrinol. Metab.,* 68, 992, 1989.
105. **Zhang, Y., Lin, J.-X., Yip, Y. K., and Vilcek, J.,** Enhancement of cAMP levels and of protein kinase activity by tumor necrosis factor and interleukin-1 in human fibroblasts: role in the induction of interleukin-6, *Proc. Natl. Acad. Sci. U.S.A.,* 85, 6802, 1988.
106. **Zuckermann, F. A. and Head, J. R.,** Murine trophoblast resists cell-mediated lysis. II. Resistance to natural cell-mediated cytotoxicity, *Cell. Immunol.,* 116, 274, 1988.

Chapter 10

Lymphohematopoietic Cytokines in the Placenta: Their Role in Reproduction

Thomas G. Wegmann
Department of Immunology
University of Alberta
Edmonton, Alberta, Canada

1. INTRODUCTION

This chapter will review information involving the maternal immune interaction with the conceptus that leads to placental growth and differentiation as well as enhanced fetal survival. In the first part of this overview I will outline the growing appreciation of this interaction as it has been developed in mice to the present stage of understanding of how lymphohematopoietic cytokines function as differentiation signals in the placenta. Thereafter, parallel observations currently being made in the human are discussed, which are yet at a premature stage of understanding, but nonetheless show promise for applications such as perinatal acquired immunodeficiency syndrome (AIDS) and, hopefully, new approaches to fertility regulation.

0-8493-8868-6/93/$0.00 + $.50

2. MURINE MATERNAL-FETAL INTERACTIONS

Over the recent past, two fundamental principles have emerged with respect to the maternal-fetal immune interaction. One is that an intact maternal immune system is not necessary for successful reproduction. Thus, mice which are doubly mutant for the SCID and beige mutations, and therefore lacking B and T cell rearrangements as well as virtually all natural killer (NK) function, nevertheless successfully reproduce.[1] In addition, two different groups have shown that mice homozygous for the β-2-microglobulin deletion, generated by homologous recombination and thus lacking almost all cell surface MHC class I expression, nevertheless show normal reproductive behavior.[2,3] Does this set of observations imply that there is no maternal immune interaction with the fetus, which enhances the survival of the latter? The answer is no. Experiments by a variety of laboratories have indicated that immunizing a number of mating combinations, which show high spontaneous fetal resorption, with paternal or third-party cells can lead to enhanced fetal survival along with increased placental size and fetal weight.[4] Drawing on our original observations involving the immune intervention which prevents the high spontaneous fetal resorption seen in CBA × DBA/2J mice,[5] Baines and colleagues reported a series of experiments in which they implicated NK-like cells at the maternal-fetal interface to be involved in the etiology of the fetal resorption. Initially they showed that there was an increased frequency of these cells in fetal-placental units subjected to the fetal resorption. Thereafter, they showed that one could intervene with antibody directed against NK cells and prevent fetal resorption by eliminating asialo-GM1 positive cells.[6] Kinsky and colleagues in Paris took these observations one step further.[7] They showed that a double-stranded RNA, poly IC, which activates NK cells, perhaps via interferon-γ stimulation, caused increased spontaneous abortion. This effect could be adoptively transferred by spleen cells from poly IC-stimulated mice and the adoptive transfer effect eliminated by pretreatment of the spleen cells with antiasialo-GM1 antibody. Incidentally, the poly IC effect works far better in inbred pregnancy than it does in hybrid pregnancy, suggesting a role for natural alloantigen recognition in resisting poly IC-induced fetal resorption. This idea was recently examined in detail in collaborative experiments done over the last year between this laboratory and Dr. B. Singh's laboratory at the University of Alberta, along with Drs. Chaouat, Kinsky, and Kapovic at Hôpital Cochin in Paris and Dr. P. Kourilsky of the Institut Pasteur (manuscript submitted). Initially we determined that poly IC-induced fetal resorption is reversible by standard alloimmunization in a number of different strain combinations, thus substantiating the hybrid effect mentioned above. In order to examine whether MHC class I antigens themselves might be involved, we did the following series of experiments. We induced poly IC-mediated fetal resorption in C57 ×

C57 matings and then attempted to reverse them using a series of Bm mutant cells. These cells differ from the parental type C57Bl/6 animal at a single class I or class II gene locus because of mutational change. BM6 is a poorly immunogenic class I mutation and provides no protection from the poly IC-induced fetal damage, whereas BM1 is a strongly immunogenic one and is protective. BM12, on the other hand, is a strongly immunogenic class II mutation and also protects. These observations have been confirmed by showing that poly IC-induced abortion can also be prevented by immunizing with L cells that have been transfected with an H-2D class I gene which shows a high level of protein expression on the cell surface. Untransfected L cells, on the other hand, are ineffective. We also have done a series of experiments with synthetic peptides, prepared by Dr. B. Singh of the University of Alberta, which represents the immunogenic domains of the MHC class I H-2K molecule. These peptides act in a similar manner in terms of preventing poly IC-mediated fetal resorption. Thus, we have established for the first time that maternal reaction against isolated MHC class I or class II antigen is sufficient to prevent fetal resorption in an experimental system in which which, although induced by poly IC, is based on spontaneous fetal resorption. There are two observations which must be noted to properly interpret these results. The first is that specificity for paternal MHC is not necessary. Third-party MHC reactivity is equally effective in preventing the fetal resorption. The second is that a nonspecific but strong immune response seems also to be sufficient in preventing the fetal resorption. Corroborating this conclusion, Toder and Strassburger have reported recently that treating CBA × DBA/2 with complete Freund's adjuvant alone, injected into the footpad, can prevent the fetal resorption seen in this strain combination.[8]

Another layer of complexity to the role of MHC in reproduction is added by recent experiments concerning the developmental regulation of MHC class I antigens in the rat placenta.[9] Gill and colleagues had previously shown that only paternal alloantigens are expressed in the rat placenta, which is curiously not the case for the mouse, where both maternal and paternal expression occurs. In a natural embryo they are expressed within the trophoblast cytoplasm but in transferred embryos they are expressed on the cell surface. In addition, surrogate mothers produce antibodies against a classical class I antigen that is coded for by the transferred embryo. Natural mothers, on the other hand, do not produce antibody of this type.[9] The mechanisms underlying the regulation of this unexpected type of MHC class I expression are as yet unclear, but clearly point to some type of gene imprinting with environmental modification. In addition, it remains to be seen whether similar observations will be made in species other than the rat.

The mechanisms by which immune intervention in the ways described above can prevent spontaneous fetal resorption remain conjectural. One consequence of such immune intervention is that both the placenta and the fetus tend to show increases in size. A striking illustration of this point is found in MRL/lpr/lpr mice. These mice show a spontaneous lupus-like syndrome involving hyperreactivity of their T cells. They also have very large placentas and extraordinarily high levels of placental phagocytosis when compared to their sister strain mice. Both parameters can be reduced dramatically by treating them with monoclonal antibodies against T cells *in vivo* during early phases of pregnancy. In addition, spleen cells from these mice, but not from sister strain mice, can be used to adoptively transfer protection against spontaneous fetal resorption in CBA mice pregnant by DBA/2J. This same maneuver also leads to an increase in placental and fetal size in the recipient mice.[10] In every strain combination which we have examined where we have treated with anti-CD4 plus anti-CD8 antibody, there is a reduction in placental size and phagocytosis, and in certain cases fetal resorption occurs. The only exception to that rule has been in three different strains of mice carrying the recessive nude mutation. In each of these cases, the placenta is small to begin with and the antibody intervention has no effect.[11] Thus, it appears that an intact immune response contributes to increased placental size, and in some cases, fetal survival.

How might these effects be mediated? One possibility is that immune stimulation leads to increased cytokine release at the maternal-fetal interface and this in turn interacts upon reproductive tissues to alter their differentiative pathways. Evidence supporting this conjecture exists. Granulocyte macrophage GM-CSF, CSF-1, and interleukin (IL)-3 have all been shown to influence trophoblast proliferation.[12] CSF-1 has been localized to uterine epithelium and is excreted in rather large quantities in the uterine fluid during early phases of pregnancy, under the control of estrogen and progesterone.[13] Receptors for CSF-1, the so-called *c-fms* protooncogene product, have been demonstrated to be present on giant cell trophoblasts and other trophoblasts as well, adjacent to the major sites of CSF-1 secretion.[14,15] Although the endocrine basis for this secretion has been well worked out, no studies have examined the immune system components that may or may not be involved. GM-CSF is released from the decidua during pregnancy.[16] *In situ* hybridizations indicate that it is made in fibroblast-like cells, endothelial-like cells, and also by monocytes within the decidua itself. In addition, cells in the spongiotrophoblast layer also seem to be producing messenger RNA for this molecule.[17] Placental GM-CSF appears to be coded for by a series of higher-molecular-weight messenger RNAs as well as the standard 1.1-kb messenger RNA molecule.[18] Additional unpublished experiments indicate that the higher-molecular-weight species code for the first two 5' exons of the GM-CSF gene but not the adjacent two exons. Further molecular biological work is necessary to characterize the detailed nature of the organ-specific expression seen for GM-CSF mRNA in the placenta. These observations have taken on additional meaning by experiments in which CBA females mated with DBA/2J mice can have dramatically reduced levels of fetal resorption if they are injected with GM-CSF or IL-3 in early phases of their pregnancy. IL-2, interferon-γ, and tumor necrosis factor (TNF)-α have the opposite effect, enhancing fetal resorption in a number of different strain combinations.[19]

Thus, there is direct evidence *in vivo* for the reproductive efficacy of these lymphohematopoietic cytokines. There are also indications that some of them may be produced by the placenta itself, perhaps by certain types of trophoblast cells. This may then explain why immune system intervention can be effective at altering placental function, because there is a commonality of cytokine utilization between the two systems. Therefore, the possibility exists for communication between the immune and reproductive systems using these cytokines which apparently function in both systems.

3. PRELIMINARY OBSERVATIONS USING HUMAN TROPHOBLAST

In collaboration with the laboratory of Dr. Larry Guilbert, we have observed that all three classical human choriocarcinomas cells, JEG, JAR, and BeWo, secrete GM-CSF and CSF-1. Antibodies specific for GM-CSF partially inhibit the proliferation of the choriocarcinoma cells, thus strongly suggesting that GM-CSF is autocrine for the growth of these cells. Antibodies against CSF-1 show no effect, but those directed against the receptor for CSF-1 also partially inhibit the proliferation. In addition, antibodies to GM-CSF eliminate the ability of human term trophoblast to syncytialize *in vitro,* a condition which can be reversed and, indeed, enhanced by adding excess GM-CSF.[23] These observations suggest that GM-CSF is involved in some fundamental way in cytotrophoblast differentiation to syncytiotrophoblast. This explains why these cytokines enhance the production of human chorionic gonadotropin and human placental lactogen from trophoblast cells in culture. This work possibly relates to that reported by Robertson and Seamark.[20] They have shown that GM-CSF promotes mouse embryo implantation in an elegant *in vitro* culture system, involving monolayers of uterine epithelium, and may therefore affect trophectoderm cell surface adhesiveness. Corroboration for the Guilbert experiments has also been obtained by Shiverick and colleagues at the University of Florida at Gainesville.[24] They have found that rat trophoblast cultures can be made to secrete certain clearly defined members of the rat placental lactogen family when they are stimulated with either GM-CSF or CSF-1. Analogously, Haimovichi et al.[21] at Harvard University have reported experiments indicating that GM-CSF inhibits mouse blastocyst attachment to fibronectin-coated wells, once again indicating a role for this molecule in modifying the properties of trophoblast membrane. Thus, it appears that what were formerly considered to be cytokines operating in the lymphohematopoietic system mediate reproductive functions by influencing the membrane properties of trophoblast and their subsequent differentiative events.

In order to clarify the situation, we need a much more detailed description of the cytokine pathways by which immunizing with paternal alloantigens and other substances leads to prevention of fetal resorption and enhancement of placental size. Understanding these pathways becomes important when one considers the phenomenon of perinatal AIDS. It has recently been shown that syncytiotrophoblast expresses CD4 molecules on the cellular surface immediately adjacent to the maternal blood stream. Gp160 can bind to this surface and the binding can be prevented by anti-CD4 monoclonal antibodies. In addition, FcγRIII receptors are also present on the surface.[22] Since GM-CSF has been implicated in releasing HIV from macrophages, it will be of some interest to determine whether this cytokine and related cytokines can affect the parameters of trophoblast differentiation which influence HIV infection and transmissibility. Since GM-CSF and CSF-1 both affect troph-oblast differentiation, this is a very real possibility indeed, and one that needs to be examined with some urgency. In collaboration with Monte Meltzer and colleagues at Walter Reed Army Hospital, we have recently shown that purified trophoblast preparations can be infected by HIV showing macrophage tropism and that this infection can be influenced by GM-CSF and CSF-1.[25] Although the experiments are preliminary, they indicate that these cytokines may well influence whether a female transmits HIV to her offspring. These preliminary experiments underscore the necessity for a better understanding of how cytokines are secreted at the maternal-fetal interface as a result of maternal-fetal immune interactions, as well as autocrine activity wihin the placenta itself, and how these cytokines influence trophoblast development and ultimately fetal survival. This should enhance our grasp of basic reproductive phenomena and allow application to such areas as perinatal AIDS and fertility regulation.

4. SUMMARY

The work reviewed here concerns the maternal immune interaction with the fetus, leading to enhanced survival and increased placental and fetal size. Recent advances indicate that major histocompatibility complex (MHC) class I and class II genes can trigger a maternal immune responsiveness that leads to increased fetal survival. This is likely based on an immunological intersection of otherwise destructive NK-like cells at the maternal-fetal interface. In addition, there is developing evidence for unusual regulation of MHC class I genes at the placental level, particularly those of the rat, in which classical class I genes are expressed only in the cytoplasm of trophoblast and not on the cell surface, with significant exceptions being found in transplanted embryos. On the effector side it is clear that the presence of maternal T cells leads to enhanced growth of the placenta and fetus because of evidence reviewed here involving deletion of immune system components. The basis for these phenomena appears to be secretion of lymphohematopoietic cytokines at the maternal-fetal interface which influence trophoblast growth and differentiation and, in particular, syncytialization. The particular cytokines involved, members of the colony-stimulating factor (CSF)-1 family, are relevant to human immunodeficiency virus (HIV) release in macrophages and, thus, may ultimately contribute to our understanding of how HIV is transmitted across the trophoblastic barrier during pregnancy. These observations also provide opportunities for novel means of regulating human fertility.

REFERENCES

1. **Croy, B. A. and Chapeau, C.,** Evaluation of pregnancy immunotrophism hypothesis by assessment of the reproductive performance of young adult mice of genotype scid/scid.bg/bg, *J. Reprod. Fertil.,* 88, 231–239, 1990.
2. **Zijlstra, M., Bix, M., Simister, N. E., Loring, J. M., Raulet, D. H., and Jaenisch, R.,** β2-microglobulin deficient mice lack CD4-8$^+$ cytolitic T cells, *Nature,* 344, 742–746, 1990.
3. **Koller, B. H., Marrack, P., Kappler, J. W., and Smithies, O.,** Normal development of mice deficient in β2M, MHC class I proteins, and CD8 plus T cells, *Science,* 248, 1227–1230, 1990.
4. **Chaouat, G., Kolb, J. P., Chaffaux, S., Riviere, M., Lankar, D., Athanassakis, I., Green, D., and Wegmann, T. G.,** The placenta and the survival of the fetal allograft, in *Immunoregulation and Fetal Survival,* Gill, T. J., III and Wegmann, T. G., Eds., Oxford University Press, New York, 1987, 239–251.
5. **Chaouat, G., Kiger, N., and Wegmann, T. G.,** Vaccination against spontaneous abortion in mice, *J. Reprod. Immunol.,* 5, 389–392, 1983.
6. **Gendron, R. L., Farookhi, R., and Baines, M. G.,** Resorption of CBA/J × DBA/2 mouse conceptuses in CBA/J uteri correlates with failure of the feto-placental unit to suppress natural killer cell activity, *J. Reprod. Fertil.,* 89, 277–284, 1990.
7. **Kinsky, R., Delage, G., Rosin, N., Thang, M. N., Hoffmann, M., and Chaouat, G.,** A murine model of NK cell mediated resorption, *Am. J. Reprod. Immunol.,* 23, 73–77, 1990.
8. **Toder, V. and Strassburger, D.,** Non-specific immunopotentiation and pregnancy loss, *Res. Immunol.,* 141, 181, 1990.
9. **Gill, T. J.,** Immunogenetics of recurrent abortions in experimental animals and in humans, in *The Immunology of the Fetus,* Chaouat, G., Ed., CRC Press, Boca Raton, FL, 1990, 293–306.
10. **Chaouat, G., Menu, E., Athanassakis, I., and Wegmann, T. G.,** Maternal T cells regulate placental size and fetal survival, *Reg. Immunol.,* 1, 143–148, 1988.
11. **Athanassakis, I., Chaouat, G., and Wegmann, T. G.,** The effects of anti-CD4 and anti-CD8 antibody treatment on placental growth and function in allogeneic and syngeneic murine pregnancy, *Cell. Immunol.,* 129, 13–21, 1990.

12. **Athanassakis, I., Bleackley, R. C., Paetkau, V., Guilbert, L., Barr, P. J., and Wegmann, T. G.**, The immunostimulatory effect of T cells and T cell lymphokines on murine fetally derived placental cells, *J. Immunol.*, 138, 37–44, 1987.

13. **Bartocci, A., Pollard, J. W., and Stanley, E. R.**, Regulation of colony stimulating factor 1 during pregnancy, *J. Exp. Med.*, 164, 956–961, 1986.

14. **Arceci, R. J., Shanahan, F., Stanley, E. R., and Pollard, J. W.**, Temporal expression and location of colony-stimulating factor 1 (CSF-1) and its receptor in the female reproductive tract are consistent with CSF-1 regulated placental development, *Proc. Natl. Acad. Sci. U.S.A.*, 86, 8818, 1989.

15. **Regenstreif, L. J. and Rossant, J.**, Expression of the *c-fms* proto-oncogene and of the cytokine, CSF-1, during mouse embryogenesis, *Dev. Biol.*, 133, 284, 1989.

16. **Wegmann, T. G. Athanassakis, I., Guilbert, L., Branch, D., Dy, M., Menu, E., and Chaouat, G.**, The role of M-CSF and GM-CSF in fostering placental growth, fetal growth, and fetal survival, *Transplant. Proc.*, 21, 566, 1989.

17. **Kanzaki, H., Crainie, M., Lin, H., Yui, J., Guilbert, L. J., and Wegmann, T. G.**, The *in situ* expression of Granulocyte-Macrophage Colony Stimulating Factor (GM-CSF) mRNA at the maternal-fetal interface, *Growth factors*, 5, 69–74, 1991.

18. **Crainie, M., Guilbert, L., and Wegmann, T. G.**, Expression of novel cytokine transcripts in the murine placenta, *Biol. Reprod.*, 43, 999–1005, 1990.

19. **Chaouat, G., Menu, E., Clark, D., Dy, M., Minkowski, M., and Wegmann, T. G.**, Control of fetal survival in CBA × DBA/2 mice by lymphokine therapy, *J. Reprod. Fertil.*, 89, 447–458, 1990.

20. **Robertson, S., Lavranos, T., and Seamark, R. F.**, *In vitro* models of the maternal-fetal interface, in *Molecular and Cellular Immunology of the Maternal-Fetal Interface*, Wegmann, T. G., Nisbett-Brown, E., and Gill, T. J., III, Eds., Oxford University Press, New York, 1991, 191–206.

21. **Haimovici, F., Hill, J. A., and Anderson, D. J.**, The effects of soluble products of activated lymphocytes and macrophages on blastocyst implantation events *in vitro*, *Biol. Reprod.*, 44, 69–75, 1991.

22. **David, F. J. E., Autran, B., Tran, H. C., Menu, E., Raphael, M., Debre, P., Hsi, B. L., Wegmann, T. G., Barre-Sinousi, F., and Chaouat, G.**, Human trophoblast cells express CD4 and are permissive for productive infection with HIV-1, *Clin. Exp. Immunol.*, 88, 10–16, 1992.

23. **Garcia-Lloret, M. et al.**, submitted.

24. **Shiverick, K.**, personal communication.

25. **Meltzer, M.**, unpublished observation.

Endocrine Regulation of the Immune System During Pregnancy

Julia Szekeres-Bartho
Department of Microbiology
Pécs University Medical School
Pécs, Hungary

Reproductive immunology is an interdisciplinary field of research. Immunological aspects of the fetal-maternal relationship have attracted the interest of reproductive biologists, endocrinologists, and immunologists for many years. However, the central question of how the fetus is protected from potentially harmful maternal attack has not yet been adequately answered.

Many observations suggest that cell-mediated immunity is altered during pregnancy. Pickard[97] and Vaughan and Ramirez[135] have demonstrated increased incidence of certain infections during pregnancy. Malignancies were also shown to be more frequent.[45,52,60,110] Skin reaction to tuberculin was reduced[72] and the survival of skin homografts was twice as long in pregnant, compared to nonpregnant, women.[2] Maternal cell-mediated immunity was shown to be regulated by serum factors[71,100] and placenta-produced factors.[19] Both pregnancy serum and placental supernatants contain pregnancy-related hormones.

Pregnancy is characterized by substantial alteration of endocrine functions. Sperm transport, gamete and ovum transport, as well as implantation, are facilitated by hormonal events, and parturition is also accompanied by marked alterations of the endocrine status.

Steroid hormones are first produced by the corpus luteum under human chorionic gonadotropin (hCG) stimulation. From the 7th week of gestation the placenta takes over steroid production and functions as a main source of steroid hormones till the end of pregnancy.

Progesterone is essential for the maintenance of pregnancy in mammals. It inhibits the contractions of myometrial smooth muscle,[73] blocks the activity of uterine collagenase,[53,61] and modifies the activity of proteolytic enzymes.[6] Its synthesis from cholesterol requires only two enzymatic steps. Pregnenolone formed this way is then transformed to progesterone. Progesterone is derived from two sources: the corpus luteum which is required for the maintenance of early pregnancy[28] and the hemochorial placenta. In humans, progesterone production gradually rises during gestation to reach a level of 3000 ng/g of placental tissue.[38] The serum concentrations of progesterone range from about 100 to 500 nM during pregnancy. Blocking of progesterone binding sites by a progesterone receptor antagonist RU-486 causes abortion in humans.[56]

The corpus luteum and the placenta also produce large amounts of estrogens. The biological significance of estrogens in the maintenance of pregnancy is not clear, since after the corpus luteum is removed, progesterone replacement alone allows pregnancy to proceed.[29]

Human chorionic gonadotropin is produced by the trophoblast in large quantities throughout gestation. This hormone plays a crucial role in the establishment and the maintenance of pregnancy. It exerts a luteotrophic effect up to the 6th to 8th week of gestation, which is essential for progesterone production by the corpus luteum. The blood level of hCG increases sharply in the first trimester of pregnancy to 160 IU/ml and then falls below 80 IU/ml. Previous studies indicated that crude hCG preparations isolated from urine of pregnant women possessed immunosuppressive activity. hCG prolonged skin allograft survival[93] and inhibited proliferation of allogeneically stimulated lymphocytes.[1,26,64] However, purified preparations of hCG possessed almost no immunosuppressive activity.[13,74,83] The same was true for human placental lactogen (hPL), which suppressed lymphocyte proliferation,[26] but after extensive purification the suppressive activity was lost.[83]

There are data that suggest sex-related differences in immune responsiveness. Males seem to have stronger cell-mediated responses than females.[106] On the other hand, females show increased capacity to produce antibodies after immunization.[4,10,32,86,104,106,114,131,136] The incidence of autoimmune disorders is higher in women during the fertile period.[31,59] These observations focused attention on the role of sex steroids in the regulation of the immune response.

Few and sometimes contradictory data are available on the effects of estrogens on the immune response. During the follicular phase an increase of peripheral blood monocytes and granulocytes was observed, and this was associated with changes in serum estradiol concentration.[76] Estrogens were also reported to augment phagocytic activity of the macrophages.[42] Estradiol enhanced the colony formation of human myelomonocytic cells.[75] This effect has been shown to be mediated by inducing the colony precursor cells to be more responsive to colony-stimulating factor (CSF).[3] Estrogens had no effect on neutrophile responsiveness in physiological concentrations,[11] nor did they affect proliferation of mitogen-stimulated cultures.[92]

Sex steroids influence both the immune cell number and function in the uterus. Four hours after ovariectomy there is a cellular infiltration in the rat placenta and this can be prevented by local administration of progesterone.[24] The number of uterine macrophages increases parallel with the fall of progesterone levels before parturition.[90] High local concentrations of progesterone are able to prolong the survival of xenogeneic and allogeneic skin grafts,[54,82,112] as well as skin grafts placed in the uterine lumen of ovariectomized ewes.[54] Also, the growth of xenogeneic tumor cells implanted in hamster uteri was prolonged by progesterone,[112] and rejection occurred immediately after cessation of steroid treatment.

Many workers have shown that progesterone blocks *in vitro* T cell activation in concentrations of 5 to 20 μg/ml.[81,88,91,107,141] Stites et al.[116] reported on different mechanisms of blocking T cell activation by progesterone and cortisol. The inhibitory effect of cortisol seems to involve monocytes, while progesterone has a direct effect on T cells. T lymphocyte proliferation requires the presence of interleukin 2 (IL-2). The production of IL-2 by a subset of T lymphocytes is induced by the macrophage-derived factor IL-1. Both glucocorticoids and progesterone were shown to block IL-1-induced proliferation;[117] however, no data are available on their effect on IL-1 production so far.

Gillis et al.[44] have demonstrated an inhibition of IL-2 production by dexamethasone, while progesterone and estradiol were without effect. Schleimer et al.[108] suggested that glucocorticoids may act both indirectly, e.g., via IL-2 production, and directly on cytotoxic T lymphocytes (CTL). In contrast to glucocorticoids, progesterone seems to interfere with IL-2 receptor binding.[134] However, to clarify this point, further experimental evidence is needed.

Suppressor cells may have an important role in the nonrejection of the fetal allograft. Clark et al.[21-23] have demonstrated nonantigen-specific suppressor cells in the decidua at the implantation site. Placental extracts can generate spleen cells with suppressive activity in the murine system.[16-18] Other workers recently reported the existence of a hormone-dependent suppressor cell population that appears in the early stages of gestation.[8,20] This kind of suppressor cell population is present in the uterus of pseudopregnant mice, as well as in mice treated with estrogen and progesterone. Furthermore, suppressor cell activity recovered from the uteri of mice varied with the stages of the estrus cycle.[9] These data suggest that steroid hormones might trigger suppressor cell generation during pregnancy. Pavia et al.[91] obtained data in mice suggesting that progesterone affects the inductive and proliferative phases of the immune responses without affecting killing by CTL, generated in the absence of steroids. Van Vlasselaer and Vandeputte,[134] on the other hand, demonstrated blocking of CTLs by progesterone at concentrations of 1 to 10 µg/ml when CTLs were preincubated with the hormone for 16 h. Cortisol required a much longer preincubation with the cells to achieve the same suppressive effect. This can be explained on the basis of IL-2 involvement in its action.

Data concerning the effect of progesterone on killing by natural killer (NK) cells are mostly negative.[70,118,133] It has to be noted, however, that in these studies nonpregnancy lymphocytes were used as a source of effector cells, and only in one of these studies was the progesterone concentration close to the physiological serum level in pregnancy. In a murine system, Furokawa et al.[39] demonstrated a decreased NK activity during pregnancy and a fluctuation of NK activity according to the estrus cycle.

Earlier we observed an immunological response of pregnancy lymphocytes to *in vitro* treatment by low concentrations of progesterone together with the lack of response, in the same conditions, of nonpregnancy lymphocytes.[120] This finding allows the assumption that higher progesterone sensitivity of pregnancy lymphocytes might be due to the presence of specific progesterone-binding sites on these cells.

Steroid hormone receptors belong to a common class of proteins of 80,000 to 100,000 molecular weight and are structurally organized in three different domains.[14,15,57,69,105,139,140] They exhibit a variable N-terminal region, a short and well-conserved cysteine-rich central domain, and a relatively well-conserved C-terminal half.[36] The C-terminal is the hormone-binding structure and it has a role in nuclear translocation. The central domain is responsible for the DNA-binding activity of the receptors.[37] The N-terminal domain is less well characterized and may have a modulatory effect on trans activation. This domain contains the antigenic determinants, and most receptor antibodies are directed against this region of the protein.[14,138] The classical model for steroid hormone action involves binding of the hormone to a cytoplasmic form of the receptor followed by a conformational change of the complex: the "transformation" step, that leads to intranuclear translocation and binding to chromatin.[63]

Unoccupied steroid hormone receptors are localized in the cytosol/cytoplasm. Upon hormone exposure they are transformed and translocated to the nuclei.[46,62,84] In recent years, data have been accumulating to indicate that, at least in some receptor systems, the receptors are predominantly localized within the nucleus.[47,49]

With monoclonal antibodies to estrogen receptor, staining was restricted to the nucleus in a wide range of estrogen target tissues in the absence of the hormone.[49,65,78,96,98] These results were interpreted as reflecting nuclear localization of the majority of the native receptor in the intact cell.[40] Similar results have been reported for progesterone receptors.[40,95] Specific high-affinity receptors have so far not been identified in resting human[88] or sheep[113] lymphocytes. Using a panel of progesterone receptor-specific monoclonal antibodies, nuclear progesterone receptors (PR) have been demonstrated in the CD8$^+$ population of peripheral pregnancy lymphocytes, while no PRs were detected in lymphocytes of nonpregnant individuals.[122,128] The percentage of PR-positive lymphocytes increased throughout gestation. Recurrent abortion, spontaneous abortion, and preterm labor, as well as labor, were associated with a fall in the number of PR-positive cells[122] (Table 1). During the process of activation neither the steroid-binding domain nor the steroid hormone itself is needed for DNA binding or transcriptional enhancement. Instead, it seems that the hormone-binding region normally prevents the domains for DNA binding and transcriptional activation from functioning. The addition of hormone relieves this inhibition.[3] The interaction between the hormone and the receptor induces conformational changes in the receptor molecule that result in higher affinity for DNA;[48,77] thus, the receptor associates with high-affinity binding sites in the chromatin. This, in turn, leads to the induction or repression of a limited number of genes, resulting in protein synthesis.

In the presence of progesterone, PR-positive lymphocytes were shown to produce a 34-kDa protein which inhibits the release of arachidonic acid.[121] This factor is a product of CD8-positive cells and acts in a species-specific manner. Immunological actions of this protein include inhibition of NK-mediated lysis (Table 2), generation of cells with suppressor phenotype and function, and inhibition of proliferation in the mixed lymphocyte reaction (MLR).[123] These phenomena are not related to altered lymphokine production. Interferon (IFN), granulocyte macrophage colony-stimulating factor (GM-CSF), IL-10, and IL-5 concentration did not show any characteristic changes in supernatants of pregnancy lymphocytes upon progesterone treatment.[143] Progesterone receptor blocker inhibits the production of this protein (Table 2), suggesting that functional PRs are needed for its production.[123] The protein appears in the serum of healthy pregnant women. Significantly lower concentrations are found in sera of women showing clinical symptoms of threatened preterm delivery and also from women with miscarriages and preterm deliveries. The serum concentration of this substance shows a good correlation with the outcome of pregnancy.[124] Lymphocyte PRs appear as early as the 10th day of human gestation, and they disappear from peripheral blood during labor.[122] Since the presence or absence of the progesterone-induced immunomodulatory factor correlates with the failure or success of gestation,[124] the regulation of lymphocyte PR seems to be of interest. Steroid hormones are potent regulators of the actual cellular level of receptors. Estrogens upregulate estrogen receptors,[85] while glucocorticoids downregulate

TABLE 1.
Percentage of Progesterone Receptor-Positive Lymphocytes in PBL from Healthy Pregnant Women of Different Gestational Ages and Women with Recurrent Abortion (RA), Spontaneous Abortion (AB), Threatened Preterm Delivery (TPD), and in Labor (L)

	Healthy Pregnant Women			RA	AB	TPD	L
	1st Trimester	2nd Trimester	3rd Trimester				
% of PR-positive cells	4 ± 0.83	5.3 ± 0.8	10 ± 1.66	0.8 ± 0.6*	1.1 ± 0.45*	1.7 ± 0.6**	0.8 ± 0.5**

* Significantly different (SD) from normal pregnant women at $p < 0.05$; **SD from normal pregnant women at $p < 0.01$.
197

TABLE 2.
Effect of Supernatants of Progesterone-Treated Pregnancy Lymphocytes or Negatively Selected Subpopulations on Natural Cytotoxicity to Human Embryonic Fibroblast Cells

Supernatants	IF	IF_{-NK}	IF_{-T4}	IF_{-T8}	$IF_{RU\ 486}$
Inhibition of natural cytotoxicity (%)	76 ± 6.3[a]	49 ± 5.4[b]	47 ± 9[b]	15 ± 5.4	2.7 ± 1.8

Note: IF, Supernatants of progesterone-treated pregnancy lymphocytes; IF_{-NK}, supernatant of HNK1-depleted progesterone-treated pregnancy lymphocytes; IF_{-T4}, supernatant of T4-depleted progesterone-treated pregnancy lymphocytes; IF_{-T8}, supernatant of T8-depleted progesterone-treated pregnancy lymphocytes; $IF_{RU\ 486}$, supernatant of progesterone + RU 486-treated pregnancy lymphocytes.

[a] Inhibition is significant at $p < 0.001$.
[b] Inhibition is significant at $p < 0.01$.

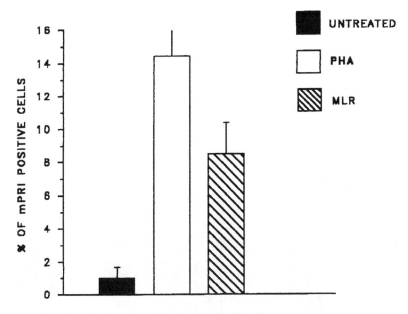

Figure 1. The effect of mitogenic or alloantigenic stimulation in progesterone receptor expression by lymphocytes of nonpregnant individuals. The bars represent the mean ± SE of 8 experiments. (*) Significantly different from nonpregnant control at $p < 0.001$.

glucocorticoid receptors.[119] Progesterone downregulates estrogen receptors.[80] Progesterone receptors are upregulated by estrogens, but downregulated by progesterone.[137]

In contrast to the classical target tissues in lymphocytes, estrogens do not induce PRs.[128] The reason for this might be the absence of estrogen receptors in peripheral human lymphocytes. However, E_2 receptors have been demonstrated in mouse spleen,[30] bovine thymus,[50] human thymic cells,[25,115] human mononuclear cells,[101] and rat macrophages.[51] By an enzyme immunoassay utilizing a rat monoclonal antibody to the human receptor, we could not demonstrate estrogen receptors in resting human lymphocytes.[122] PRs are induced, on the other hand, by *in vitro* mitogenic or alloantigenic stimulation of nonpregnancy lymphocytes (Figure 1).[128] *In vivo* allogeneic stimulation has similar effects, as shown by the high ratio of PR-positive cells in peripheral blood lymphocytes (PBL) of liver transplanted and blood transfused patients (Figure 2).[125]

Studies on transfected cell lines showed that polymorphic class I as well as class II HLA antigens induced PRs in nonpregnancy lymphocytes, whereas cells transfected with a murine monomorphic class I antigen (Be 37) did not. Furthermore, the presence of murine monomorphic major histocompatibility complex (MHC) products downregulated phytohemagglutinin (PHA)-induced PR expression. HLA-G- (a recently discovered class I monomorphic antigen present in the trophoblast)[35,68] transfected cell lines, on the other hand, did

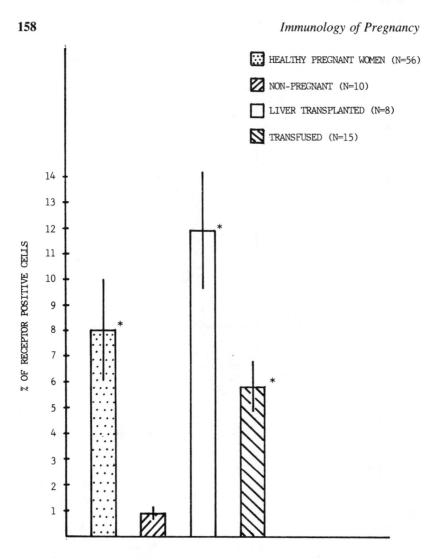

Figure 2. Progesterone receptors in peripheral blood lymphocytes of liver transplanted and transfused patients. The bars represent mean ± SEM of individuals. (*) Significantly different from healthy nonpregnant controls at p <0.001. (From Szekeres-Bartho, J. et al., *Immunol. Lett.*, 22, 259, 1989. With permission of Elsevier Science.)

not downregulate PHA-induced progesterone receptor expression in normal human lymphocytes. These findings suggest that lymphocyte progesterone-binding sites—at least as far as their regulation is concerned—are different from the classical progesterone receptors.

The above data allow the assumption that in pregnancy antigenic stimulation by the fetus might be involved in the induction of PRs but the tissue representing the appropriate antigen is still to be identified. Trophoblast, a tissue of embryonic origin and in close contact with maternal blood throughout gestation, might be a possible candidate. Maternal immune response to paternal,[94] neonatal,[103] or placental[142] alloantigens is well documented. During normal human pregnancy there is no direct contact between the fetus and maternal blood. Trophoblast, the barrier between the maternal and fetal sides, does not express classical polymorphic HLA antigens, but it expresses trophoblast-specific antigens,[7,43] trophoblast leukocyte cross-reactive antigens,[79] and monomorphic class I HLA antigens.[102]

The role of placental cells in local immunoregulation is well established. As a function of placental differentiation and maturation, trophoblast cells might change their antigen presentation, and thus exert a regulatory effect on lymphocyte PR expression. Indeed, syncytiotrophoblast villous surface membranes or trophoblast-enriched cells from 1st trimester placentas induced PRs in lymphocytes of nonpregnant individuals, while villous surface membranes or trophoblast-enriched cells from term placentas did not, and even downregulated PHA-induced lymphocyte PR expression (Table 3). Thus, aging trophoblast cells might begin to express surface structures that regulate PR expression.

Antihormones or hormone antagonists are compounds that prevent an endogenous hormone from exerting its biological effects by blocking the cellular hormone receptors. They bind with high affinity to the progesterone receptor to inhibit the action of the hormone.[5,33,34] The antihormone should be characterized by high specificity, high affinity for, and slow dissociation rate from the receptor in order to ensure effective competition with the native hormone, by absence finally of any agonistic activity. Among the steroid antagonists, antiprogestins are closest to the "ideal" compound. None of them are fully specific for progesterone receptors, all of them also bind to a certain extent to glucocorticoid receptors and possess antiglucocorticoid activity *in vitro* and *in vivo*.[55] ZK 98734, a new antiprogestational steroid, is 3 to 10 times more potent as an abortificient and possesses a lower antiglucocorticoid activity than RU 486 in animal models.[12,87,99]

Administration of progesterone receptor blockers in early pregnancy may lead to abortion.[56,67,111] In some patients this treatment fails to terminate pregnancy.[27,67] This provides a suitable *in vivo* model to investigate immunologic and other effects of progesterone separately in the same system. In an attempt to clarify the role of immunological mechanisms in the maintenance of pregnancy, lymphocyte function in successful pregnancy terminations was compared to that in failure cases. Among 5- to 6-week pregnant women treated with antiprogesterone for pregnancy termination, good and poor responders were found.

Lymphocytes from high responders reacted with a rapid increase of cytotoxic activity and a fall in progesterone sensitivity and progesterone-binding capacity; whereas in low responders, lymphocyte function did not change considerably during the treatment. Serum concentration of SP-1 decreased in both groups during the treatment, reflecting a block of trophoblastic receptors.[58] Cessation of pregnancy correlated better with the block

TABLE 3.
Induction and Regulation of PR Expression in Nonpregnancy Lymphocytes by Placental Cells and Villous Surface Membranes (STPM) Isolated from 1st-Trimester and Term Placentas

Treatment of Lymphocytes	None	5 Days Incub. with 1st Trim. Plac. Cells	5 Days Incub. with Term Plac. Cells	48 h PHA	48 h PHA + 1st Trim Plac. Cells	48 h PHA + Term Plac. Cells	48 h PHA + 1st Trim STPM	48 h PHA + Term STPM
PR-positive cells (%)	0.8 ± 0.1	14 ± 1.5*	1.3 ± 0.2	32 ± 1.2	42 ± 6	3.2 ± 1**	30 ± 1.7	4.5 ± 1.5**

* SD from untreated nonpregnancy lymphocytes at *p* <0.001.
** SD from PHA-induced nonpregnancy lymphocytes at *p* <0.001.

of lymphocyte PRs than with trophoblastic PR block, suggesting that the block of lymphocyte PRs may play a role in pregnancy termination.[126]

In vitro data obtained with human cells suggest a correlation between the rate of PR expression and the success or failure of pregnancy, but provide no direct evidence for their role in maintaining normal gestation. However, data obtained in murine models suggest that the progesterone-induced protein is not only immunomodulatory *in vitro,* but also antiabortive *in vivo,* thus being biologically significant.

Earlier studies by Gendron and Baines[41] suggest an NK involvement in murine resorptions. Adoptive transfer of high NK activity spleen cells from poly (I) poly (C 12U) treated mice is abortogenic in pregnant BALB/c mice.[66]

In vivo administration of supernatants from progesterone-treated pregnancy spleen cells corrected the increased resorption rates, while supernatants of progesterone-treated nonpregnancy spleen cells were without effect (Figure 3).[129] Treatment of pregnant BALB/c mice with 2 mg/kg of RU 486 resulted in 100% abortion. The supernatant of progesterone-treated pregnancy spleen cells counteracted the abortive effect of the antiprogesterone, while control supernatants did not (Figure 4).[130] The supernatant of progesterone-treated pregnancy spleen cells also corrected the spontaneously high resorption rates in CBA/J × DBA/2 matings.[127]

Recently Toder et al.[132] have shown that the increased resorption in the CBA/J × DBA/2 combination was reduced by complete Freund adjuvant (CFA) treatment of the pregnant females. In our hands, progesterone-treated spleen cells from DBA-pregnant CBA females did not produce any immunologic blocking factor. This is in line with the hypothesis that an appropriate antigenic stimulation is required for lymphocyte progesterone receptor induction.

These data allow the following conclusions: following stimulation by the fetus, CD8$^+$ lymphocytes from pregnant women develop progesterone receptors (PR). Progesterone stimulates PR-positive lymphocytes to release an immunomodulatory protein which (1) blocks NK-mediated lysis; (2) induces cells with suppressor phenotype and function; and (3) prevents both spontaneous and induced fetal resorptions in mice.

PR-positive lymphocytes disappear from blood during human labor and this correlates with the ability of term placental cultures to block the induction of PR-positive lymphocytes by PHA.

In this chapter, an attempt to summarize the data available on the putative role of immuno-endocrinological interactions in the maintenance and cessation of pregnancy was made. Other chapters of this book show that the mechanism contributing to the success of gestation is extremely complex, involving gene regulation of antigen expression and presentation, the complicated network of cytokine action, etc. Despite the convincing evidence for

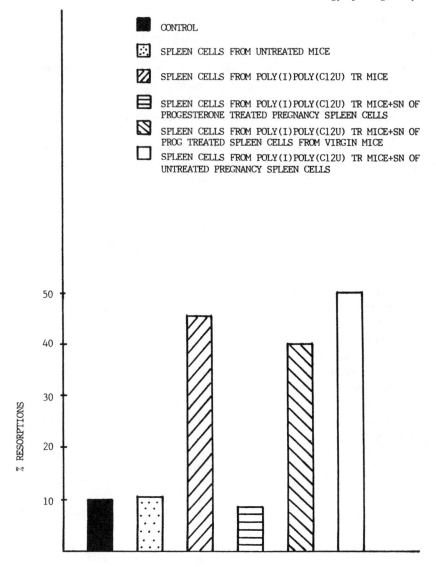

Figure 3. The effect of supernatants from progesterone-treated pregnancy spleen cells on NK-mediated resorption.

each of these pathways, one has to be aware that none of them is exclusive. Future prospects for reproductive immunology would be a synthesis of the data accumulated so far, and a presentation of a clear picture of the sequence of events resulting in successful gestation.

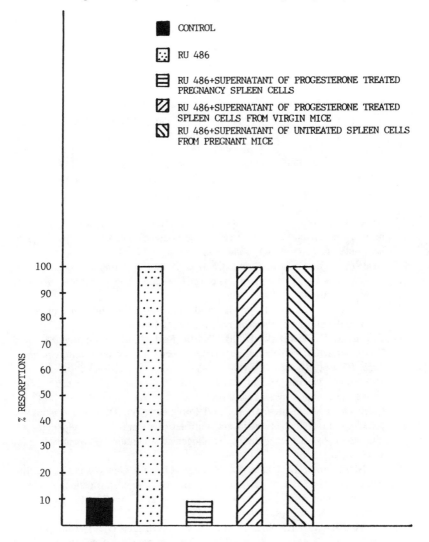

Figure 4. The effect of supernatants from progesterone-treated pregnancy spleen cells on progesterone receptor block-induced abortion.

REFERENCES

1. **Adcock, E. W., Teasdale, F., August, C. S., Cox, S., Mescia, G., Battaglia, F. O., and Naughton, M. C.,** Human chorionic gonadotropin: its possible role in maternal lymphocyte suppression, *Science,* 108, 845, 1973.
2. **Andersen, R. H. and Monroe, C. W.,** Experimental study of the behavior of adult human skin homografts during pregnancy, *Am. J. Obstet. Gynecol.,* 84, 1096, 1962.

3. **Barak, V., Biran, S., Halimi, M., and Treves, A.,** The effect of estradiol on human myelomonocytic cells. II. Mechanism of enhancing activity on colony formation, *J. Reprod. Immunol.,* 9, 355, 1986.

4. **Batchelor, J. R.,** Hormonal control of antibody formation, in *Regulation of the Antibody Response,* Cinader, B., Ed., Charles C Thomas, Springfield, IL, 1968, 276.

5. **Baulieu, E. E.,** RU 486: an antiprogestin steroid with contragestive activity in women, in *The Antiprogestin Steroid RU 486 and Human Fertility Control,* Baulieu, E. E. and Segal, S. J., Eds., Plenum Press, New York, 1985, 1–25.

6. **Beier, H. M.,** Hormonal stimulation of protease inhibitor activity in endometrial secretion during early pregnancy, *Acta Endocrinol.,* 63, 141, 1970.

7. **Billington, W. D. and Bell, S. C.,** Immunobiology of mouse trophoblast, in *Biology of Trophoblast,* Loke, Y. W. and Whyte, A., Eds., Elsevier, Amsterdam, 1983, 571.

8. **Brierley, J. and Clark, D. A.,** Identification of trophoblast independent, hormone dependent suppressor cell in the uterus of pregnant and pseudopregnant mice, *Fed. Proc.,* 44, 1884, 1985.

9. **Brierley, J. and Clark, D. A.,** Characterization of hormone-dependent suppressor cells in the uterus of mated and pseudopregnant mice, *J. Reprod. Immunol.,* 10, 201, 1987.

10. **Butterworth, M., McClellan, B., and Allansmith, M.,** Influence of sex on immunoglobulin in levels, *Nature,* 214, 1224, 1967.

11. **Buyon, J. P., Korchak, H. M., Rutherford, L. E., Ganguly, M., and Weissmann, G.,** Female hormones reduce neutrophil responsiveness *in vitro,* *Arch. Rheum.,* 27, 623, 1984.

12. **Bygdeman, M. and Swahn, M. L.,** Progesterone receptor blockage. Effect on uterine contractility and early pregnancy, *Contraception,* 32, 45, 1985.

13. **Caldwell, J. L., Stites, D. P., and Fudenberg, H. H.,** Human chorionic gonadotropin effects of crude and purified preparations on lymphocyte responses to phytohaemagglutinin and allogeneic stimulation, *J. Immunol.,* 115, 1249, 1975.

14. **Carlstedt-Duke, J., Okret, S., Wrange, O., and Gustafsson, J. A.,** Immunological analysis of the glucocorticoid receptor: identification of a third domain separated from the steroid-binding and DNA binding domains, *Proc. Natl. Acad. Sci. U.S.A.,* 79, 4260, 1982.

15. **Carlstedt-Duke, J., Stromstedt, P. E., Wrange, O., Bergmann, T., Gustafsson, J. A., and Jornvall, H.,** Domain structure of the glucocorticoid receptor protein, *Proc. Natl. Acad. Sci. U.S.A.,* 84, 4437, 1987.

16. **Chaouat, G., Chaffaoux, S., Duchet-Suchaux, M., and Voisin, G.,** Immunoactive products of mouse placenta. I. Immunosuppressive effects of crude and water soluble extracts, *J. Reprod. Immunol.,* 2, 127, 1980.

17. **Chaouat, G. and Kolb, J. P.,** Immunoreactive products of murine placenta. II. Afferent suppression of maternal cell-mediated immunity by supernatants from short term cultures of murine trophoblast enriched cell suspensions, *Ann. Immunol. (Inst. Pasteur),* 135C, 205, 1984.

18. **Chaouat, G. and Chaffraux, S.,** Placental products induce suppressor cells of graft-versus-host reaction, *Am. J. Reprod. Immunol. Microbiol.,* 6, 107, 1984.

19. **Chaouat, G.,** Placental immunoregulatory factors, *J. Reprod. Immunol.,* 10, 179, 1987.

20. **Clark, D. A., McDermott, M. R., and Szewczuk, M. R.,** Impairment of host-versus-graft reaction in pregnant mice. II. Selective suppression of cytotoxic T cell generation correlates with soluble suppressor activity and with successful allogeneic pregnancy, *Cell. Immunol.,* 52, 106, 1980.

21. **Clark, D. A., Slapsys, R. M., Croy, B. A., Koeck, J., and Rossant, J.,** Local active suppression by suppressor cells in the decidua: a review, *Am. J. Reprod. Immunol.,* 5, 78, 1984.

22. **Clark, D. A., Slapsys, R. M., Croy, B. A., and Rossant, J.,** Immunoregulation of host-versus-graft responses in the uterus, *Immunol. Today,* 5, 111, 1984.

23. **Clark, D. A., Chaput, A., Walker, C., and Rosenthal, K. L.,** Active suppression of host-versus-graft reaction in pregnant mice. IV. Soluble suppressor activity obtained from decidua of allopregnant mice blocks response to IL-2, *J. Immunol.,* 134, 1659, 1985.

24. **Clemens, L. E., Contopoulos, A. N., Ortiz, S., Stites, D. P., and Siiteri, P. K.,** Inhibition by progesterone (P) of leucocyte migration *in vivo* and *in vitro,* in Abstracts of the 59th Annual Meeting of the Endocrine Society, Abstract No. 237, 175, 1977.

25. **Cohen, J. H. M., Danel, L., Cordier, G., Saez, S., and Revillard, J. P.,** Sex steroid receptors in peripheral T cells: absence of androgen receptors and restriction of estrogen receptors to OKT8 positive cells, *J. Immunol.,* 131, 2767, 1983.

26. **Contractor, S. F. and Davies, H.,** Effect of human chorionic somatomammotropin and human chorionic gonadotropin on phytohaemagglutinin induced lymphocyte transformation, *Nature,* 243, 284, 1973.

27. **Couzinet, B., LeStrat, N., Ulmann, A., Baulieu, E. E., and Schaison, G.,** Termination of early pregnancy by the progesterone antagonist Ru 486 (mefipristone), *N. Engl. J. Med.,* 315, 1565, 1986.

28. **Csapo, A. I.,** The see-saw theory of parturition, in *The Fetus and Birth,* Ciba Foundation Symp. 47 (New Series), Elsevier, Excerpta Medica, North Holland, Amsterdam, 1977, 159.

29. **Csapo, I. A. and Wiest, W. G.,** An examination of the quantitative relationship between progesterone and the maintenance of pregnancy, *Endocrinology,* 85, 735, 1969.

30. **Defletsen, M. A., Smith, B. C., and Dickerman, H. W.,** A high-affinity low-capacity receptor for estradiol in normal and anaemic mouse spleen cytosols, *Biochem. Biophys. Res. Commun.,* 76, 1151, 1977.

31. **Dubois, E. L. and Tuffanelli, D. L.,** Clinical manifestations of systemic lupus erythematosus. Computer analysis of 520 cases, *JAMA,* 190, 104, 1964.

32. **Eidinger, G. and Garrett, T. J.,** Studies of the regulatory effects of sex hormones on antibody formation and stem cell differentiation, *J. Exp. Med.,* 136, 1098, 1972.

33. **Elger, W., Beier, S., Chwalisz, K., Fahnrich, M., Hasan, S. H., Henderson, D., Neef, G., and Rohde, R.,** Studies on the mechanism of action of progesterone antagonists, *J. Steroid Biochem.,* 12, 835, 1986.

34. **Elger, W., Fahnrich, M., Beier, S., Quing, S. S., and Chwalisz, K.,** Endometrial and myometrial effects of progesterone antagonists in pregnant guinea pigs, *Am. J. Obstet. Gynecol.,* 157, 1065, 1987.

35. **Ellis, S. A., Sargent, I. L., Redman, C. W. G., and McMichael, A. J.,** Evidence for a novel HLA antigen found on human extravillous trophoblast and choriocarcinoma cell line, *Immunology,* 59, 595, 1986.

36. **Evans, R. M.,** The steroid and thyroid receptor superfamily, *Science,* 240, 889, 1988.

37. **Evans, R. M. and Hollenberg, S. M.,** Zinc fingers: guilt by association, *Cell,* 52, 1, 1988.

38. **Ferre, F., Uzan, M., Jolivet, A., Jassens, Y., Tanguy, G., Sureau, C., and Cedard, L.,** Influence of the oral administration of micronized progesterone on plasma and tissue steroid levels in human pregnancy, *Acta Physiol. Hung.,* 65, 44, 1985.

39. **Furokawa, K., Itoh, K., Okamura, K., Kumagai, K., and Suzuki, M.,** Changes in the NK cell activity during the estrus cycle and pregnancy in mice, *J. Reprod. Immunol.,* 6, 353, 1984.

40. **Gasc, J.-M., Renoir, J.-M., Radanyi, C., Joab, I., Tuohimaa, P., and Baulieu, E. E.,** Progesterone receptor in the chick oviduct: an immunohistochemical study with antibodies to distinct receptor components, *J. Cell. Biol.,* 99, 1193, 1984.

41. **Gendron, R. and Baines, M.,** Infiltrating decidual natural killer cells are associated with spontaneous abortion in mice, *Cell. Immunol.,* 113, 262, 1988.

42. **George, W. D., Partridge, W., and Burn, J. I.,** Macrophage activity and hormonal responsiveness in mammary cancer, *Br. J. Surg.,* 60, 317, 1973.

43. **Ghani, A., Kunz, W. H., and Gill, T. J.,** Pregnancy induced monoclonal antibody to a unique fetal antigne, *Transplantation,* 37, 503, 1984.

44. **Gillis, S., Crabtree, G., and Smithy, K.,** Glucocorticoid induced inhibition of T cell growth factor production. I. The effect on mitogen induced lymphocyte proliferation, *J. Immunol.,* 123, 1624, 1979.

45. **Gleicher, N., Cohen, C. J., and Deppe, G.,** Familial malignant melanoma of the female genitalia, *Obstet. Gynecol. Surv.,* 34, 1, 1979.

46. **Gorski, J., Toft, D., Shyamala, G., Smith, D., and Notides, A.,** Hormone receptors: studies on the interaction of estrogen with the uterus, *Recent Prog. Horm. Res.,* 24, 45, 1968.

47. **Gorski, J., Welshons, W. V., Sakai, D. et al.,** Evolution of a model of estrogen action, *Recent Prog. Horm. Res.,* 42, 297, 1986.

48. **Green, S., Walter, P., Kumar, V. et al.,** Human oestrogen receptor DNA: sequence, expression and homology to v-erb A, *Nature,* 320, 134, 1986.

49. **Greene, G. L., Sobel, N. B., King, W. J. et al.,** Immunochemical studies of estrogen receptors, *J. Steroid Biochem.,* 20, 51, 1984.

50. **Grossman, C. J., Sholiton, L. J., and Nathan, P.,** Rat thymic estrogen receptor. I. Preparation, location and physiological properties, *J. Steroid Biochem.,* 11, 1233, 1979.

51. **Gulshan, S., McCruden, A. B., and Stimson, W. H.,** Oestrogen receptors in macrophages, *Scand. J. Immunol.,* 31, 691, 1990.

52. **Gustaffsson, D. C. and Kottmeyer, H. L.,** Carcinoma of the cervix, associated with pregnancy, *Acta Obstet. Gynecol. Scand.,* 41, 1, 1962.

53. **Halme, J. and Woessner, J. F.**, Effect of progesterone on collagen breakdown and tissue collagenolytic activity in the involuting rat uterus, *J. Endocrinol.*, 66, 357, 1975.

54. **Hansen, P. J., Bazer, F. W., and Segerson, E. C.**, Skin graft survival in the uterine lumen of ewes treated with progesterone, *Am. J. Reprod. Immunol. Microbiol.*, 12, 48, 1986.

55. **Henderson, D.**, Antiprogestational and antiglucocorticoid activities of some novel 11 beta-aryl substituted steroids, in *Pharmacology and Clinical Uses of Inhibitors of Hormone Secretion and Action*, Furr, B. J. A. and Wakeling, A. E., Eds., Bailliere Tindall, London, 1987, 184–211.

56. **Herrmann, W., Wyss, R., Riondel, A., Philibert, D., Teutsch, G., Sakiz, E., and Baulieu, E. E.**, Effet d un steroide anti-progesterone chez la femme: interruption du cycle menstruel et de la grossesse au debut, *Compt. Rend. Acad. Sci. (Paris)*, 294, 933, 1982.

57. **Hollenberg, S. M., Giguere, V., Segui, P., and Evans, R. M.**, Colocalization of DNA binding and transcriptional activation functions in the human glucocorticoid receptor, *Cell*, 49, 39, 1987.

58. **Horne, C. H. W., Towler, C. M., Pugh-Humphreys, R. G. P., Thompson, A. W., and Bohn, H.**, Pregnancy-specific beta 1 glycoprotein—a product of the syncytiotrophoblast, *Experientia*, 32, 1197, 1976.

59. **Inman, R. D.**, Immunologic sex differences and the female predominance in systemic lupus erythematosus, *Arthr. Rheum.*, 21, 849, 1978.

60. **Janerich, D. T.**, The influence of pregnancy on breast cancer risk. It is endocrinological, or immunological?, *Med. Hypotheses*, 6, 1149, 1980.

61. **Jeffrey, J. J. and Koob, T. J.**, Hormonal regulation of colagen catabolism by the uterus, *Endocrinol. Excerpta Medica Int. Congr. Ser.*, 273, 1115, 1973.

62. **Jensen, E. V. and DeSombre, E. R.**, Mechanism of action of the female sex steroids, *Annu. Rev. Biochem.*, 41, 203, 1972.

63. **Jensen, E. V., Suzuki, T., Kawashima, T., Stumpf, W. E., Jungblut, P. W., and DeSombre, E. R.**, A two step mechanism for the interaction of estradiol with rat uterus, *Proc. Natl. Acad. Sci. U.S.A.*, 59, 632, 1968.

64. **Kaye, M. D. and Jones, W. R.**, Effect of human chorionic gonadotropin on *in vitro* lymphocyte transformation, *Am. J. Obstet. Gynecol.*, 109, 1029, 1971.

65. **King, W. J. and Greene, G. L.**, Monoclonal antibodies localize estrogen receptor in the nuclei of target cells, *Nature*, 307, 745, 1984.

66. **Kinsky, R., Delage, G., Rosin, N., Thang, M. N., Hoffmann, M., and Chaouat, G.**, A murine model for NK-mediated resorption, *Am. J. Reprod. Immunol.*, 23, 73, 1990.

67. **Kovacs, L., Sas, M., Resch, B., Ugocsai, G., Swahn, M. L., Bygdemann, M., and Rowe, P. J.**, Termination of very early pregnancy by RU 486—an antiprogestational compound, *Contraception*, 29, 399, 1984.

68. **Kovacs, S., Main, E. K., Librach, C., Stubblebine, M., Fischer, S. J., and DeMars, R.**, A class I antigen expressed on human trophoblasts, *Science*, 248, 220, 1990.

69. **Kumar, V., Green, S., Staub, A., and Chambon, P.**, Localization of the estradiol binding and putative DNA binding domains in the human oestrogen receptor, *EMBO J.*, 5, 2231, 1986.

70. **Langhoff, E. and Ladefoged, J.,** The immunosuppressive potency of various steroids on peripheral blood lymphocytes, T cells, NK and K cells, *Int. J. Immunopharmacol.*, 7, 483, 1985.

71. **Leikin, S.,** Depressed maternal lymphocyte responses to phytohaemagglutinin in pregnancy, *Lancet*, 2, 43, 1972.

72. **Lichtenstein, M. R.,** Tuberculin reaction in tuberculosis during pregnancy, *Am. Rev. Tuberc. Pulm. Dis.*, 48, 89, 1942.

73. **Lye, S. J. and Porter, D. G.,** Demonstration that progesterone blocks uterine activity in the ewe *in vivo* by a direct action on the myometrium, *J. Reprod. Fertil.*, 52, 87, 1978.

74. **Maes, R. F. and Claverie, N.,** The effect of preparations of human chorionic gonadotropin on lymphocyte stimulation and immune response, *Immunology*, 33, 351, 1977.

75. **Maoz, H., Kaiser, N., Halimi, M., Barak, V., Haimovitz, A., Weinstein, D., Simon, A., Yagel, S., Biran, S., and Trevers, A. J.,** The effect of estradiol on human myelomonocytic cells. I. Enhancement of colony formation, *J. Reprod. Immunol.*, 7, 325, 1985.

76. **Mathur, S., Mathur, R. S., Goust, J. M., Williamson, H. O., and Fudenberg, H. H.,** Cyclic variations in white cell subpopulations in the human menstrual cycle: correlation with progesterone and estradiol, *Clin. Immunol. Immunopathol.*, 13, 246, 1978.

77. **Maxwell, B. L., McDonnel, D. P., Conneely, O. M. et al.,** Structural organization and regulation of the chicken estrogen receptor, *Mol. Endocrinol.*, 1, 25, 1987.

78. **McClellan, M. C., West, N. B., Tacha, D. E., Greene, G. L., and Brenner, R. M.,** Immunocytochemical localization of estrogen receptors in the macaque reproductive tract with monoclonal antiestrophilins, *Endocrinology*, 114, 1001, 1984.

79. **McIntyre, J. A. and Faulk, W. P.,** Allotypic trophoblast lymphocyte cross reactive (TLX) cell surface antigens, *Hum. Immunol.*, 4, 27, 1982.

80. **Milgrom, E., Thi, L., Atger, M. et al.,** Mechanisms regulating the concentration and conformation of progesterone receptors in the uterus, *J. Biol. Chem.*, 248, 6366, 1973.

81. **Mori, T., Kobayashi, H., Nashimoto, H., Suzuki, A., and Nishimura, T.,** Inhibitory effect of progesterone and 20-alpha hydroxypregn-4-n-3-one on the phytohaemagglutinin-induced transformation of human lymphocytes, *Am. J. Obstet. Gynecol.*, 127, 151, 1977.

82. **Moriyama, I. and Sugawa, T.,** Progesterone facilitates implantation of xenogeneic cultured cells in hamster uterus, *Nature New Biol.*, 236, 150, 1972.

83. **Morse, J. H., Stearns, G., Arden, J., Agosto, M. G., and Canfield, R. E.,** The effects of crude and purified human choriogonadotropin on *in vitro* stimulated human lymphocyte cultures, *Cell. Immunol.*, 25, 178, 1976.

84. **Mueller, G. C., Vonderhaar, B., Kim, U. H., and LeMahieu, M.,** Estrogen action: an inroad to cell biology, *Recent Prog. Horm. Res.*, 28, 1, 1972.

85. **Muldoon, T. G.,** Regulation of steroid hormone receptor activity, *Endocr. Rev.*, 1, 339, 1980.

86. **Myers, M. J. and Petersen, B. H.,** Estradiol induced alterations of the immune system. I. Enhancement of IgM production, *Int. J. Immunopharmacol.*, 7, 207, 1985.

87. **Neef, G., Beier, S., Elger, W., Henderson, D., and Wiechert, R.,** New steroids with antiprogestational and antiglucocorticoid activities, *Steroids,* 44, 349, 1984.

88. **Neifeld, J. P., Lippman, L. E., and Toromey, D. C.,** Steroid hormone receptors in normal human lymphocytes. Induction of glucocorticoid receptor activity by PHA stimulation, *J. Biol. Chem.,* 252, 2972, 1977.

89. **Neifeld, J. P. and Toromey, D. C.,** Effects of steroid hormones on phytohaemagglutinin stimulated human peripheral blood lymphocytes, *Transplantation,* 27, 309, 1979.

90. **Padykula, H. A. and Tansey, T. R.,** The occurrence of uterine stromal and intraepithelial monocytes and heterophils during normal late pregnancy in the rat, *Anat. Rec.,* 193, 329, 1979.

91. **Pavia, C., Siiteri, P. K., Perlman, J. D., and Stites, D. P.,** Suppression of murine allogeneic cell interactions by sex hormones, *J. Reprod. Immunol.,* 1, 33, 1979.

92. **Pavonen, T., Andersson, L. C., and Adlercreutz, H.,** Sex hormone regulation of *in vitro* immune response. Estradiol enhances human B cell maturation via inhibition of suppressor T cells in pokeweed mitogen-stimulated cultures, *J. Exp. Med.,* 154, 1935, 1981.

93. **Pearse, W. H. and Kaiman, H.,** Human chorionic gonadotropin and skin allograft survival, *Am. J. Obstet. Gynecol.,* 98, 573, 1967.

94. **Pence, H., Petty, E. M., and Rocklin, R. E.,** Suppression of maternal responsiveness to paternal antigens by maternal plasma, *J. Immunol.,* 114, 525, 1985.

95. **Perrot-Applanat, M., Logeat, F., Groyer-Picard, M. T., and Milgrom, E.,** Immunocytochemical study of mammalian progesterone receptor using monoclonal antibodies, *Endocrinology,* 116, 1473, 1985.

96. **Pertschuk, L. P., Eisenberg, K. B., Carter, A. C., and Feldman, J. G.,** Immunohistologic localization of estrogen receptors in breast cancer with monoclonal antibodies, *Cancer,* 55, 1513, 1985.

97. **Pickard, R. E.,** Varicella pneumonia in pregnancy, *Am. J. Obstet. Gynecol.,* 100, 504, 1968.

98. **Press, M. F., Nousek-Goebl, N., King, W. J., Herbst, A. L., and Greene, G. L.,** Immunohistochemical assessment of estrogen receptor distribution in the human endometrium throughout the menstrual cycle, *Lab. Invest.,* 51, 495, 1984.

99. **Puri, C. P., Kholkute, S. D., Pongubala, J. M. R., Patil, R. K., Elger, W. A. G., and Jayaraman, S.,** Effect of antiprogestin ZK 98.734 on the ovarian cycle, early pregnancy, and on its binding to progesterone receptors in the myometrium of marmoset Callithrix jacchus, *Biol. Reprod.,* 38, 528, 1988.

100. **Purtilo, D. T., Hallgren, H. M., and Yunis, E. J.,** Depressed maternal lymphocyte response to PHA in human pregnancy, *Lancet,* 2, 43, 1978.

101. **Ranelletti, F. O., Piantelli, M., Carbone, A., Rinelli, A., Scambia, G., Panici, P. B., and Mancuso, S.,** Type II estrogen binding sites and 17 beta hydroxysteroid dehydrogenase activity in human peripheral blood mononuclear cells, *J. Clin. Endocrinol. Metab.,* 67, 888, 1988.

102. **Redman, C. W. G., McMichael, A. J., Stirrat, G. M. et al.,** Class I major histocompatibility complex antigens on human extravillous trophoblast, *Immunology,* 52, 457, 1984.

103. **Rocklin, R. E., Zuckerman, J. R., Alpert, E. et al.**, Effect of multiparity on human maternal hypersensitivity to fetal antigen, *Nature*, 241, 130, 1973.

104. **Rowley, M. J. and Mackay, R. I.**, Measurement of antibody producing capacity in man. I. The normal response to flagellin from Salmonella adelaide, *Clin. Exp. Immunol.*, 5, 407, 1969.

105. **Rusconi, S. and Yamamoto, K. R.**, Functional dissection of the hormone and DNA binding activities of the glucocorticoid receptor, *EMBO J.*, 6, 1309, 1987.

106. **Santoli, D., Trinchieri, G., Zmijewsky, C. M., and Koprowsky, H.**, HLA-Related control of spontaneous and antibody-dependent cell-mediated cytotoxic activity in humans, *J. Immunol.*, 117, 765, 1976.

107. **Schiff, R. I., Mercier, D., and Bukley, R. H.**, Inability of gestational hormones to account for the inhibitory effects of pregnancy plasmas on lymphocyte responses *in vitro*, *Cell. Immunol.*, 20, 69, 1975.

108. **Schleimer, R., Jaques, A., Shiu, H., Lichtenstein, L., and Plaut, M.**, Inhibition of T-cell mediated cytotoxicity by anti-inflammatory steroids, *J. Immunol.*, 132, 266, 1984.

109. **Screpanti, I., Gulino, A., and Pasqualini, J. R.**, The fetal thymus of guinea pig as an estrogen target organ, *Endocrinology*, 111, 1552, 1982.

110. **Shiu, H. M., Schottenfeld, D., McLean, B., and Fortner, J. G.**, Adverse effect of pregnancy on melanoma, *Cancer*, 37, 181, 1976.

111. **Shoupe, D., Mishell, D. R., Jr., Brenner, P. F., and Spitz, I. M.**, Pregnancy termination with high and medium dosage regimen of RU 486, *Contraception*, 33, 455, 1986.

112. **Siiteri, P. K., Febres, F., Clemens, L. E., Chang, R. J., Gondos, B., and Stites, D. P.**, Progesterone and the maintenance of pregnancy: is progesterone nature's immunosuppressant?, *Ann. N.Y. Acad. Sci.*, 286, 384, 1977.

113. **Staples, L. D. and Heap, R. B.**, Studies on steroids and proteins in relation to the immunology of pregnancy in the sheep, in *Immunological Aspects of Reproduction in Mammals*, Chrighton, D. B., Ed., Butterworths, London, 1984, 195.

114. **Stern, K. and Davidson, I.**, Effect of estrogen and cortisol on immune haemoantibodies in mice of inbred strains, *J. Immunol.*, 74, 479, 1955.

115. **Stimson, W. H.**, Oestrogen and human T lymphocytes: presence of specific receptors in the T suppressor cytotoxic subset, *Scand. J. Immunol.*, 28, 345, 1988.

116. **Stites, D. P., Bugbee, S., and Siiteri, P. K.**, Differential actions of progesterone and cortisol on lymphocyte and monocyte interaction during lymphocyte activation. Relevance to immunosuppression in pregnancy, *J. Reprod. Immunol.*, 5, 215, 1983.

117. **Stites, D. P. and Siiteri, P. K.**, Steroids as immunosuppressants in pregnancy, *Immunol. Rev.*, 75, 117, 1983.

118. **Sulke, A. N., Jones, D. B., and Wood, P. J.**, Hormonal modulation of natural killer activity *in vitro*, *J. Reprod. Immunol.*, 7, 105, 1985.

119. **Svec, F.**, Glucocorticoid receptor regulation, *Life Sci.*, 36, 2359, 1985.

120. **Szekeres-Bartho, J., Hadnagy, J., and Pacsa, A. S.**, The suppressive effect of progesterone on lymphocyte cytotoxicity: unique progesterone sensitivity of pregnancy lymphocytes, *J. Reprod. Immunol.*, 7, 121, 1985.

121. **Szekeres-Bartho, J., Kilar, F., Falkay, G., Csernus, V., Torok, A., and Pacsa, A. S.**, Progesterone-treated lymphocytes of healthy pregnant women release a factor inhibiting cytotoxicity and prostaglandin synthesis, *Am. J. Reprod. Immunol. Microbiol.*, 5, 15, 1985.

122. **Szekeres-Bartho, J., Reznikoff-Etievant, M. F., Varga, P., Pichon, M. F., Varga, T., and Chaouat, G.**, Lymphocytic progesterone receptors in human pregnancy, *J. Reprod. Immunol.*, 16, 239, 1989.

123. **Szekeres-Bartho, J., Autran, B., Debre, P., Andreu, G., Denver, L., and Chaouat, G.**, Immunoregulatory effects of a suppressor factor from healthy pregnant women's lymphocytes after progesterone induction, *Cell. Immunol.*, 122, 281, 1989.

124. **Szekeres-Bartho, J., Varga, P., and Pejtsik, B.**, ELISA test for detecting an immunological blocking factor in human pregnancy serum, *J. Reprod. Immunol.*, 16, 19, 1989.

125. **Szekeres-Bartho, J., Weill, B. J., Mike, G., Houssin, D., and Chaouat, G.**, Progesterone receptors in lymphocytes of liver-transplanted and transfused patients, *Immunol. Lett.*, 22, 259, 1989.

126. **Szekeres-Bartho, J., Szabo, J., and Kovacs, L.**, Alteration of lymphocyte reactivity in women treated with the progesterone receptor blocker ZK 98734, *Am. J. Reprod. Immunol.*, 21, 46, 1989.

127. **Szekeres-Bartho, J. and Chaouat, G.**, A lymphocyte derived progesterone induced blocking factor corrects resorption in a murine abortion system, *Am. J. Reprod. Immunol.*, 23, 26, 1990.

128. **Szekeres-Bartho, J., Szekeres, Gy., Debre, P., Autran, B., and Chaouat, G.**, Reactivity of lymphocytes to a progesterone receptor-specific monoclonal antibody, *Cell. Immunol.*, 125, 273, 1990.

129. **Szekeres-Bartho, J., Kinsky, R., and Chaouat, G.**, The effect of a progesterone-induced immunologic blocking factor on NK mediated resorption, *Am. J. Reprod. Immunol.*, 24, 105, 1990.

130. **Szekeres-Bartho, J., Kinsky, R., and Chaouat, G.**, A progesterone-induced immunologic blocking factor corrects high resorption rate in mice treated with antiprogesterone, *Am. J. Obstet. Gynecol.*, 163, 1320, 1990.

131. **Terres, G., Morrison, S. L., and Habricht, G. S.**, A quantitative difference in the immune response between male and female mice, *Proc. Soc. Exp. Biol. Med.*, 127, 664, 1968.

132. **Toder, V., Strassburger, D., Irlin, I., Carp, H., Pecht, M., and Trainin, N.**, Nonspecific immunopotentiators and pregnancy loss: complete Freund adjuvant reverses high fetal resorption rate in CBA/J × DBA/2 mouse combination, *Am. J. Reprod. Immunol.*, 24, 63, 1990.

133. **Uksila, J.**, Human NK cell activity is not inhibited by pregnancy and cord serum factors and female steroid hormones *in vitro*, *J. Reprod. Immunol.*, 7, 111, 1985.

134. **Van Vlasselaer, P. and Vandeputte, M.**, Effect of sex steroids and trophoblast culture supernatants on the cytotoxic activity in mice, in *Pregnancy Proteins in Animals*, Han, J., Ed., Walter de Gruyter, Berlin, 1986, 482.

135. **Vaughan, J. E. and Ramirez, H.**, Coccidioidmycosis as a complication of pregnancy, *Calif. Med.*, 74, 121, 1951.

136. **Von Haam, E. and Rosenfeld, I.**, The effect of estrone on antibody production, *J. Immunol.*, 43, 109, 1942.

137. **Walters, M. R. and Clark, J. H.,** Cytosol and nuclear compartmentalization of progesterone receptors of the rat uterus, *Endocrinology,* 103, 601, 1978.

138. **Westphal, H. M., Moldenhauer, G., and Beato, M.,** Monoclonal antibodies to the rat liver glucocorticoid receptor, *EMBO J.,* 1, 1467, 1982.

139. **Wrange, O. and Gustafsson, J. A.,** Separation of the hormone and DNA binding sites of the hepatic glucocorticoid receptor by means of proteolysis, *J. Biol. Chem.,* 253, 856, 1978.

140. **Wrange, O., Okret, S., Radojcac, M., Carlstedt-Duke, J., and Gustafsson, J. A.,** Characterization of the purified activated glucocorticoid receptor from rat liver cytosol, *J. Biol. Chem.,* 259, 4534, 1984.

141. **Wyle, F. A. and Kent, J. R.,** Immunosuppression by sex steroid hormones. I. The effect upon PHA and PPD stimulated lymphocytes, *Clin. Exp. Immunol.,* 27, 407, 1977.

142. **Youtanokorn, V. and Matangkasombut, P.,** Specific plasma factors blocking human maternal cell-mediated immune reaction to placental antigens, *Nature (New Biol.),* 242, 110, 1973.

143. **Wegmann, T. G.,** personal communication.

Chapter

12

Natural and Experimental Animal Models of Reproductive Failure

Malcolm G. Baines and Robert L. Gendron
Department of Microbiology and Immunology
McGill University
Montreal, Quebec, Canada

1. REPRODUCTIVE FAILURE

1.1. Introduction

While the immunological contradictions posed by mammalian reproduction have long puzzled and intrigued immunologists, a comprehensive understanding of the causes of spontaneous abortion have evaded the insights of those who study embryonic development.[64,65,70] Many excellent texts and reviews exist, but a considerable difficulty is encountered when one attempts to determine the impact of the different causes of fetal losses.[44,113] One significant reason for this dearth of information is simply the lack of model systems amenable to experimental manipulation which could reveal the evidence needed to solve these questions. Due to the lack of appropriate test

8868-6/93/$0.00 + $.50

systems, most of the clinical studies have been retrospective in nature and the data produced have often been contradicted by data obtained from prospective or experimental studies. Furthermore, several fundamental misconceptions may have misled the focus of reproductive research for many years.[20] This review will identify available models of spontaneous abortion and show where experimental data from model systems may provide new insights into the causes of pregnancy failure.

1.2. Embryo Resorption vs. Fetal Abortion

A definition of terms is essential before one starts an ordered discussion of the experimental models which may be appropriate for the study of mechanisms and causes of spontaneous abortion. Until the questions are clear, it is difficult to select appropriate models for analysis. In this review, it is assumed that there is no need for experimental models of preimplantation loss or early embryonic loss which involve either anatomic or endocrine anomalies of the maternal reproductive system. The primary focus of this review will be upon immunological defects (Table 1). It is clear that the pathophysiology of early embryo loss or resorption, occurring within 7 to 14 days following implantation, is fundamentally different from spontaneous fetal abortions, which occur later during the period of human fetal morphogenesis (>6 weeks).[70] The former appears to result from placental failure or a failure to suppress the maternal rejection response, while the latter may be largely due to defects in maternal physiology or fetal development. In the human, both of these types of abortion primarily occur within the first trimester of pregnancy, though in other species where offspring are born at a less mature stage of development, this event may occur at any time until the fetus is anatomically complete or delivered, whichever is the sooner (Table 2). A simple proportioning of the gestation period is therefore an inappropriate way to compare abortions in different species, since it is not the speed of embryonic development which is the determining parameter, but rather the speed of the normal maternal innate or adaptive immune response, which is relatively constant for all warm-blooded species. Studies of genetic effects controlled by genes like the *Ped* gene in mice indicate that the rate of preimplantation development is also an MHC-linked trait which may significantly affect the success of early preembryo growth.[147] Therefore, in this review, human early embryo loss will be defined as losses occurring after implantation but before 6 weeks from the last menstrual period and spontaneous fetal abortion will describe losses after 6 weeks (Table 2).[27,28,30,45]

1.3. Early Spontaneous Preembryonic Resorption

Peri-implantation preembryonic resorption usually occurs without the expulsion of any products of conception and, therefore, usually occurs unnoticed by the maternal host. It has been estimated that between 24 and 62%

TABLE 1.
Common Causes of Clinically Recognized
Spontaneous Abortion

Fetomaternal Pathology	Spontaneous (%)	Recurrent[a] (%)
Population abortion rate	12–17	<1
Fetal genetic defects	40–60	20–35
Fetal intrauterine infection	3–10	Rare
Maternal uterine defects	2–3	23–44
Maternal endocrine defects	3–15	5–35
Maternal immunological factors	0–35	10–45
Other medical causes[b]	1–2	?
Unknown causes	1–3	?
Parental genetic anomaly[c]	0.2–0.4	2–10

[a] Women who have experienced three or more consecutive spontaneous abortions. Age is known to increase the incidence of genetic and uterine defects and possibly also autoimmune-mediated losses.

[b] Other medical causes include hemorrhage, hypoxia, hypertension, diabetes, intrauterine growth retardation, placenta previa, or trauma.

[c] Based on an observed genetic anomaly rate in newborns of 0.6%, 1/3 of which (0.2%) show no phenotypic markers while 2/3 show morphogenetic changes. Gamete genetic anomaly may be higher as sperm genetic defects were found to be 8% in normal males.

Data compiled from standard texts and recent research publications. Balasch et al., 1989; Boyd, 1989; Brambati et al., 1986; Branch, 1987; Canadian Collaborative Study, 1989; Claytonsmith et al., 1990; Confino and Gleicher, 1990; Cubberly, 1987; Cunningham et al., 1989; Drugan et al., 1990; Dudley and Branch, 1989; Filkins and Russo, 1985; Gill, 1986, 1988; Gladen, 1990; Hafez, 1984; Hall, 1987; Johnson et al., 1990; Kochenour, 1987; Levgur et al., 1990; Liu et al., 1987; Mardh, 1989; Mowbray, 1987; Petitti, 1987; Redman and Sargent, 1986; Reed et al., 1989; Reznikoff-Eteviant, 1988; Salat-Baroux, 1988; Simpson, 1990; Stabile et al., 1987; Thaler and McIntyre, 1990; Varga et al., 1989; Warburton, 1986, 1987.

of all human conceptions fail during the period between 3 and 6 weeks from the last menstrual period (Table 2).[52,95,152] Outbred animal pregnancy models also show loss rates between 25 and 40%.[71,80] Where human and animal products of conception are available for study at this stage, there is evidence that, in most cases, embryonic development appears normal but placental development fails.[9,131,132] Thus, the studies of early occult resorption of placenta and embryo indicate that the failure of placental development may be a major factor in preembryonic losses.

Studies of a murine model of early embryonic loss have supported the contention that embryonic loss is related to the failure of placental development.[60,131] Histological examination of these conceptions in abortion-prone mice reveals that the embryo initially implants and appears to develop normally. In a minority of cases, the placenta develops and the embryo dies

TABLE 2.
Estimates of Pregnancy Outcome vs. Gestational Age[a]

Pregnancies Studied	Gestational Age in Weeks			Perinatal Death	Viable Neonate
	0–5	6–11	12–24		
All conceptions					
Embryo/fetal fate	Abort	Abort	Abort	SB/ND[b]	Living
Observed frequency	24–62%	10–25%	2–5	0.5–1%	25–35%
Estimated average	50%	13%	3%	1%	33%
Aborted pregnancies[d]					
Genetic defects	27%	54%	12–48%	4–6%	
Uterine defects	?	15%	25–30%	?	
Endocrine defects	?	23%	?	?	
I/U infection[c]	?	?	3–10%	?	
Immunological causes	?	?	10–22%	?	
Other medical causes	?	?	1–2%	?	
Unknown causes	?	?	1–3%	?	

[a] Gestational age from last normal menstrual period (PLNMP).
[b] SB/ND, stillbirth or neonatal death.
[c] I/U, intrauterine.
[d] 12–17% of pregnancies clinically verified at 6 weeks subsequently abort.

Data compiled from standard texts and recent research publications. Balasch et al., 1989; Boyd, 1989; Brambati et al., 1986; Branch, 1987; Canadian Collaborative Study, 1989; Claytonsmith et al., 1990; Confino and Gleicher, 1990; Cubberly, 1987; Cunningham et al., 1989; Drugan et al., 1990; Dudley and Branch, 1989; Filkins and Russo, 1985; Gill, 1986, 1988; Gladen, 1990; Hafez, 1984; Hall, 1987; Johnson et al., 1990; Kochenour, 1987; Levgur et al., 1990; Liu et al., 1987; Mardh, 1989; Mowbray, 1987; Petitti, 1987; Redman and Sargent, 1986; Reed et al., 1989; Reznikoff-Etievant, 1988; Salat-Baroux, 1988; Simpson, 1990; Stabile et al., 1987; Thaler and McIntyre, 1990; Varga et al., 1989; Warburton, 1986, 1987.

leaving an empty sac, but in most cases the fetus appears normal while the development of the placenta may be impaired. The first signs of impending problems appear to be a progressive infiltration of the basal decidua by large granular lymphocytes with a natural killer (NK) cell phenotype.[39,41,55,61] Normally these NK-like cells appear only transiently within 24 to 48 hours after implantation and disappear prior to the establishment of placental blood flow.[39,41,130] In implantations that subsequently resorb, the infiltration progressively approaches and invades the trophoblast-decidual interface and eventually the embryo itself.[60] Placental development is impaired and the vascular spaces become hemorrhagic and thrombosed. The terminal stages of infiltration are associated with the local production of tumor necrosis factor and embryonic death.[19,63] Whether the fundamental cause of fetal loss is due to the stimulation of the maternal rejection response or the absence of fetally derived regulatory signals which directly or indirectly suppress the maternal response, is still not clear at this time, though the latter scenario is favored.

1.4. Later Spontaneous Embryonic and Fetal Abortion

The distinction between early embryo resorption and fetal abortion of clinically recognized pregnancies is important, because the latter occurs after the development of a fully functional placenta. In this case the subsequent expulsion of the products of conception provides clear evidence that the pregnancy has terminated. Most later spontaneous fetal abortions occur before the 16th week of human gestation.[110,146] Though abortions occurring after the 6th week of pregnancy account for only 10 to 17% of all clinically documented pregnancies, the majority of these have been assumed to be due to fetal genetic or other abnormalities (Table 1).[53,146] Certainly, there is karyotypic and morphological evidence that a large proportion of aborted embryos are genetically or developmentally abnormal and their death may predate the expulsion of the placental tissues by some considerable time.[87] While 4 to 14% of elective pregnancy terminations show empty embryonic sacs, over 80% of spontaneous "empty sac" abortions occur between 6 and 12 weeks.[104] Thus, some later losses may be primarily due to intrauterine embryonic death followed some time later by the expulsion of the empty trophoblastic capsule implying that the trophoblast is the more important source of pregnancy-enhancing factors.

2. CAUSES AND MECHANISMS OF SPONTANEOUS ABORTION

2.1. Introduction

In attempting to list the major causes of spontaneous abortion, it was found that the majority of the data identified fetal abortions occurring after

6 weeks. While the frequency of spontaneous fetal abortion after 6 weeks may be less than one quarter of the rate of early preembryonic abortion or less than one sixth of all losses, many studies ignore the most significant fraction of these events (Table 2). The most commonly accepted causes and their approximate frequency are listed on Table 1. Since retrospective studies provided most of the data for these figures, the assumption that these are the only, or even the major, contributing factors is somewhat speculative. Furthermore, the tabular data is combined from several sources which do not agree on many points. The tables are presented in an attempt to identify important areas for further discussion and research on fetal losses.

2.2. Common Causes of Fetal Wastage in Human Pregnancies

The most controversial causes of abortions are those of a presumed genetic etiology. Studies have indicated that 50 to 60% of fetuses aborted between 4 and 14 weeks show chromosomal abnormalities.[53,65,66,101,146] However, there are several problems with the acquisition of this data which confuse its interpretation. The establishment of the embryonic karyotype requires the growth of viable embryo-derived cells, which may be difficult to obtain when one is dealing with aborted tissues. There may be inadvertent *in vitro* selection of cytogenetic data. Cells grown from previously anoxic and often necrotic fetal tissues could have suffered reoxygenation-associated chromosomal damage during culture. The respiratory burst which accompanies reoxygenation is known to favor the production of superoxide and oxyradicals which can directly cause DNA breakages.[133,143]

Furthermore, maternal age, genetic anomalies, or a history of repetitive abortion is associated with an increased rate of fetal genetic anomaly (Table 1). Studies of the incidence of chromosomal breakages in chorionic villus cells obtained from normal pregnancies and the termination of healthy pregnancies have indicated that 4 to 8% of these tissues also show karyotypic anomalies (Table 3).[15] The fact that the anomaly rate in newborns is only 0.6% indicates that genetically abnormal embryos are preferentially aborted. Though little data exist concerning resorptions before 5 weeks, it would appear from some studies that the genetic anomaly rate is not significantly higher than the 4 to 8% rate of "normal" pregnancies (Table 3). The assumption that the products of conception from repetitive aborters is genetically abnormal is called into question when many women benefit from immunotherapy (see below). True genetic anomalies would be expected to be unresponsive to treatment. Therefore, the contribution of genetic factors to later fetal wastage still requires more research before a firm conclusion can be drawn as to their role as a primary cause of spontaneous abortion.

If one were to focus upon abortions of clearly immune etiology, then these would include isoimmune, alloimmune, and autoimmune responses.[13,22,102] It has long been known that isoantibody responses to fetal erythrocyte antigens can cause fetal death due to the passage of hemolytic

TABLE 3.
Frequency of Embryonic Karyotypic Abnormalities in Pregnancies Studied

Source of Tissues	Gestational Age in Weeks			Perinatal Death	Viable Neonate
	0–5	6–11	12–24		
Viable pregnancies	5–9%	4–6%	2–4%	N/A	0.6%
Induced abortion	?	4–6%	N/A	N/A	N/A
Spontaneous abortion	27%	50–60%	12–48%	5%	N/A
Repeated abortion	?	?	3–8%	?	N/A

Note: Karyotype for normal pregnancies determined from fetal chorionic villus sampling, amniocentesis, or from neonatal or adult blood lymphocytes. Normal pregnancies verified by human chorionic gonadotropin (hCG) assay and sonography. N/A, not available or not applicable.

Data compiled from standard texts and recent research publications. Balasch et al., 1989; Boyd, 1989; Brambati et al., 1986; Branch, 1987; Canadian Collaborative Study, 1989; Claytonsmith et al., 1990; Confino and Gleicher, 1990; Cubberly, 1987; Cunningham et al., 1989; Drugan et al., 1990; Dudley and Branch, 1989; Filkins and Russo, 1985; Gill, 1986, 1988; Gladen, 1990; Hafez, 1984; Hall, 1987; Johnson et al., 1990; Kochenour, 1987; Levgur et al., 1990; Liu et al., 1987; Mardh, 1989; Mowbray, 1987; Petitti, 1987; Redman and Sargent, 1986; Reed et al., 1989; Reznikoff-Eteviant, 1988; Salat-Baroux, 1988; Simpson, 1990; Stabile et al., 1987; Thaler and McIntyre, 1990; Varga et al., 1989; Warburton, 1986, 1987.

antibodies across the placenta. However, this cause of fetal death has been greatly reduced by the use of passive immunization of high-risk gravid women with anti-Rho antibodies (Anti-D) to prevent isoimmunization. Moreover, no suitable natural animal models for this form of fetal demise are known to exist. Furthermore, there is no convincing evidence that conventional alloimmune responses jeopardize pregnancies and considerable experience which shows that alloimmune responses may enhance fetal survival (see immunotherapy below). However, the role of autoimmunity in fetal abortion, in particular anti-phospholipid antibodies and lupus anticoagulant have been well documented.[13,120] Between 11 and 46% of women with systemic lupus erythematosus (SLE) aborted their conceptuses and there was a clear association between abortion and the titer of lupus anti-coagulant (LAC) or anti-cardiolipin (ACL) antibodies.[13,50,100] This rate of abortion clearly exceeded the expectations for women without ACL or LAC antibodies (Table 2). Though the major fraction of autoimmune disease-associated abortions occurred after 13 weeks, the primary target of the autoantibodies also appeared to be the placenta. Frequent findings in the placenta include intervillous thrombosis, infarction, and necrosis, but the pathophysiology is by no means clear. Abortion can be induced in experimental animals (BALB/c mice) inoculated with ACL or LAC antibodies, but the interpretation may be confused by the use of a human antibody in a xenogeneic murine host.[14] Nevertheless, this model provides a means for determining the specific cytopathology of autoimmune abortion.

2.3. Current Theories to Explain Fetal Survival

A discussion of current theories of fetal acceptance largely focus upon two mechanisms; resistance and suppression. The former refers to the resistance of the fetus and placental tissues to maternal specific or nonspecific effectors,[85,154] while the latter refers to the local active suppression of maternal responsiveness by either fetally or maternally derived suppressive cells or factors. Suppressor cells can regulate the activation of both major histocompatibility complex (MHC)-specific and nonspecific killer cells which cause abortion.[24,25,63] However, research on these subjects is still not conclusive and many questions remain to be answered. The majority of current research utilizes the *in vitro* culture of maternal and fetal tissues in order (1) to determine whether the fetal tissues stimulate maternal lymphocytes; (2) to understand how feto-placental tissues resist maternal effectors; and (3) to understand how fetal or maternal suppressor cells or factors regulate maternal responses to fetal antigens. A second approach is to examine these effectors *in situ* in normal conceptions in humans and experimental animals. Immunodeficient animals provide a useful environment in which to assess the contributions of the components of the immune system to fetal acceptance. Individual strains of animals exist which lack one or more components of the innate resistance (complement, NK cells, macrophages) or acquired immune system (T cells, B cells, or both). The ultimate approach is to study the success or failure of reproduction in human patients and representative experimental models. While fetal wastage in humans is a serious problem, the relatively low incidence of spontaneous abortion of documented pregnancies and the very early occurrence of occult fetal resorption make useful studies difficult from both a practical and ethical point of view. What is needed are several reproducible experimental models of fetal wastage in which the cell biology and immunology of spontaneous abortion can be investigated.

2.4. Alloimmunization Therapy of Spontaneous Abortion in Humans

As stated above, alloimmunization of the maternal host with paternal tissue antigens rarely caused the termination of an established pregnancy.[4,118] Conversely, there were indications that the maternal immune system normally recognized the presence of paternal MHC antigens during pregnancy and often induced alloimmunity to fetal antigens resulted in an increase in placental weight and fetal weight, indicating a beneficial effect of specific immunity.[10,77,89] This was supported by evidence from human pregnancies which appeared to indicate that the sharing of MHC antigens between mother and father was associated with suboptimal reproductive performance and even an increased incidence of pregnancy-induced hypertension (eclampsia) and spontaneous abortion.[7,8,73] However, the fact that both genetically isolated human populations with partial sharing of MHC alleles (Hutterites), and inbred animals with complete MHC identity appear to reproduce normally brings this assumption into question.[106] Further studies of this issue using congenic mouse strains could help to resolve this contradiction.

In any event, the assumption that alloimmunity to paternal MHC alleles was beneficial has led to the institution of deliberate alloimmunization of women who habitually abort, in order to enhance maternal immunity to fetal MHC antigens.[16,34,47,59,128a,137] Immunization of habitual aborters with either their husbands' lymphocytes or pooled allogeneic lymphocytes appears to improve fetal survival.[16,67,98] It is still not clear whether the active component of the maternal response to the therapy is a blocking antibody or an activated suppressor cell, though it is clear that the effect need not be systemic but can be confined to the uterus.[10,18,27] This is the first example, in the field of reproduction, of the successful transfer of an active immunotherapeutic protocol from an experimental animal model to human clinical practice. The further development of these forms of therapy would be greatly enhanced by the availability of appropriate experimental models of spontaneous abortion-prone pregnancies in which to test improved alloimmunization protocols.

2.5. Ideal Features of an Experimental Model

In general, a useful model of spontaneous abortion should be as identical as possible, in terms of causes, effector mechanisms, and pathophysiology, to human spontaneous abortion. In addition, it would be convenient if the species were small, prolific, inexpensive, and had a short gestation period. Furthermore, the placental physiology and endocrinology should be as similar to that of the human as possible. Finally, control of the diverse genetic parameters which can also effect the outcome of pregnancy is essential. As indicated below, for these and other reasons, the murine models of spontaneous abortion using inbred and congenic parental strains enjoy a considerable advantage.

3. NATURAL MODELS OF SPONTANEOUS ABORTION

3.1. Introduction

The frequencies of conception losses are highly variable. The average loss rates for most species appear to fall between 30 and 50% of all conceptions. The human loss rates may fall slightly above this value and certainly inbred species appear to fall well below. An understanding of these events can be obtained from a survey of the various natural models of embryo and fetal loss.

3.2. Spontaneous Abortion in Interspecies Matings

While interspecies matings occasionally occur naturally, it must be recognized that it is not the normal state of affairs, and as such is considered here as an experiment of nature. The most common interspecies matings are documented between the female horse (mare) and male donkey (jack) which results in the production of an interspecies hybrid mule. As with most viable interspecies hybrids, the mule is usually sterile. However, there are occasional reports that female mules have been successfully mated with a male horse (stallion), producing viable offspring. The reciprocal cross of a stallion with a female donkey (jenny), though less successful for physiological reasons, can also produce living offspring (hinny). Other species can interbreed and, rarely, produce live offspring, such as the shoat (sheep × goat) and several others within the dog or cat families, though most interspecies matings result in early embryonic death and resorption without any live births. Little is known concerning the mechanisms of embryo loss, though the causes are assumed to be genetic. Almost invariably, interspecies offspring are infertile even when mated to the parental species because of errors in gamete formation (meiotic block). Differences in the number of chromosomes and the location of homologous gene loci between paternal and maternal genomes, cause nondisjunction errors during the meiotic divisions which are necessary to produce a haploid set of chromosomes within the gametes.

Such interspecies matings between the larger domestic species, while occasionally producing useful livestock, are neither efficient on the farm nor useful to those researchers who study reproduction in the laboratory. Unless one has access to a breeding farm and large-scale veterinary facilities, the size of the species, the cost of the materials, and the long gestation periods make such species virtually useless for experimental purposes. Unfortunately, most of the convenient laboratory species do not readily interbreed and few, if any, produce living interspecies progeny. This is probably due more to the lack of experimental attempts rather than the scarcity of species. The unique contributions of Rossant, Croy, and Clark in developing the murine interspecies mating model between *Mus musculus* and *Mus caroli* provided a novel opportunity for the examination of the factors leading to successful interspecies pregnancies. Though the technical skills required to produce viable offspring have precluded the general use of this model, the results produced by these investigators have revolutionized our understanding of the immunobiology of reproduction.[37,119,119a]

Prior to the existence of the murine interspecies mating models, it was widely held that fetal losses were mostly due to genetic abnormalities.[44] The role of the trophoblast was considered to be that of a simple barrier between mother and fetus with or without major endocrine properties in the human and mouse, respectively.[85] Rossant and colleagues showed that an intact *Mus caroli* blastocyst or *(Mus musculus × Mus caroli)* hybrid blastocyst in the *M. musculus* female invariably begins to resorb at day 9.5 of pregnancy and no conceptuses successfully come to term.[119a] The construction of chimeric embryos demonstrated that a *Mus caroli* embryo could survive to term inside a *Mus musculus* trophoblastic capsule or placenta. The surviving feto-placental units successfully induced a maternal suppressor cell response within the decidua which prevented the infiltration of the xenogeneic embryos by maternal lymphocytes.[24] Therefore, the trophoblast was not simply a physical barrier, since maternal *Mus musculus* mononuclear cells could traverse the *Mus caroli* barrier but not the *Mus musculus* barrier. Rather, the trophoblast was apparently involved in the species specific recruitment of maternal non-T suppressor lymphocytes within the decidua, which both prevented the maternal allospecific rejection response and enhanced placental development. Without the benefit of a compatible trophoblast capable of inducing a local suppressive response, the *Mus caroli* embryos were quickly recognized by the maternal lymphocytes as foreign, and were invaded within 5 days of implantation by nonspecific killer cells of both the T cell and NK lineage.[26,38,39,41,57,58] The fact that *Mus caroli* embryos are rejected by both the NK-deficient Beige mouse and the T- cell- and B cell-deficient SCID mouse leads one to question whether any immune mechanism is involved.[35,39,40] However, recent studies have revealed that both strains have residual natural defense mechanisms which can be augmented during early pregnancy.[26,30] These effector cells appear to be NK-like in that they can weakly kill both NK targets and trophoblast target cell lines in a non-MHC-restricted manner.[39,57,58] Furthermore, these animals have normal macrophages (MØ) and there may be an element of cooperation between NK cells and macrophages.[63] In fact, the direct cause of embryo loss appears initially to be the destruction of the placental trophoblast and only secondarily, the death of the embryo.[35]

This *Mus musculus* × *Mus caroli* model is in some ways similar to the CBA♀ × DBA♂ spontaneous resorption model described in detail below. However, they do differ in one significant feature. Whereas alloimmunization of the maternal CBA♀ mouse with the tissue antigens of the paternal MHC genotype (DBA♂ or BALB/c♂) results in unchanged or even improved reproductive performance, the immunization of *Mus musculus* females with *Mus caroli* tissue antigens accelerates the maternal T cell-mediated response directed against the *Mus caroli* embryos.[26] This indicates that the maternal immunoregulation that normally enhances embryonic survival is generally neither inducible, nor operative across species barriers. Further examination of the interspecies mating model may substantiate this hypothesis.

3.3. Spontaneous Abortion in Intraspecies Matings

Two basic avenues exist for the investigation of spontaneous abortions: the discovery of natural matings that spontaneously abort vs. the genetic manipulation of species to create genetic defects that cause fetal wastage. Whereas the latter is the surer approach, it assumes that the defect created by the investigator is reflective of the normal problems which cause abortion. The fortuitous discovery of natural models of spontaneous abortion, on the other hand, ensures that the hand of man has not inadvertently manipulated the system in an inappropriate way.

Until relatively recently, no convenient laboratory models of spontaneous abortion existed which met all or most of the criteria listed above. Clark was the first investigator to recognize that the mating of CBA♀ × DBA♂ mice resulted in an unusually high loss of the embryos in first pregnancies.[23] Between 25 and 50% of the embryos in such matings spontaneously resorb by day 12 of gestation and the frequency of resorption appears to increase with the age of the CBA♀ maternal mouse.[17,23] Though it was demonstrated that these aborting pregnancies were deficient in a decidual suppressor cell necessary for maternal immunoregulation, progress in the development of this model has proceeded rapidly. A major breakthrough was achieved, by Kiger and colleagues when they demonstrated that CBA♀ could be vaccinated against embryo resorption by preimmunization with BALB/c♂ or ♀ spleen cells (BALB/c and DBA/2 are both H2d).[17,89] Subsequently, Gendron showed that the effector cells associated with fetal resorption in these mice were not T cells, as was previously hypothesized, but elements of the innate resistance system.[60] While confirming that CBA♀ × DBA♂ implantation sites were deficient in both NK inhibitory cells and a lipophilic inhibitory factor, it was also shown that the presumptively resorbing embryos were being infiltrated by both NK-like cells and macrophages.[62] Modulation of the activity of the asialo GM1-positive class of lymphocytes had a direct effect on the frequency of embryo loss, confirming their importance.[46,90] Finally, though these NK-like cells contain perforin, the NK cell cytolytic effector molecule, the majority of researchers have failed to show that these NK-like cells are indeed cytotoxic *in vivo*.[39,55,109,130,156] However, the *in vitro* culture of these cells with interleukin-2 (IL-2) activates a potent cytolytic function which can destroy trophoblast cells that are normally resistant to NK cells.[48,74,93,154,155] Successful pregnancies contain locally active suppressor cells which inhibit IL-2 activity and the activation of NK cells.[62,108,127]

The question concerning the *in vivo* function of these NK-like cells remains to be conclusively answered. However, the *in vivo* depletion of NK cells, using anti-asialo GM1 antisera, markedly reduced embryonic losses, indicating that the NK-like cells were essential to the initiation of embryonic resorption.[46,63] Moreover, the *in vivo* activation of NK cytotoxic function or the adoptive transfer of *in vitro* activated NK or lymphokine-activated killer (LAK) cells to abortion-resistant gravid mice could directly induce fetal losses in otherwise normal matings.[46,90] A role for NK-like cells in abortion appears clear and preliminary data indicate that the embryotoxic factor active during embryonic resorption may be tumor necrosis factor (TNF)-α. Exogenous TNF-α can induce resorption and the treatment of gravid CBA♀ with inhibitors of the TNF-α expression and function can prevent embryonic losses.[19,63] Both MØ and NK cells can produce TNF-α, though the former cells are considered to be the major source.[76] In addition, NK cells can produce interferon gamma, or macrophage activation factor which is important for the priming of MØ for TNF-α production.[107] It appears possible that embryo resorption may be mediated by macrophage-derived TNF-α, facilitated by the NK-like cells serving a role as an essential "helper" cell.[83]

The nature of the feto-placental target of the TNF-α is also unknown at this time. However, TNF-α is known to have a major function as an antiangiogenic factor due to its cytolytic effect on microvascular endothelial cells.[123,128,148] In addition, trophoblast cells express TNF receptors and exogenous TNF causes both a direct placental and embryonic cytopathic effect.[19,51,79,84] In tumor growth models, the endothelial damage induced by TNF-α initiates platelet aggregation and thrombus formation in the tumor foci, thereby terminating their normal blood supply, causing ischemia and necrosis. This picture is generally consistent with the hemorrhage, thrombosis, and necrosis grossly evident within the resorbing CBA♀ × DBA♂ embryos at day 9 to 10 of pregnancy. Thus, the major effect of TNF-α might be expected to be the direct cytolysis of trophoblast cells, though TNF-α may also damage the maternal endothelial cells within the decidua and ectoplacental cone, thereby indirectly preventing normal placental development.[124]

The final word on spontaneous abortion must be that additional models are required to fully explore its causes and mechanisms. Appropriate models probably exist within the animal resources which are available to researchers, if we could only identify them. Chaouat has discovered that the C57B1/10♀ × C57Bl/10.A♂ murine strain combination also aborts with high frequency.[18a] Furthermore, the trait can be segregated by appropriate backcross matings, thereby creating additional murine models. Clark has recently shown that C3H♀ × DBA/2♂ matings also result in a 26% embryo loss rate.[31] Many other strains of mice show increasing embryo losses with age, as do other species, including man.[80,110] Swine are known to resorb about a third of their embryos about 1 week after implantation, which occurs at day 17 of pregnancy.[82] The time course of this event in swine, dated from the day of implantation, is similar to that of early embryo resorption in mice. Swine could therefore be an appropriate species to supply for study much larger quantities of the regulatory cells and factors than are obtainable from mice.

A survey of domestic species show that the loss of 20 to 40% of fertile embryos within 7 to 14 days after implantation is not unusual. Rather, the very low loss rates of 5 to 10% seen in most inbred mouse matings appears to be the exception, and not the rule. Swine provide an ideal model, though similar data can be obtained from cattle, horses, cats, dogs, rabbits, and other species. In the two weeks between implantation on day 7 following insemination and day 20, over 30% of swine embryos are resorbed. Only 3% of more developed fetal swine are subsequently aborted or are stillborn. The pig therefore provides another model for the study of early embryo loss. Although even small varieties of this species are not well suited to the small research laboratory, it is clearly an important domestic resource and the improvement of embryonic survival in swine could well boost the efficiency of the pork production industry.

3.4. Creation of New Models for the Study of Spontaneous Abortion

Now that we have a better hypothetical model to explain the survival of the ''fetal graft'', one approach to the analysis of the mechanisms responsible for fetal enhancement is to obtain strains of experimental animals deficient in some of the mediators essential for fetal acceptance. Naturally immunodeficient animals are one group of experimental animals for these studies. Another example of such an animal model is the osteopetrotic mouse (op/op).[151] This strain of mouse has a total inability to produce colony-stimulating factor (CSF)-1, and as a result is incapable of restructuring bone and has a very poor breeding performance associated with early embryo loss. Exogenous supplementation of CSF restores bone resorption in the op/op mouse but reproduction was not examined.[54] This strain could provide an appropriate model for the testing of the immunotrophism theory which holds that optimal fetal and placental growth is dependent on T cell-derived cytokines.[2,3,149] If indeed the interaction between maternal CSF-1 and trophoblast CSF-1 receptor (*c-fms*) is essential for placental development, this mouse could provide a useful model for answering this question by exogenously supplementing the gravid mouse with CSF-1. Alternatively, if no natural mutants exist for a desired cytokine or factor, one could now create them through the use of current molecular genetic technologies to either "knock out" or specifically enhance the expression of the genetic loci under investigation.[33a,94a]

Another approach is to alter the cytological composition of embryos in a manner similar to that described by Rossant and Croy.[119a] A reexamination of the data by Surani and co-workers[131,132] of the mechanisms of failure of parthenogenetic eggs appears to provide an ideal model for the study of placental failure. When parthenogenetic embryos (embryos from a chemically activated unfertilized ovum) or gynogenetic embryos (embryos from an unfertilized ovum to which a female pronucleus was transferred), are transferred to normal recipients, the embryos initially implant and develop, but subsequently resorb at day 10 of pregnancy. Furthermore, the observed defect is clearly localized to placental development while the embryos appear relatively normal, if somewhat small for their stage of development.[131] If a male pronucleus (either *X* or *Y*) is transferred to the unfertilized ovum, creating an androgenetic embryo, normal implantation, placental development, and viable offspring are produced. Recent studies involving the creation of fusion chimeras between either androgenetic (viable) or parthenogenetic (resorption prone) embryos and normally fertilized embryos, showed that by day 10, the androgenetic cells were exclusively found in the trophoblast and yolk sac while the parthenogenetic cells were found in the embryo and yolk sac mesoderm.[132] Only the fusion of normal embryos with normal embryos or parthenogenetic embryos produced chimeric offspring, but the contribution of parthenogenetic cells to extra-embryonic tissues was negligible. The implication of these studies is that the paternal chromosomes are responsible for placental development either due to a selective growth advantage or due to a negative selection against maternal chromosomes at the feto-maternal interface. This novel data may provide further support for the concept that alloantigenicity at the placental interface, rather than identity, is essential to the optimal development of the placenta and subsequent protection of the fetus. Mechanistically, the male pronuclear genome could either be capable of providing the correct signals to the maternal decidual cells or receiving the correct signals for placental development, whereas the maternal pronuclear genome could be inactive to cytokine signals. To date, there is no evidence to indicate whether embryo failure in this model is ultimately effected either by placental insufficiency or by a maternal immune or innate resistance response. Chimeric mice can also be used as the maternal host in order to investigate the cellular interactions in the developing placenta.[86] These models provide an outstanding opportunity for the further examination of the genetic and immunologic factors which determine placental development.

4. EXPERIMENTAL MODELS OF INDUCED ABORTIONS

4.1. Introduction

The previous paragraph introduced the topic of the creation of models of spontaneous abortion which occurs without any exogenous inducer of abortion. The fundamental question is whether any abortion is truly spontaneous, or whether some, or even all, are induced by either endogenous or exogenous factors which may or may not be currently detectable to the observer. Is a spontaneous abortion directly caused by a fetal genetic defect which results in a failure to express an appropriate response, or is the gravid female actively responding to an inductive fetal stimulus which precipitates the abortion? These questions too, at this time are unanswerable, other than to state that it is also possible to exogenously induce abortion, thereby creating model systems for examining the mechanisms which actually cause fetal demise.

4.2. Abortion Induced by Progesterone Antagonists

The most common model of induced abortion, or more correctly, the inhibition of normal implantation of fertilized ova, is provided by the action of contraceptive hormone supplements or intrauterine devices. As these hormonal models interfere with embryo development, attachment, and implantation before the embryo has had any significant time to interact with the maternal immune system, these models will not be considered further in this review. A related model involves the termination of an established pregnancy using the antiprogesterone drug, RU 486 or mifepristone.[126,129] This new abortogenic compound is a useful clinical and research tool, because it can effectively induce abortion between the 5th and 10th weeks of pregnancy or later with little or no harmful side effects. The action of this drug is to block the interaction between progesterone (PG) and the progesterone receptor (PGR) on maternal target cells. It was shown that maternal lymphocytes express progesterone receptors and that PG induced these cells to produce an immunosuppressive 34-kDa glycoprotein.[134,135] One of the effects of RU 486, in addition to the induction of abortion, was to block the production of the immunosuppressive 34-kDa suppressive factor. Preliminary data indicates that the infusion of the 34-kDa suppressive factor into either RU-486 or poly-innosinic:cytidylic acid (pI:C)-treated mice, partially prevented embryonic loss.[135,136] This model could provide new insights into the role of PG in the enhancement of fetal survival.

4.3. Abortion Induced by Lymphokines or Lymphokine Modulation

Two significant papers have contributed to our understanding of the potential roles for lymphokines in the development of the feto-placental unit. First, the demonstration by Wegmann that the depletion of the maternal T cell population prior to implantation significantly reduced feto-placental weight, implying that the growth of the placenta in particular was dependent on T cell-derived cytokines.[2,3] Growth could be restored by infusions of CSF-1, granulocyte monocyte colony-stimulating factor (GM-CSF), or IL-3, cytokines produced by T cells.[2] Furthermore, spontaneous abortion was prevented by exogenous GM-CSF.[19] CSF-1 was seen in metrial gland cells, decidual stroma, and uterine epithelium, while GM-CSF was seen in decidual endothelial cells, fibroblasts, and lymphoid cells.[150] These and other observations led the authors to propose a role for immunotrophism in the cytokine-induced promotion of placental and possibly fetal development.[149] As stated above, the osteopetrotic mouse would appear to provide an ideal model for the investigation of the principles of immunotrophism.[151]

Just as IL-2 can enhance autologous defense mechanisms in the fight against malignant disease, so can these same mechanisms cause the rejection of the fetal graft. Lala and colleagues have shown that the stimulation of LAK cells during early pregnancy has a negative effect on fetal survival.[93] This effect is greatly increased to the point where entire litters are aborted by a single treatment with IL-2 when the females are pretreated with indomethacin or aspirin to diminish the level of arachidonic acid metabolites produced by the cyclooxygenase pathway.[108] Prostaglandin E_2 is normally a potent inhibitor of NK cell and LAK activation by tumor or fetal grafts, and the prevention of its production allows exogenous IL-2 to optimally stimulate the LAK precursors.[92,108,122] When this is coupled with the demonstrated NK-activating effects of indomethacin, it is not surprising that the production of these extremely active cytolytic cells results in the demise of the feto-placental unit.[144] It has also been shown that the induction of other cytokines such as interferons alpha and beta by inoculation with pI:C also results in fetal death in nonabortion-prone strains.[46,90]

Furthermore, cytokines such as interferon gamma (IFN-γ), IL-1, IL-2, CSF-1, and TNF-α have been shown to have a direct embryotoxic effect *in vitro* but the relevance to *in vivo* events has not been proven.[79,139] Finally, macrophage-derived monokines also have a deleterious effect on embryonic viability. While it appears consistent with other studies that exogenous TNF-α can cause fetal death, it is perhaps surprising that the intracerebroventricular (ICV) injection of interleukin 1 beta (IL-1β) can also cause precipitate embryonic loss.[42] Since TNF-α and IL-1β are often synergistic in their effects, these results could indicate that IL-1β may induce local TNF-α, causing fetal demise.[76,124] The focus of the effects of TNF-α may be the placenta, since it has been shown that TNF-α can directly inhibit trophoblast growth due, in part, to the fact that placental trophoblast cells express receptors for many cytokines, including TNF-α.[51,83] It was therefore significant that the ICV IL-1β treatment was observed to markedly impair development of the ectoplacental cone into a definitive placenta.[42]

4.4. Inhibition of Lymphokine Activities Prevents Spontaneous Abortion

Where a model provides an elevated spontaneous abortion rate, the role of cytokines can be studied by either direct inhibition of their action or blocking of the appropriate receptor. Such experiments have not been greatly successful to date, as the immune system has an enormous capacity to counteract such treatments. In this regard, the attempts to abrogate LAK and cytotoxic T lymphocytes (CTL) activation by anti-IL-2 receptor (IL-2R) antibodies were also unsuccessful.[40] Similarly, antibodies to immunotrophic cytokines (CSF-1, GM-CSF, etc.) have only had modest effects.[19] However, pretreatment of mice with the TNF-α-inhibiting drug pentoxifylline significantly reduced both lipopolysaccharide (LPS)-induced abortions in outbred mice and spontaneous abortions in CBA/j ♀ mice, confirming the importance of TNF-α in inducing abortion.[63]

4.5. Abortions Induced by Lipopolysaccharides or Endotoxin

Most mouse strains, whether inbred or outbred, do not show high rates of spontaneous abortion. However, we have shown that treatment of pregnant mice with the interferon inducer pI:C or LPS can induce even normal syngeneic or outbred embryos to be resorbed.[46,63] Furthermore, these embryos also show the decidual NK-like cellular infiltrates and augmented systemic NK activity associated with spontaneous abortion.[60,90] It has previously been shown that the injection of relatively large doses of LPS during late gestation can induce fetal abortion.[21,114,153] Endotoxin ingestion or injection causes acute hyperthermia and other metabolic alterations which often lead to abortion in pregnant sheep, swine, and other animals.[78,103,105]

It should be recalled that IL-1β induces hyperthermia and therefore, one of the mechanisms of ICV IL-1β may be to arrest trophoblast growth by a form of heat shock response. The reasons for the abortogenic effects of LPS are unclear, but the observation of immunoglobulin passage from maternal ovine blood to fetal fluids following LPS inoculation clearly indicates endothelial damage, a feature often ascribed to TNF-α.[111] It is well known that the challenge of primed MØ with relatively low doses of LPS triggers the production and release of TNF-α. Therefore, the further examination of the immunobiology of LPS-induced abortions could provide another valuable model for the analysis of the immunosuppressive mechanisms essential for fetal survival and the effector mechanisms leading to spontaneous abortion.

As stated above, previous authors have inoculated relatively high doses of LPS during later pregnancy to induce abortion. In our recent studies, we noted that during early pregnancy, the embryo is exquisitely sensitive to minute doses of LPS.[63] The effect of doses of LPS as low as 0.1 μg per mouse causes abortion of the entire contents of the uterus within 24 h. The different dose ranges of LPS effective in early and later pregnancy provides a tool to selectively examine its abortion-inducing effects. The effects of low-dose LPS appear to be absolutely limited to the implantation sites, as no other tissues appear to be affected. This may indicate a number of factors of importance to fetal survival, including the possibility that trophoblasts may be sensitive to heat shock responses. Implantation may be associated with the local priming of decidual MØ which have the potential to release TNF when appropriately challenged. Furthermore, we have confirmed that the resorbing embryos in LPS-induced abortion were quickly infiltrated by ASGM1[+] cells and MØ, and that depletion of the maternal NK population, as described above, significantly improved fetal survival in both spontaneous and LPS-induced abortion models, directly implicating either maternal NK-like cells and/or MØ.[63] This model suggests that exogenous sources of LPS or Gram-negative organisms may threaten fetal survival during early pregnancy. Therefore, LPS provides us with another means for modulating pregnancy outcome and examining the mechanisms responsible for fetal resorption.[5]

4.6. Induction of Abortion by the Abrogation of Suppression

The abortogenic effects of treatment of gravid mice with agents that inhibit cyclooxygenase activity have been discussed above in relation to the induction of LAK activity by IL-2. The blocking of the production of the inhibitory arachidonic acid metabolite prostaglandin E_2 has a direct stimulatory effect on NK or LAK activity and an indirect negative effect on fetal survival.[144] Even in the absence of exogenous IL-2, indomethacin can induce a significant elevation in fetal losses.[93,122] While there is no clinical evidence that indomethacin augments embryo losses in human pregnancies, the occult nature of this event may conceal whatever impact the abrogation of prostaglandin E production may have on human embryonic survival.

An alternative approach to the modulation of pregnancy outcome has been through the infusion of specific antibodies. Both alpha-fetoprotein (AFP) and transforming growth factor beta (TGF-β) have been postulated to inhibit the maternal response to the fetoplacental unit.[1,29,81,141] While it is undeniable that the injection of anti-AFP into gravid mice causes fetal abortion, it is by no means clear how these factors enhance early fetal survival.[99] AFP has been shown to induce the expression of a natural suppressor cell activity in the maternal decidua and the spleen of newborn mice. The depletion of these cells in maternal tissues by passive immunization of gravid mice with a monoclonal antibody to the suppressor cell induced abortion.[69] The recent demonstration that the decidual suppressor factor is related to TGF-β may indicate that maternal TGF-β may be important as a suppressor before the fetus develops the ability to produce significant amounts of AFP.[29]

Recent studies by Tartakovsky and Gorelik[138] have shown that maternal immunization against a syngeneic regressor tumor cell may also jeopardize fetal survival, though by a less well-understood mechanism. The antitumor response could modulate suppressor cell activity or induce an immune response to oncofetal antigens. Further work is needed on this model in order to fully understand the mechanisms involved.

Finally, the modulation of the production of enhancing antibodies could also create a model for studying abortion. In human pregnancies, the absence of serum blocking antibodies or retro-placental globulins has been linked to spontaneous abortion.[55a,116,117] Whereas attempts to cause abortion by depleting or inhibiting the production of enhancing antibodies have been unsuccessful, the reverse may be effective. The transfusion of retroplacental globulins into habitual aborters or the immunization against paternal MHC antigens or TLX antigens may enhance fetal survival.[8,67,88,98] These factors seem irrelevant to most laboratory species, perhaps due in part to their short gestation period. Blocking antibodies could be required to inhibit the maternal alloimmune response to paternal MHC antigens by either masking paternal epitopes or by suppressing allotype expression by trophoblast cells. In murine pregnancy, the early lack of MHC expression by the murine embryo followed by its limited expression in the placenta, may leave very little time for the initiation of an effective alloimmune response between days 10 and 18 of pregnancy.

5. CONCLUDING STATEMENTS ON ANIMAL MODELS OF ABORTION

There is no doubt that many models of spontaneous and induced abortion exist and that many more await discovery. While it is by no means clear at this time whether the major causes of embryonic loss or fetal death are genetic or immunological, the only expedient approach to resolving this controversy is through the use of appropriate animal models. It is also only through the use of such models that rational therapeutic protocols can be developed. It is conceivable that the majority of early losses could be prevented by an appropriate means of immunotherapy. The final consideration is to attempt to rationalize the evolutionary advantages of the observed high rates of conception loss. Could this be an inevitable consequence of a reproductive system which stringently selects for healthy offspring, thereby sparing the females the unnecessary hazards of gestating and delivering a malformed fetus unsuited to perpetuating the species? Would the therapeutic prevention of early embryo losses lead to an increase in the birth of offspring with genetic or morphological malformations? The answers to these and other questions will be conclusively obtained only through the investigation of experimental models of spontaneous pregnancy failure.

REFERENCES

1. **Altman, D. J., Schneider, S. L., Thompson, D. A., Cheng, H. L., and Tomasi, T. B.,** A transforming growth factor-beta-2 (TGF-beta-2)-like immunosuppressive factor in amniotic fluid and localization of TGF-beta-2 messenger RNA in the pregnant uterus, *J. Exp. Med.,* 172, 1391–1401, 1990.
2. **Athanassakis, I., Bleackley, R. C., Paetkau, V., Guilbert, L., Barr, P. J., and Wegmann, T. G.,** The immunostimulatory effect of T cells and T cell lymphokines on murine fetally derived placental cells, *J. Immunol.,* 138, 37–45, 1987.
3. **Athanassakis, I., Chaouat, G., and Wegmann, T. G.,** The effects of anti-CD4 and anti-CD8 antibody treatment on placental growth and function in allogeneic and syngeneic murine pregnancy, *Cell. Immunol.,* 129, 13–21, 1990.
4. **Baines, M. G., Millar, K. G., and Pross, H. F.,** Allograft enhancement during normal murine pregnancy, *J. Reprod. Immunol.,* 2, 141–149, 1980.
5. **Baines, M. G. and Gendron, R. L.,** Are both endogenous and exogenous factors involved in spontaneous foetal abortion?, *Res. Immunol.,* 141, 154–158, 1990.
6. **Balasch, J.,** Alloimmune and autoimmune mechanisms in recurrent spontaneous abortion, *Immunologia,* 8, 111–121, 1989.
7. **Beer, A. E., Quebbeman, J. F., Ayers, J. W. T., and Haines, R. F.,** Major histocompatibility complex antigens, maternal and paternal immune responses and chronic habitual abortions in humans, *Obstet. Gynecol.,* 141, 987–1000, 1981.
8. **Beer, A. E.,** Immunopathologic factors contributing to recurrent spontaneous abortions in humans, *Am. J. Reprod. Immunol.,* 4, 182–185, 1983.
9. **Bieber, F. R. and Driscoll, S. G.,** Evaluation of spontaneous abortion and malformed fetus, in *Diseases of the Fetus and Newborn,* Reed, G. B., Claireux, A. E., and Bain, A. D., Eds., Chapman and Hall, London, 1989, 59–70.
10. **Bobe, P., Chaouat, G., Stanislawski, M., and Kiger, N.,** Immunogenetic studies of spontaneous abortion in mice. II. Antiabortive effects are independent of systemic regulatory mechanisms, *Cell. Immunol.,* 98, 447–486, 1986.
11. **Boyd, M. E.,** Spontaneous abortion, *Can. J. Surg.,* 32, 260–264, 1989.
12. **Brambati, B., Simoni, G., and Fabro, S.,** Chorionic villus sampling, *Clin. Biochem. Anal.,* 21, 1–23, 1986.
13. **Branch, D. W.,** Immunologic disease and fetal death, *Clin. Obstet. Gynecol.,* 30, 295–311, 1987.
14. **Branch, D. W., Dudley, D. J., Mitchell, M. D., Creighton, K. A., Abbott, T. M., Hammond, E. H., and Daynes, R. A.,** Immunoglobulin G fractions from patients with antiphospholipid antibodies cause fetal death in BALB/c mice: a model for autoimmune fetal loss, *Am. J. Obstet. Gynecol.,* 163, 210–206, 1990.

15. **Canadian Collaborative CVS Amniocentesis Clinical Trial Group,** Multicenter randomized clinical trial of chorion villus sampling and amniocentesis, *Lancet,* 2, 1–6, 1989.

16. **Carp, H. J. A., Toder, V., Gazit, E., Orgad, S., Mashiach, S., Nebel, L., and Serr, D. M.,** Immunization by paternal leukocytes for prevention of primary habitual abortion—results of a matched controlled trial, *Gynecol. Obstet. Invest.,* 29(1), 16–21, 1990.

17. **Chaouat, G., Kiger, N., and Wegmann, T. G.,** Vaccination against spontaneous abortion in mice, *J. Reprod. Immunol.,* 5, 389–392, 1983.

18. **Chaouat, G. and Monnot, P.,** Systemic active suppression is not necessary for successful allopregnancy, *Am. J. Reprod. Immunol.,* 6, 5–8, 1984.

18a. **Chaouat, G., Clark, D. A., and Wegmann, T. G.,** Genetic aspects of the CBA × DBA/2 and B10 × B10.A models of murine pregnancy failure and its prevention by lymphocyte immunisation, in *Early Pregnancy Loss, Mechanisms and Treatment,* Beard, R. W. and Sharp, F., Eds., Peacock Press, Ashton-under-Lyme, England, 1988, 89–102.

19. **Chaouat, G., Menu, E., Clark, D. A., Dy, M., Minkowski, M., and Wegmann, T. G.,** Control of fetal survival in CBA × DBA/2 mice by lymphokine therapy, *J. Reprod. Fertil.,* 89, 447–458, 1990.

20. **Chaouat, G. and Wegmann, T. G.,** 30th Forum in immunology—the immunology of spontaneous abortion, *Res. Immunol.,* 141, 153–228, 1990.

21. **Chedid, L., Boyer, F., and Parant, M.,** Etude de l'action abortive des endotoxines injectees a la souris gravide normale, castree ou hypophysectomisee, *Ann. Inst. Pasteur,* 102, 77–84, 1962.

22. **Christiansen, O. B., Lauritsen, J. G., Andersen, E. S., and Grunnet, N.,** Autoimmune associated recurrent abortions, *Hum. Reprod.,* 4, 913–917, 1989.

23. **Clark, D. A., McDermott, M. R., and Szewczuk, M. R.,** Impairment of host-vs-graft reaction of pregnant mice. II. Selective suppression of cytotoxic T-cell generation correlates with successful allogeneic pregnancy, *Cell. Immunol.,* 52, 106–118, 1980.

24. **Clark, D. A., Slapsys, R. M., Croy, B. A., and Rossant, J.,** Suppressor cell activity in uterine decidua correlates with successor failure of murine pregnancies, *J. Immunol.,* 131, 540–542, 1983.

25. **Clark, D. A., Chaput, A., Walker, C., and Rosenthal, K. L.,** Active suppression of host-vs-graft disease in pregnant mice. VII. Soluble suppressor activity obtained from decidua of allopregnant mice blocks the response to IL-2, *J. Immunol.,* 134, 1659–1665, 1985.

26. **Clark, D. A., Croy, B. A., Rossant, J., and Chaouat, G.,** Immune presensitization and local intrauterine defences as determinants of success or failure of murine interspecies pregnancies, *J. Reprod. Fertil.,* 77, 633–643, 1986.

27. **Clark, D. A., Chaouat, G., Guenet, J.-L., and Kiger, N.,** Local active suppression and successful vaccination against spontaneous abortion in CBA/J mice, *J. Reprod. Immunol.,* 10, 79–87, 1987.

28. **Clark, D. A., Croy, G. A., Wegmann, T. G., and Chaouat, G.,** Immunological and para-immunological mechanisms in spontaneous abortion: recent insights and future directions, *J. Reprod. Immunol.,* 12, 1–13, 1987.

29. **Clark, D. A., Falbo, M., Rowley, R. B., Banwatt, D., and Stedronska-Clark, J.,** Active suppression of host-vs-graft reaction in pregnant mice. IX. Soluble suppressor activity obtained from allopregnant mouse decidua that blocks the cytolytic effector response to IL-2 is related to transforming growth factor-beta, *J. Immunol.,* 141, 3833–3841, 1988.

30. **Clark, D. A. and Chaouat, G.,** What do we know about spontaneous abortion mechanisms?, *Am. J. Reprod. Immunol.,* 19, 28–38, 1989.

31. **Clark, D. A., Drake, B., Head, J. R., Stedronskaclark, J., and Banwatt, D.,** Decidua-associated suppressor activity and viability of individual implantation sites of allopregnant C3H mice, *J. Reprod. Immunol.,* 17, 253–264, 1990.

32. **Claytonsmith, J., Farndon, P. A., McKeown, C., and Donnai, D.,** Examination of fetuses after induced abortion for fetal abnormality, *Br. Med. J.,* 300, 295–297, 1990.

33. **Confino, E. and Gleicher, N.,** Pregnancy wastage with abnormal autoimmunity, *Immunol. Allergy Clin. North Am.,* 10, 103–108, 1990.

33a. **Cosgrove, D., Gray, D., Derich, A., Kaufman, J., Benoist, C., and Mathis, D.,** Mice lacking MHC class II molecules, *Cell,* 66, 1051–1066, 1991.

34. **Cowchock, F. S., Smith, J. B., David, S., Scher, J., Batzer, F., and Corson, S.,** Paternal mononuclear cell immunization therapy for repeated miscarriage—predictive variables for pregnancy success, *Am. J. Reprod. Immunol.,* 22, 12–17, 1990.

35. **Crepeau, M. A. and Croy, B. A.,** Evidence that specific cellular immunity cannot account for death of Mus caroli embryos transferred to Mus musculus with severe combined immune deficiency disease, *Transplantation,* 45, 1104–1110, 1988.

36. **Crepeau, M. A., Yamashiro, S., and Croy, B. A.,** Morphological demonstration of the failure of Mus caroli trophoblast in the Mus musculus uterus, *J. Reprod. Fertil.,* 86, 277–288, 1989.

37. **Croy, B. A., Rossant, J., and Clark, D. A.,** Histological and immunological studies of post implantation death of mus caroli embryos in the mus musculus uterus, *J. Reprod. Immunol.,* 4, 277–294, 1982.

38. **Croy, B. A., Rossant, J., and Clark, D. A.,** Recruitment of cytotoxic cells by ectopic grafts of xenogeneic, but not allogeneic, trophoblast, *Transplantation,* 37, 84–90, 1984.

39. **Croy, B. A., Gambel, P., Rossant, J., and Wegmann, T. G.,** Characterization of murine decidual natural killer (NK) cells and their relevance to the success of pregnancy, *Cell. Immunol.,* 93, 315–327, 1985.

40. **Croy, B. A., Crepeau, M., Yamashiro, S., and Clark, D. A.,** Further studies on the transfer of Mus caroli embryos to immunodeficient Mus musculus, in *Reproductive Immunology: Materno-Fetal Relationship,* Chaouat, G., Ed., INSERM Colloque, Paris, 1987, 101–112.

41. **Croy, B. A., Waterfield, A., Wood, W., and King, G. J.,** Normal murine and porcine embryos recruit NK cells to the uterus, *Cell. Immunol.,* 115, 471–480, 1988.

42. **Croy, B. A. and Summerlee, A. J. S.,** Intracerebroventricular administration of a single small dose of HrII-1-beta is sufficient to initiate murine pregnancy failure, *Res. Immunol.,* 141, 195–202, 1990.

43. **Cubberly, D. A.,** Diagnosis of fetal death, *Clin. Obstet. Gynecol.,* 30, 259–277, 1987.

44. **Cunningham, F. G., MacDonald, P. C., and Gant, N. F.,** *Complications of Pregnancy: Abortion,* Williams Obstetrics, 18th ed., Appleton and Lange, Norwalk, CT, 1989, 489–509.

45. **Daya, S., Rosenthal, K. L., and Clark, D. A.,** Immunosuppressor factor(s) produced by decidua-associated suppressor cells: a proposed mechanism for fetal allograft survival, *Am. J. Obstet. Gynecol.,* 156, 344–350, 1987.

46. **de Fougerolles, A. R. and Baines, M. G.,** Modulation of the natural killer cell activity in pregnant mice alters the spontaneous abortion rate, *J. Reprod. Immunol.,* 11, 146–153, 1987.

47. **Denegri, J. F., Altin, M., McConnachie, P., Peterson, J., Benny, W. B., Zouves, C. G., and Wilson, D.,** Immunotherapy of primary immunological aborters: rationale for the use of pooled cryopreserved purified normal peripheral blood mononuclear cells, *Am. J. Reprod. Immunol. Microbiol.,* 12, 65–70, 1986.

48. **Drake, B. L. and Head, J. R.,** Murine trophoblast can be killed by lymphokine-activated killer cells, *J. Immunol.,* 143, 9–15, 1989.

49. **Drugan, A., Koppitch, F. C., Williams, J. C., Johnson, M. P., Moghissi, K. S., and Evans, M. I.,** Prenatal genetic diagnosis following recurrent early pregnancy loss, *Obstet. Gynecol.,* 75, 381–384, 1990.

50. **Dudley, D. J. and Branch, D. W.,** New approaches to recurrent pregnancy loss, *Clin. Obstet. Gynecol.,* 32, 520–532, 1989.

51. **Eades, D. K., Cornelius, P., and Pekal, P. H.,** Characterization of the tumor necrosis factor receptor in human placenta, *Placenta,* 9, 247–251, 1988.

52. **Edmonds, D. K., Lindsay, K. S., Miller, J. F., Williamson, E., and Wood, P. J.,** Early embryonic mortality in women, *Fertil. Steril.,* 38, 447–453, 1982.

53. **Eiben, B., Bartels, I., Bahrporsch, S., Borgmann, S., Gatz, G., Gellert, G., Goebel, R., Hammans, W., Hentemann, M., Osmers, R., Rauskolb, R., and Hansmann, I.,** Cytogenetic analysis of 750 spontaneous abortions with the direct-preparation method of chorionic villi and its implications for studying genetic causes of pregnancy wastage, *Am. J. Hum. Genet.,* 47, 656–663, 1990.

54. **Felix, R., Cecchini, M. G., and Fleisch, H.,** Macrophage colony stimulating factor restores *in vivo* bone resorption in the OP/OP osteopetrotic mouse, *Endocrinology,* 127, 2592–2594, 1990.

55. **Ferry, B. L., Starkey, P. M., Sargent, I. L., Watt, G. M. O., Jackson, M., and Redman, C. W. G.,** Cell populations in the human early pregnancy decidua—natural killer activity and response to interleukin-2 of Cd56-positive large granular lymphocytes, *Immunology,* 70, 446–452, 1990.

55a. **Fiddes, T. M., O'Reilly, D. B., Cetrulo, C. L., Miller, W., Rudders, R., Osband, M., and Rocklin, R. E.,** Phenotypic and functional evaluation of suppressor cells in normal pregnancy and in chronic aborters, *Cell. Immunol.,* 97, 407–419, 1986.

56. **Filkins, K. and Russo, J. F.,** Human prenatal diagnosis, *Clin. Biochem. Anal.,* 18, 1–40, 1985.

57. **Gambel, P., Rossant, J., Hunziker, R. D., and Wegmann, T. G.,** Decidual cells in murine pregnancy and pseudopregnancy—origin and natural killer cell activity, *Transplant. Proc.,* 17, 905–909, 1985.

58. **Gambel, P., Croy, B. A., Moore, W. D., Hunziker, R. D., Wegmann, T. G., and Rossant, J.,** Characterization of immune effector cells present in early murine decidua, *Cell. Immunol.,* 93, 303–315, 1985.

59. **Gatenby, P. A., Moore, H., Cameron, K., Doran, T. J., and Adelstein, S.,** Treatment of recurrent spontaneous abortion by immunization with paternal lymphocytes: correlates with outcome, *Am. J. Reprod. Immunol.,* 19, 21–28, 1989.

60. **Gendron, R. L. and Baines, M. G.,** Infiltrating decidual natural killer cells are associated with spontaneous abortion in mice, *Cell. Immunol.,* 113, 261–268, 1988.

61. **Gendron, R. L. and Baines, M. G.,** Morphometric analysis of the histology of spontaneous fetal resorption in a murine pregnancy, *Placenta,* 10, 309–318, 1989.

62. **Gendron, R. L., Farookhi, R., and Baines, M. G.,** Resorption of CBA/J × DBA/2 mouse conceptuses in CBA/J uteri correlates with failure of the feto-placental unit to suppress natural killer cell activity, *J. Reprod. Fertil.,* 89, 277–284, 1990.

63. **Gendron, R. L., Nestel, F. P., Lapp, W. S., and Baines, M. G.,** Lipopolysaccharide-induced fetal resorption in mice is associated with the intrauterine production of tumour necrosis factor-alpha, *J. Reprod. Fertil.,* 90, 395–402, 1990.

64. **Gill, T. J., III,** Immunity and pregnancy, *Crit. Rev. Immunol.,* 5, 201–229, 1985.

65. **Gill, T. J., III,** Immunological and genetic factors influencing pregnancy and development, *Am. J. Reprod. Immunol. Microbiol.,* 10, 117–121, 1986.

66. **Gill, T. J., III,** Immunological and genetic factors influencing pregnancy, in *Physiology of Reproduction,* Knobil, E., Neill, J. C., Ewing, C. L., Markert, C. L., Greenwald, G. S., and Pfaff, D. W., Eds., Raven Press, New York, 1988, 2023–2043.

67. **Gilmansachs, A., Luo, S. P., Beer, A. E., and Beaman, K. D.,** Analysis of anti-lymphocyte antibodies by flow cytometry or microlymphocytotoxicity in women with recurrent spontaneous abortions immunized with paternal leukocytes, *J. Clin. Lab. Immunol.,* 30, 53–59, 1989.

68. **Gladen, B.,** Risk factors for spontaneous abortion and its recurrence, *Am. J. Epidemiol.,* 131, 570–571, 1990.

69. **Gronvik, K.-O., Hoskin, D. W., and Murgita, R. A.,** Monoclonal antibodies against murine neonatal and pregnancy-associated natural suppressor cells induce resorption of the fetus, *Scand. J. Immunol.,* 25, 533–541, 1987.

70. **Hafez, E. S. E.,** Spontaneous abortion, *Adv. Reprod. Health Care,* 1, 1–351, 1984.

71. **Hafez, E. S. E.,** *Reproduction in Farm Animals,* Lea & Febiger, Philadelphia, 1987.

72. **Hall, B. D.,** Nonchromosomal malformations and syndromes associated with stillbirth, *Clin. Obstet. Gynecol.,* 30, 278–283, 1987.

73. **Head, J. R., Drake, B. L., and Zuckermann, F. A.,** Major histocompatibility antigens on trophoblast and their regulation: implications in the maternal-fetal relationship, *Am. J. Reprod. Immunol. Microbiol.,* 15, 12–19, 1987.

74. **Head, J. R.,** Can trophoblast be killed by cytotoxic cells? *In vitro* evidence and *in vivo* possibilities, *Am. J. Reprod. Immunol.,* 20, 100–106, 1989.

75. **Heikinheimo, O., Ylikorkala, O., and Lahteenmaki, P.,** Antiprogesterone Ru-486—a drug for non-surgical abortion, *Ann. Med.,* 22, 75–84, 1990.

76. **Herrmann, F., Gebaauer, G., Lindemann, A., Brach, M., and Mertels-mann, R.,** Interleukin-2 and interferon-gamma recruit different subsets of human peripheral blood monocytes to secrete interleukin-1-beta and tumour necrosis factor-alpha, *Clin. Exp. Immunol.,* 77, 124–130, 1989.

77. **Hetherington, C. M., Humber, D. P., and Clarke, A. G.,** Genetic and immunological aspects of litter size in the mouse, *J. Immunogenet.,* 3, 245–252, 1976.

78. **Hilbelink, D. R., Chen, L. T., and Bryant, M.,** Endotoxin-induced hyperthermia in pregnant golden hamsters, *Teratogen. Carcinogen. Mutagen,* 6, 209–217, 1986.

79. **Hill, J. A., Haimovici, F., and Anderson, D. J.,** Products of activated lymphocytes and macrophages inhibit mouse embryo development *in vitro, J. Immunol.,* 139, 2250–2254, 1987.

80. **Holinka, C. F., Tseng, Y. C., and Finch, C. E.,** Reproductive aging in C57Bl/6J mice: plasma progesterone, viable embryos and resorption frequency throughout pregnancy, *Biol. Reprod.,* 20, 1201–1211, 1979.

81. **Hoskin, D. W., Gronvik, K.-O., Hooper, D. C., Reilly, B. D., and Murgita, R. A.,** Altered immune response patterns in murine syngeneic pregnancy: presence of natural null suppressor cells in maternal spleen identifiable by monoclonal antibodies, *Cell. Immunol.,* 120, 42–61, 1989.

82. **Hughes, P. E.,** *Reproduction in the Pig,* Butterworths, London, 1980.

83. **Hunt, J. S.,** Cytokine networks in the uteroplacental unit: macrophages as pivotal regulatory cells, *J. Reprod. Immunol.,* 16, 1–17, 1989.

84. **Hunt, J. S., Soares, M. J., Lei, M.-G., Smith, R. N., Wheaton, D., Atherton, R. A., and Morrison, D. C.,** Products of lipopolysaccharide-activated macrophages (tumor necrosis factor-alpha, transforming growth factor-beta) but not lipopolysaccharide modify DNA synthesis by rat trophoblast cells exhibiting the 80-kDa lipopolysaccharide-binding protein, *J. Immunol.,* 143, 1606–1614, 1989.

85. **Hunziker, R. D., Gamble, P., and Wegmann, T. G.,** Placenta as a selective barrier to cellular traffic, *J. Immunol.,* 133, 667–672, 1984.

86. **Johnson, S. R. and Lala, P. K.,** Three methods for producing fertile hemopoietic chimeras in mice, *Am. J. Anat.,* 185, 1–8, 1989.

87. **Johnson, M. P., Drugan, A., Koppitch, F. C., Uhlmann, W. R., and Evans, M. I.,** Postmortem chorionic villus sampling is a better method for cytogenetic evaluation of early fetal loss than culture of abortus material, *Am. J. Obstet. Gynecol.,* 163, 1505–1510, 1990.

88. **Kajino, T., McIntyre, J. A., Faulk, W. P., Deng, S. C., and Billington, W. D.,** Antibodies to trophoblast in normal pregnant and secondary aborting women, *J. Reprod. Immunol.,* 14, 267–283, 1988.

89. **Kiger, N., Chaouat, G., Kolb, J. P., Wegmann, T. G., and Guenet, J. L.,** Immunogenetic studies of spontaneous abortion in mice: preimmunization of females with allogeneic cells, *J. Immunol.,* 134, 2966–2970, 1985.

90. **Kinsky, R., Delage, G., Rosin, N., Thang, M. N., Hoffmann, M., and Chaouat, G.,** A murine model of NK cell mediated resorption, *Am. J. Reprod. Immunol.,* 23, 73–77, 1990.

91. **Kochenour, N. K.,** Other causes of fetal death, *Clin. Obstet. Gynecol.,* 30, 312–320, 1987.
92. **Lala, P. K.,** Similarities between immunoregulation in pregnancy and in malignancy—the role of prostaglandin-E2, *Am. J. Reprod. Immunol.,* 20, 147–152, 1989.
93. **Lala, P. K., Scodras, J. M., Graham, C. H., Lysiak, J. J., and Parhar, R. S.,** Activation of maternal killer cells in the pregnant uterus with chronic indomethacin therapy, IL-2 therapy, or a combination therapy is associated with embryonic demise, *Cell. Immunol.,* 127, 368–381, 1990.
94. **Levgur, M., Rodriguez, L. J., Smith, K. D., and Steinberger, E.,** Risk factors for pregnancy loss apparent at conception in infertile couples, *Int. J. Fertil.,* 35, 51–57, 1990.
94a. **Liao, N. S., Bix, M., Zijlstra, M., Jaenisch, R., and Raulet, D.,** MHC class-I deficiency-susceptibility to natural killer (NK) cells and impaired NK activity, *Science,* 253, 199–202, 1991.
95. **Lippman, A. and Farookhi, R.,** The Montreal pregnancy study: an investigation of very early pregnancies, *Can. J. Public Health,* 77, 157–163, 1986.
96. **Liu, D. T. Y., Symonds, E. M., and Golbus, M. S.,** *Chorionic Villus Sampling,* Year Book Medical Publishers, Chicago, 1987.
97. **Mardh, P. A.,** Infertility and related problems due to infections, *Serono Symp. Pub.: Unexplained Infertil. Basic Clin. Aspects,* 62, 191–195, 1989.
98. **McIntyre, J. A., Coulam, C. B., and Faulk, W. P.,** Recurrent spontaneous abortion, *Am. J. Reprod. Immunol.,* 21, 100–104, 1989.
99. **Mizejewski, G. J. and Vonnegut, M.,** Mechanism of fetal demise in pregnant mice immunized to murine alpha-fetoprotein, *Am. J. Reprod. Immunol.,* 5, 32–38, 1984.
100. **Moncayo, R., Moncayo, H., Steffens, U., Soelder, E., Kersting, A., and Dapunt, O.,** Serum levels of anticardiolipin antibodies are pathologically increased after active immunization of patients with recurrent spontaneous abortion, *Fertil. Steril.,* 54, 619–623, 1990.
101. **Mowbray, J. F.,** Genetic and immunological factors in human recurrent abortion, *Am. J. Reprod. Immunol. Microbiol.,* 15, 138–141, 1987.
102. **Mowbray, J. F.,** Autoantibodies, alloantibodies and reproductive success, *Curr. Opinion Immunol.,* 2, 761–764, 1990.
103. **Naylor, J. M. and Kornfeld, D. S.,** Relationship between metabolic changes and clinical signs in pregnant sheep given endotoxin, *Can. J. Vet. Res.,* 50, 402–409, 1986.
104. **Nishimura, H. and Shiota, K.,** Early embryonic death; pathology and associated factors, *Adv. Reprod. Health Care,* 1, 115–131, 1984.
105. **Norman, J. O. and Elissade, M. H.,** Abortion in laboratory animals induced by Moraxella bovis, *Infect. Immun.,* 24, 427–433, 1979.
106. **Ober, C., Elias, S., O'Brien, E., Kostyu, D. D., Hauck, W. W., and Bombard, A.,** HLA sharing and fertility in Hutterite couples: evidence for prenatal selection against compatible fetuses, *Am. J. Reprod. Immunol. Microbiol.,* 18, 111–116, 1988.
107. **Ortaldo, J. R.,** Cytokine production by CD3-large granular lymphocytes, in *Functions of the Natural Immune System,* Reynolds, C. W. and Wiltrout, R. H., Eds., Plenum Press, New York, 1989, 299–321.

108. **Parhar, R. S., Yagel, S., and Lala, P. K.,** PGE2-Mediated immunosuppression by first trimester human decidual cells block activation of maternal leukocytes in the decidua with potential anti-trophoblast activity, *Cell. Immunol.,* 120, 61–75, 1989.

109. **Parr, E. L., Young, L. H. Y., Parr, M. B., and Young, J. D. E.,** Granulated metrial gland cells of pregnant mouse uterus are natural killer-like cells that contain perforin and serine esterases, *J. Immunol.,* 145, 2365–2372, 1990.

110. **Petitti, D. B.,** The epidemiology of fetal death, *Clin. Obstet. Gynecol.,* 30, 253–358, 1987.

111. **Poitras, B. J., Miller, R. B., Wilkie, B. N., and Bosu, W. T. K.,** The maternal to fetal transfer of immunoglobulins associated with placental lesions in sheep, *Can. J. Vet. Res.,* 50, 68–73, 1986.

112. **Redman, C. W. G. and Sargent, I. L.,** Immunological disorders of human pregnancy, *Oxford Rev. Reprod. Biol.,* 8, 223–266, 1986.

113. **Reed, G. B., Bain, M. D., and Voland, J.,** Overview of antenatal and neonatal period, in *Diseases of the Fetus and Newborn*, Reed, G. B., Claireux, A. E., and Bain, A. D., Eds., Chapman and Hall, London, 1989, 3–39.

114. **Reider, R. F. and Thomas, L.,** Studies of the mechanisms involved in the production of abortion by endotoxin, *J. Immunol.,* 84, 189–193, 1960.

115. **Reznikoff-Etievant, M.-F.,** Immunology of abortions, *Reprod. Nutr. Dev.,* 28, 1615–1629, 1988.

116. **Riggio, R. R., Haschemeyer, R., Cheigh, J., Suthanthiran, M., Tapia, L., Stubenbord, W., and Stenzel, K. H.,** Enhanced allograft survival rates with the adjunctive use of a pregnancy serum derivative—past experience and proposed use with cyclosporine, *Transplant. Proc.,* 17, 2760–2763, 1985.

117. **Rocklin, R. E., Kitzmiller, J., and Garvoy, M. R.,** Maternal-fetal relation. II. Further characterisation of an immunologic blocking factor that develops during pregnancy, *Clin. Immunol. Immunopathol.,* 22, 305–315, 1982.

118. **Roe, R. and Bell, S.,** Humoral immune responses in murine pregnancy. II. Kinetics and nature of the response in females preimmunized against paternal alloantigens, *Immunology,* 46, 23–31, 1982.

119. **Rossant, J. and Frels, W. I.,** Interspecific chimeras in mammals: successful production of live chimeras between Mus musculus and Mus caroli, *Science,* 208, 419–421, 1980.

119a. **Rossant, J., Croy, B. A., Clark, D. A., and Chapman, V. M.,** Interspecific hybrids and chimeras in mice, *J. Exp. Zool.,* 228, 223–233, 1983.

120. **Rote, N. S., Dostaljohnson, D., and Branch, D. W.,** Anti-phospholipid antibodies and recurrent pregnancy loss: correlation between the activated partial thromboplastin time and antibodies against phosphatidylserine and cardiolipin, *Am. J. Obstet. Gynecol.,* 163, 575–584, 1990.

121. **Salat-Baroux, J.,** Recurrent spontaneous abortion, *Reprod. Nutr. Dev.,* 28, 1555–1569, 1988.

122. **Scodras, J. M., Parhar, R. S., Kennedy, T. G., and Lala, P. K.,** Prostaglandin-mediated inactivation of natural killer cells in the murine decidua, *Cell. Immunol.,* 127, 352–367, 1990.

123. **Shalaby, M. R., Laegreid, W. W., Ammann, A. J., and Liggit, H. D.,** Tumor necrosis factor-alpha-associated uterine endothelial injury *in vivo:* influence of dietary fat, *Lab. Invest.,* 61, 564–571, 1989.

124. **Silen, M. L., Firpo, A., Morgello, S., Lowry, S. F., and Francus, T.,** Interleukin-1 alpha and tumor necrosis factor alpha cause placental injury in the rat, *Am. J. Pathol.,* 135, 239–244, 1989.

125. **Simpson, J. L.,** Incidence and timing of pregnancy losses—relevance to evaluating safety of early pregnatal diagnosis, *Am. J. Med. Genet.,* 35, 165–173, 1990.

126. **Sitrukware, R., Thalabard, J. C., Deplunkett, T. L., Lewin, F., Epelboin, S., Mowszowicz, I., Yaneva, H., Tournaire, M., Chavinie, J., Mauvais-jarvis, P., and Spitz, I. M.,** The use of the antiprogestin Ru486 (Mifedpristone)—as an abortifacient in early pregnancy—clinical and pathological findings—predictive factors for efficacy, *Contraception,* 41, 221–243, 1990.

127. **Slapsys, R. and Clark, D. A.,** Active suppression of host versus graft reaction in pregnant mice. V. Kinetics, specificity and *in vivo* activity of non-T suppressor cells localized to the genital tract of mice during first pregnancy, *Am. J. Reprod. Immunol.,* 3, 65–71, 1983.

128. **Slungaard, A., Vercellotti, G. M., Walker, G., Nelson, R. D., and Jacob, H. S.,** Tumor necrosis factor-alpha-cachectin stimulates eosinophil oxidant production and toxicity towards human endothelium, *J. Exp. Med.,* 171, 2025–2041, 1990.

128a. **Smith, J. B. and Cowchock, F. S.,** Immunological studies in recurrent spontaneous abortion: effects of immunization of women with paternal mononuclear cells on lymphocytotoxic and mixed lymphocyte reaction blocking antibodies and correlation with sharing of HLA and pregnancy outcome, *J. Reprod. Immunol.,* 14, 99–115, 1988.

129. **Somell, C. and Olund, A.,** Induction of abortion in early pregnancy with Mifepristone, *Gynecol. Obstet. Invest.,* 29, 13–15, 1990.

129a. **Stabile, I., Campbell, S., and Grudzinskas, J. G.,** Ultrasonic assessment of complications during first trimester of pregnancy, *Lancet,* 2, 1237–1240, 1987.

130. **Stewart, I. and Mukhtar, D. D. Y.,** The killing of mouse trophoblast cells by granulated metrial gland cells *in vitro, Placenta,* 9, 417–427, 1988.

131. **Surani, M. A. H., Barton, S. C., and Norris, M. L.,** Development of reconstituted mouse eggs suggests imprinting of the genome during gametogenesis, *Nature,* 308, 548–550, 1984.

132. **Surani, M. A. H., Barton, S. C., Howlett, S. K., and Norris, M. L.,** Influence of chromosomal determinants on development of androgenetic and parthenogenetic cells, *Development,* 103, 171–178, 1988.

133. **Sussman, M. S. and Bulkley, G. B.,** Oxygen derived free radicals in reperfusion injury, *Meth. Enzymol.,* 186, 711–723, 1990.

134. **Szekeres-Bartho, J., Kilar, F., Falkay, G., Csernus, V., Torok, A., and Pacsa, A. S.,** The mechanism of the inhibitory effect of progesterone on lymphocyte cytotoxicity. I. Progesterone-treated lymphocytes release a substance inhibiting cytotoxicity and prostaglandin synthesis, *Am. J. Reprod. Immunol. Microbiol.,* 9, 15–19, 1985.

135. **Szekeres-Bartho, J., Chaouat, G., and Kinsky, R.,** A progesterone-induced blocking factor corrects high resorption rates in mice treated with antiprogesterone, *Am. J. Obstet. Gynecol.,* 163, 1320–1322, 1990.

136. **Szekeres-Bartho, J., and Chaouat, G.,** Lymphocyte-derived progesterone-induced blocking factor corrects resorption in a murine abortion system, *Am. J. Reprod. Immunol.,* 23, 26–28, 1990.
137. **Takakuwa, K., Goto, S., Hasegawa, I., Ueda, H., Kanazawa, K., Takeuchi, S., and Tanaka, K.,** Result of immunotherapy on patients with unexplained recurrent abortion—a beneficial treatment for patients with negative blocking antibodies, *Am. J. Reprod. Immunol.,* 23, 37–41, 1990.
138. **Tartakovsky, B. and Gorelik, E.,** Immunization with a syngeneic regressor tumor causes resorption in allo-pregnant mice, *J. Reprod. Immunol.,* 13, 113–123, 1988.
139. **Tartakovsky, B.,** CSF-1 Induces resorption of embryos in mice, *Immunol. Lett.,* 23, 65–69, 1989.
140. **Thaler, C. J. and McIntyre, J. A.,** Fetal wastage and nonrecognition in human pregnancy, *Immunol. Allergy Clin. North Am.,* 10, 79–102, 1990.
141. **van Oers, N. S. C., Cohen, B. L., and Murgita, R. A.,** Isolation and characterization of a distinct immunoregulatory isoform of alpha-fetoprotein produced by the normal fetus, *J. Exp. Med.,* 170, 811–827, 1989.
142. **Varga, P. J., Szereday, Z., Artner, A., and Szekeres-Bartho, J.,** Early pregnancy loss, premature and low birth weight delivery, and increased maternal lymphocyte cytotoxicity, *Am. J. Reprod. Immunol.,* 19, 136–140, 1989.
143. **VonSonntag, C. and Schuchmann, H. P.,** Radical mediated DNA damage in presence of oxygen, *Meth. Enzymol.,* 186, 511–520, 1990.
144. **Voth, R., Storch, E., Huller, K., and Kirchner, H.,** Activation of cytotoxic activity in cultures of bone marrow derived macrophages by indomethacin, *Eur. J. Immunol.,* 17, 145–148, 1987.
145. **Warburton, D. and Byrne, J.,** Estimation of the prevalence of chromosomal anomalies expressed in chorionic villus samples processed, *Clin. Biochem. Anal.,* 21, 23–30, 1986.
146. **Warburton, D.,** Chromosomal causes of fetal death, *Clin. Obstet. Gynecol.,* 30, 268–277, 1987.
147. **Warner, C. M., Brownwell, M. S., and Ewoldsen, M. A.,** Why aren't embryos immunologically rejected by their mothers?, *Biol. Reprod.,* 38, 17–31, 1988.
148. **Warner, S. J. C. and Libby, P.,** Human vascular smooth muscle cells: target for and source of tumor necrosis factor, *J. Immunol.,* 142, 100–110, 1989.
149. **Wegmann, T. G.,** Placental immunotropism: maternal T cells enhance placental growth and function, *Am. J. Reprod. Immunol. Microbiol.,* 15, 67–71, 1987.
150. **Wegmann, T. G.,** The cytokine basis for cross-talk between the maternal immune and reproductive systems, *Curr. Opinion Immunol.,* 2, 765–769, 1990.
151. **Wiktor-Jedrzejczak, W., Bartocci, A., Ferrante, A. W., Ahmed-Ansari, A., Sell, K. W., Pollard, J. W., and Stanley, E. R.,** Total absence of colony stimulating factor 1 in the macrophage deficient osteopetrotic (op/op) mouse, *Proc. Natl. Acad. Sci. U.S.A.,* 87, 4828–4832, 1990.
152. **Wilcox, A. J. Weinberg, C. R., O'Connor, J. F., Baird, D. D., Schlatterer, J. P., Canfield, R. E., Armstrong, E. G., and Nisula, B. C.,** Incidence of early loss of pregnancy, *New Engl. J. Med.,* 319, 189–194, 1988.

153. **Zahl, P. A. and Bjerknes, C.,** Induction of decidual placental hemorrhage in mice by the endotoxins in certain Gram negative bacteria, *Proc. Soc. Exp. Biol. Med.,* 54, 329–332, 1943.

154. **Zuckerman, F. A. and Head, J. R.,** Murine trophoblast resists cell-mediated lysis. I. Resistance to allospecific cytotoxic T lymphocytes, *J. Immunol.,* 139, 2856–2865, 1987.

155. **Zuckermann, F. A. and Head, J. R.,** Murine trophoblast resists cell-mediated lysis. II. Resistance to natural cell-mediated cytotoxicity, *Cell. Immunol.,* 116, 274–287, 1988.

156. **Baines, M. G.,** unpublished data.

Chapter

13

The Immunology of Preeclampsia

C. W. G. Redman and I. L. Sargent
Nuffield Department of Obstetrics and Gynaecology
John Radcliffe Hospital
Oxford, England

1. THE CLINICAL FEATURES OF ECLAMPSIA AND PREECLAMPSIA

Preeclampsia is a common and dangerous complication of human pregnancy. It remains the most important cause of maternal death in many westernized countries. Eclampsia is distinguished from preeclampsia by the additional complication of maternal *grand-mal* seizures. Although the problems become clinically apparent only in the second half of pregnancy, during labor, or in the first few days after delivery, it is believed that they originate during the first trimester.

Preeclampsia complicates some cases of hydatidiform mole[35,136,165] where the uterus contains only disordered placental tissue. Thus, a fetus is not necessary, only the placenta. The illness always ultimately regresses when the uterus is emptied of placental tissue, which confirms that the placenta is its cause.

Theories that implicated the placenta in the pathogenesis of preeclampsia began to be developed around the beginning of the century[75-77] in relation to the newly discovered process of trophoblast deportation into the maternal circulation,[164] then to that of chorionic villus necrosis secondary to acute placental infarction.[205] The placental theories have been developed by others[89] and it has slowly become clearer that the central process in preeclampsia is a relative insufficiency of the uteroplacental circulation.

Because the primary cause of preeclampsia is unknown (although it is localized to the placenta) the condition is recognized as a syndrome—a cluster of features that occur together. Maternal hypertension and proteinuria are those by which the disease is usually defined, but the syndrome is more extensive, with involvement of the maternal liver, coagulation and nervous systems,[148] and more polymorphic, with considerable variation between cases.

There is also a preeclamptic fetal syndrome, being the consequences of failure of the fetal supply line with secondary intrauterine growth retardation and respiratory insufficiency. Individuals differ in the extent to which the maternal and fetal syndromes are expressed: some may have severe maternal involvement with a relatively normal fetus, others the converse.

By focusing on the placental pathologies that cause the syndrome, we begin to realize that preeclampsia is but one manifestation of a broader group of clinical disorders, all secondary to closely linked, or identical, placental problems, including cases of fetal growth retardation without maternal hypertension and even some cases of early miscarriage.

2. WHY IMMUNE MECHANISMS COULD BE IMPORTANT IN PREECLAMPSIA

The reason why immune mechanisms are invoked to explain the pathogenesis of preeclampsia is that it is primarily a disorder of first pregnancy[120] and a change of partner increases the risk in parous women.[33,46,84] Whereas the first-pregnancy preponderance could have other explanations, the apparent partner specificity, which is still an unconfirmed observation, can be explained only by an immune process. It implies that preeclampsia is a disorder of incompatibility between mother and fetus and arises from deficient maternal immune accommodation to the "fetal allograft".

The current hypothesis depends on the concept of immunoregulation, by postulating that in normal pregnancy the mother develops an obligatory immune response to her genetically incompatible fetus which prevents its otherwise inevitable immune rejection. Previous exposure to alloantigens shared by the fetus is, in this context, deemed to be beneficial. In other words, **preimmunization** is considered to ameliorate the adverse effects of maternal-fetal incompatibility so that the first-pregnancy preponderance of preeclampsia can be explained.

Preimmunization is a central (and contentious) issue concerning the prevention of recurrent spontaneous abortions. In relation to preeclampsia, previous exposure to paternal antigens in a pregnancy ending in induced abortion appears to confer some protection,[167,182] although not everyone can detect this effect.[28] Prior exposure to paternal antigens on sperm may bestow similar protection, because in some studies,[106,122] but not all,[127] the incidence of preeclampsia is higher among women who use barrier methods of contraception. Conception by donor insemination creates the converse situation of little or no prior exposure where the incidence of preeclampsia might be predicted to be unduly high. Unfortunately there are no good controlled studies, although the largest uncontrolled study showed an apparently high incidence of preeclampsia.[132] A previous blood transfusion is also protection.[47]

There are certain atypical presentations of preeclampsia associated with an unusually large trophoblast mass: with hydatidiform mole;[35] placental hydrops;[89] or multiple pregnancy.[120] In these circumstances it is postulated that the immunoregulatory mechanisms of normal pregnancy are overwhelmed by the size of the antigenic load of the placenta, particularly as moles are entirely androgenetic in origin.[97] In other preeclamptic pregnancies, not associated with these factors, overload may result from increased trophoblast deportation—that is, the exfoliation of trophoblast fragments into the maternal circulation.[34,88]

The immune hypotheses for recurrent spontaneous abortion and preeclampsia are essentially the same. An absolute failure of maternal immune regulation would lead to early fetal rejection and abortion. Preeclampsia is presumed to involve a relative failure of the same processes—although pregnancy continues, it is compromised. Inadequate maternal immune adaptation to the conceptus would be more likely in the first than in a later pregnancy, so explaining the first-pregnancy preponderance of preeclampsia.

3. PLACENTAL ISCHEMIA IS A KEY EVENT IN THE DEVELOPMENT OF PREECLAMPSIA

There is no placental lesion that is specific to preeclampsia, but certain changes are more common or extensive than normal—including syncytial sprouts, proliferation of the cytotrophoblast, infarcts,[51] and focal syncytial necrosis with diminished and distorted microvilli.[94]

The common factor for all these features appears to be hypoxia, in that there is evidence that this can stimulate proliferation of cytotrophoblast[52,83,126,195] and the formation of syncytial sprouts,[7] as well as damaging the syncytial microvilli.[121] The most obvious macroscopic features of many preeclamptic placentas are infarcts;[118,201,206] Young[205] thought that they were the cause of eclampsia. However, there is now agreement that there may be infarcts without preeclampsia and, conversely, preeclampsia without infarcts.[118] The infarctions relate directly to occlusions of the maternal spiral arteries.[24,199]

The concept " . . . that a diffuse hypoxia or relative maternal ischemia of the placenta is the proximate or precipitating cause of preeclampsia and of the associated placental dysfunctions"[137] is reinforced by the results of animal experiments.

Spontaneous "toxemias" occur in various animal species, including the guinea pig and sheep,[9,48,166] but they are unlike the human condition. "Preeclampsia" has been reported in a chimpanzee[181] and possible eclampsia in both a gorilla[10] and a chimpanzee,[95] but even in primates there is no equivalent problem that has been clearly defined.

However, hypertension or a preeclamptic-like illness can be induced by surgical restriction of the uteroplacental blood supply in the rabbit,[15,200] dog,[1,61,71,72,109,203] or baboon.[30,78] Whereas some of the reports have proved hard to replicate, the baboon model is convincing because it has been demonstrated by two groups, both of which have shown the induction of renal glomerular endotheliosis which is one of the more characteristic lesions of preeclampsia.[144]

The concept that placental ischemia mediates preeclampsia leads to a two-stage model for its pathogenesis. In the first stage, one or more processes impede the uteroplacental circulation; in the second stage, the fetus and mother develop pathology secondary to the ischemic placenta. The presumed mechanism of the second stage is that one or more factors are released from the ischemic placenta to enter the maternal circulation to cause the maternal illness. Immune processes have been invoked in both stages, although they can only be primary in the first—if these concepts (yet to be proven) are correct.

Two problems affect the spiral arteries in the uteroplacental circulation of the placentas from cases of preeclampsia. The first is deficient placentation; the second is an obstructive lesion called acute atherosis.

3.1. Placentation and Preeclampsia

A key feature of placentation, a process completed during the first half of human pregnancy, is invasion of the spiral arteries by cytotrophoblast. To establish perfusion of the intervillous space, trophoblast must "break in" to, or perforate, the maternal circulation. The spiral arteries are eroded from without as trophoblast cells insinuate themselves into their walls. The invasive trophoblast penetrates to the decidual-myometrial junction by 12 weeks but continues inwards, until about 18 weeks, into the deeper myometrial segments of the arteries.[67] Then, for reasons that are not understood, the process ceases with disappearance of many of the trophoblast cells by term.

Trophoblast infiltration of spiral arteries induces major structural or "physiological" changes in the distal segments of the spiral arteries, which permit the greatly expanded uteroplacental blood flow of the second half of pregnancy.[25] The remodeled segments of the arteries lose all muscular and elastic elements in their walls, and become widely dilated, tortuous fibrous tubes. Within the walls are scattered cytotrophoblast cells, which may in places replace the endothelial lining.[25] Neither the basal arteries nor the placental bed veins show evidence of the same processes.

An important feature in pregnancies that are complicated eventually by preeclampsia is that endovascular migration is inhibited, being restricted to the decidual tips of the spiral arteries. The myometrial segments of the spiral arteries retain their musculoelastic structure, have a smaller caliber and, when examined in placental bed biopsies taken at delivery, are devoid of the usual remnants of infiltrating cytotrophoblast.[26,155]

Similar changes are a feature of some cases of intrauterine growth retardation[41,169] and of abortion.[100] If poor placentation is the primary pathology of preeclampsia, it originates long before there is clinical disease. The inference is that in its most severe form, poor placentation causes abortion, but with less severe problems the pregnancy continues with the later evolution of two syndromes—maternal and fetal, secondary to placental ischemia. This concept suggests a possible link between preeclampsia and spontaneous abortions that are immunologically mediated. It also implies that some cases of intrauterine growth retardation without maternal hypertension, that would not now be labeled as preeclampsia, are in fact different variants of the same disease.

Thus, the first stage of the pathogenesis of preeclampsia is determined by the way in which fetal and maternal tissues coexist, the mutual tolerance which permits the paradoxical survival of the fetal allograft. Clearly, immune mechanisms may have a primary role to play.

3.2. Acute Atherosis

The second defect in the spiral arteries is "acute atherosis", a lesion first defined by Hertig.[69] It begins with focal disruption of the endothelium, proliferation of the modified smooth muscle cells of the intima, and medial necrosis.[154] Intracellular lipid is the main feature of the lesion and affects two cell types—myointimal and macrophage. The affected arteries may become partially or completely blocked.[154,206] The changes begin to regress after delivery and within a few weeks begin to resemble typical atherosclerosis.[206]

The cause of acute atherosis is not known, although it is clear that it is not, as was once thought, a result of maternal hypertension. The lesion is not observed in other hypertensive states, nor does it correlate with the severity or duration of maternal hypertension.[99] Indeed, it is not specific to preeclamptic pregnancies. As does the problem of deficient placentation, it may also underlie some cases of intrauterine growth retardation without maternal hypertension.[41,169]

It is also not exclusively a problem of the second half of pregnancy, the time when it has been most extensively studied. Acute atherosis is found in the arteries from curettings taken at therapeutic or spontaneous abortions, more commonly in primiparous than multiparous women.[117] The relation with parity suggests involvement in the pathogenesis of preeclampsia, but clearly, longitudinal studies are not possible to determine if acute atherosis is in fact a much earlier lesion of the disease than hitherto thought.

Hence, the time course of the evolution of acute atherosis is not clear. That it occurs in the first half of pregnancy suggests that it may be related to placentation. However the infarction and other gross pathology secondary to the obstruction of the spiral arteries are clinically more evident at the end of pregnancy, in the second stage of the disease.

Immunoglobulin and complement components are deposited in the lesions, whereas they are not found in the decidual vessels of normotensive women nor those with chronic hypertension.[103] The immunoglobulin is largely IgG according to one report,[83] IgM according to another,[111] but both agree that the complement components include C3. Similarly, in acute atherosis in the arteries of aborted first- and second-trimester pregnancies there are mural deposits of C3 in primiparous women.[116] These observations have led to the suggestion that acute atherosis is an immunologically mediated lesion.

An early histological feature of acute atherosis is endothelial damage and this may be but one aspect of a more generalized problem because there is evidence of maternal endothelial damage elsewhere: in the characteristic renal lesion of preeclampsia, glomerular endotheliosis,[144] as well as in other vessels.[168] This has led to the hypothesis that the maternal syndrome of preeclampsia results from diffuse endothelial damage[153] and preliminary evidence for a circulating factor toxic to cultured endothelium has been found.[156] The existence of this factor remains to be confirmed and its nature is undefined. The report that preeclampsia is associated with endothelial autoantibodies[147] suggests a possible immune mechanism.

This raises the issue of whether at least some of the manifestations of preeclampsia result from autoimmunity, triggered in some way by the state of pregnancy. It is, however, difficult to suppose that autoimmune processes could be primary, because how could the first-pregnancy preponderance and partner specificity be explained?

4. IN WHICH STAGE OF PREECLAMPSIA MIGHT IMMUNE MECHANISMS OPERATE?

Until the importance of deficient placentation in the genesis of preeclampsia was realized, it was considered that the illness at the end of pregnancy (the second stage) might itself represent a breakdown of immune regulation, with a partial "rejection" of the fetus by the mother. Thus, in many studies, evidence for these disturbances was sought in terms of changes in peripheral blood or by direct examination of the placenta.

However, since it is now known that the disease may result from failure in placentation, the key abnormalities may be developing during the first half of pregnancy. So, it has to be considered what immune mechanisms could be operating at this time and how they can be studied. This presents two problems. First, little is known about what controls placentation in normal gestation. Second, if there is deficient placentation it is clinically inapparent when it develops, so those who have it cannot be distinguished immediately from those who do not; even if they could, the problems in the placenta could not be studied directly without terminating the pregnancy.

Our knowledge of the mechanisms of maternal tolerance of the fetal allograft is rudimentary and that concerning preeclampsia is virtually confined to facts about its inheritance and some data concerning the relevance of the HLA system which, for obvious reasons, should play a central role in the immune relations between mother and fetus.

5. GENETIC FACTORS AND MATERNAL-FETAL INCOMPATIBILITY

Preeclampsia runs in families and its occurrence can be explained by postulating a recessive maternal gene with an estimated population frequency of about 25%.[32,37] Since the disorder may be partner-specific, paternally derived gene products should be relevant as with rhesus disease; but the familial pattern does not exclude a paternal contribution because the complex genetics of maternal/fetal incompatibility disorders can, under some conditions, simulate straightforward maternal inheritance.[139]

The observation of an exceptionally high incidence of preeclampsia in an inbred family[23] might be explained by the operation of the putative recessive preeclampsia gene, but could otherwise result from increased histocompatibility between partners, as with recurrent abortion.

Results of other studies do not contribute to a consistent picture. Less, not more, preeclampsia has been noted in an inbred community in Turkey.[178] It has also been suggested that preeclampsia is more likely with male than female fetuses[194] and with dizygous rather than monozygous twin pregnancies,[177] pointing to excessive maternal-fetal incompatibility as a contributory factor. Neither of these observations has been confirmed in later studies.[96,125] Preeclampsia is not associated with blood group ABO incompatibilities.[66,138]

6. PREECLAMPSIA AND THE HLA SYSTEM

There are a number of loosely related issues. First, is HLA incompatibility (or compatibility) one of the factors in a disturbed immune relationship between mother and fetus that causes or predisposes to preeclampsia? Second, how is fetal HLA expressed on the tissue that matters—namely, the fetal trophoblast—that is exposed to the maternal immune system? Third, is one or more of the maternal genes causing preeclampsia located in the major histocompatibility complex (MHC) on chromosome 6, so that the familial occurrence of preeclampsia is HLA linked?

Excessive HLA compatibility between partners has been considered to underlie immunologically mediated recurrent abortions,[55] although it is not consistently observed, a topic which has been previously reviewed.[150] The same association has been claimed in preeclamptic couples,[19,90] although others cannot confirm the finding.[92] Recently, preeclampsia has been associated with increased maternal-fetal sharing of HLA-DR4,[101] which has reactivated the concept.

An excess of HLA homozygosity, particularly at the B locus[151] was also not confirmed,[92] although a similar pattern was reported in women with recurrent spontaneous abortions.[93] If the association were real it would have the effect of reducing incompatibility between mother and fetus without increasing the degree of antigen sharing.

The emphasis on HLA incompatibility as a possible determinant of success of the fetal allograft is historical rather than logical—the concept arising from the belief that the fetal allograft should be like other allografts. In fact, the engrafted tissue is trophoblast which does not express HLA-A, -B, -C, or -D, the polymorphic strong histocompatibility determinants. Instead, some forms of trophoblast, particularly those in direct contact with maternal tissues rather than blood, express a novel monomorphic HLA antigen—HLA-G.[44] HLA-G has no known function, immune or otherwise, but, it must be supposed, is involved in some way in interactions with maternal cells in the decidua.

The absence of HLA on syncytiotrophoblast, the fetal tissue forming the major interface with the mother, precludes the possibility that maternal T cells, cytotoxic or helper, can respond directly to trophoblast (reviewed elsewhere[152]). This explains why maternal sensitization to fetal HLA is a sporadic event,[162] possibly the result of random breaks in the integrity of the syncytiotrophoblast either temporarily exposing underlying placental stromal cells or permitting small feto-maternal bleeds, known to provoke rhesus sensitization. The lack of classical HLA may increase the susceptibility of trophoblast to nonadaptive immunity, for example, mediated by natural killer (NK) cells,[119] and HLA-G may provide a neutral signal that suppresses NK activity as class I MHC antigen expression seems to do.

Third, HLA may be a marker for closely linked genes which predispose to, or cause, preeclampsia and account for its familial incidence. Although preeclampsia has been associated with HLA-DR4,[101,171] the converse finding of a significant **negative** association with preeclampsia has also been reported.[73] More recently, analysis of the restriction fragment length polymorphisms of HLA DR beta in informative pedigrees[202] has shown that the putative preeclampsia gene(s) are not HLA linked.

In summary, there is little consistent evidence that HLA genes are involved in preeclampsia, although maternal-fetal incompatibility could still be relevant. HLA antigens are not the only determinants of immune reactivity, so there is still the need to define more closely how the maternal immune system recognizes and responds to the fetus in normal pregnancy, as well as those destined to be complicated by preeclampsia.

Virtually all of the rest of our knowledge of immune disturbances in preeclampsia relates to the second stage of disease, in particular, to changes in peripheral blood cells, immunoglobulins, and the complement system. However, before these are summarized, it is appropriate (in relation to a placental disease) to consider whether the histopathology of the placentas of preeclamptic women suggests immunological disturbances.

7. IMMUNE CAUSES FOR THE PLACENTAL PATHOLOGY

The concepts so far discussed would lead to the expectation that at delivery the placenta of a preeclamptic women would show features more of ischemia than immunologically mediated processes. This is, in general, the case, although some reports seek to emphasize the possibility that immune damage is occurring in the placenta during the second stage of the illness.

Preeclamptic placentas contain more intense deposits of C1q, C3d, and C9, distributed in the same way as in normal placentas: patchily in the larger fetal stem vessels (C1q and C9); or focally in the trophoblast basement membrane (C3d and C9). There are no differences in the amount or distribution of C4 and C6.[172] A quantitative rather than qualitative difference in distribution was also seen using an antibody detecting C9 bound to the cytolytic terminal complement complex.[188] These observations provide some evidence for an inflammatory process, but none that it is immunologically mediated. It could still be the result, for example, of ischemic tissue damage.

There is more evidence of a possible immune process in the lesion of chronic villitis of unknown origin.[6] The tertiary and terminal villi are infiltrated with a mixture predominantly of histiocytes and lymphocytes, among which there may also be fibroblasts, polymorphonuclear leukocytes, plasma cells, and multinucleate giant cells. All of one villus, or a cluster of villi, are diffusely involved; there may be secondary obliterative vasculitis of the fetal vessels and perivillous deposition of fibrin occluding the intervillous space. In a proportion of cases, the intervillous space may also contain inflammatory cells and the decidua, focal lymphocytic infiltrates.[159]

Although the problem is associated with preeclampsia,[112,158] it has been more closely linked to intrauterine growth retardation.[5,53,113] Since it is one of the theses of this chapter that both clinical syndromes may be separate consequences of a single, primary placental disturbance, this need not be evidence that the villitis is merely an inconstantly associated feature. Nevertheless, it is questioned that the associations with preeclampsia or intrauterine growth retardation exist at all,[108] and on the present evidence it is hard to conclude that this sort of lesion demonstrates that a disturbance of maternal immune tolerance of the placenta underlies preeclampsia. Thus, although the processes affecting the maternal spiral arteries may have immune origins, there is little convincing evidence of direct immune pathology in the placenta.

Most of the changes in peripheral blood components in preeclampsia were sought in relation to the concept that the second stage of the illness is immunologically mediated. This does not fit the model being presented here. If the placental ischemia theory is correct then any changes detected would be secondary, perhaps contributing to the total pathology but not essential for its initiation. However, the observations concerning peripheral blood leukocytes, immunoglobulins, and complement components will be briefly examined.

7.1. Peripheral Blood Leukocytes

During normal pregnancy, there is a significant leukocytosis, owing mainly to an increased number of neutrophils,[21,142] but also of monocytes.[143] The absolute numbers of lymphocytes, particularly T cells, are either unchanged[36,38,143] or reduced slightly.[27,129,175,185] Although some have suggested that normal pregnancy is associated with a relative reduction of CD4[+] helper T cells,[175,197] this has not been confirmed.[31,129,185]

In preeclampsia the composition of peripheral blood leukocytes is largely unchanged. No consistent pattern emerges from various reports. There have been suggestions that the proportion of T cells is reduced,[176] and that of T-helper cells is increased,[130] or, conversely, reduced;[13] the numbers of monocytes have been reported to be increased[60,176]—but not in all studies.[130]

7.2. Maternal Cell-Mediated Immunity in Preeclampsia

There is also no clear evidence that immune cell function is altered in peripheral blood. At first, evidence of maternal sensitization to paternal or fetal HLA was sought with the hypothesis that preeclampsia resulted from alloimmune rejection of the conceptus. Abnormal sensitization was found in three studies: measuring leukocyte migration inhibitory factor (LIF) production after culture with pooled placental antigen;[192] in 6-d mixed lymphocyte reactions (MLR) with paternal cells;[65] and in phytohemagglutin-stimulated coculture of maternal and fetal cells.[56] In contrast, depressed one-way MLR between maternal and paternal or fetal cells[90] or normal two-way responses[39] were also reported. We reexamined the question by determining the time courses of the maternal-paternal one-way MLR.[161] No evidence for maternal sensitization was found in the immediate postpartum period, and in particular there were no paternal-specific cytotoxic cells.[149] However, we observed an unpredicted and unexplained suppression, in the control reciprocal culture, of the paternal response to maternal stimulator cells. Comparable suppression was not seen when paternal cells were stimulated by the cells of an HLA-identical nonpregnant sister of the preeclamptic spouse. Thus, the pattern was a feature of the pregnancy, not of the preeclamptic woman's tissue type. This was confirmed by reversion to normal, 6 months later. Thus, abnormal maternal immune cell reactivity specific for preeclampsia can be demonstrated, but the mechanisms and significance remain obscure.

There has been one report of significant increases in serum interleukin 2 concentrations in preeclampsia interpreted as evidence for maternal immune cell stimulation by fetal alloantigens.[184] Another, of increased but otherwise undefined mitogenic activity, measured with fibroblasts, has been presented as possible evidence for maternal endothelial cell damage, perhaps secondary to increased release of platelet-derived growth factor, a product of endothelium as well as platelets.[131]

Studies of peripheral blood NK cell activity have yielded conflicting results. Significantly increased,[193] unchanged,[70,133] or decreased[2] activities have been reported in preeclampsia.

7.3. Polymorphonuclear Cell Function in Normal and Preeclamptic Pregnancies

Not only are the numbers of peripheral blood neutrophils increased during normal pregnancy, but their functions are altered. Phagocytosis of latex particles[110] or opsonized zymosan[170] is increased when assessed by chemiluminescence which measures the production of certain free radicals derived from oxygen, stimulated by phagocytosis; but that of candida is unaltered when assessed visually.[43] There is significantly greater metabolic activation, in terms of glucose oxidation, during phagocytosis by leukocytes from pregnant than from nonpregnant women.[128]

Spontaneous migration in autologous plasma is also enhanced in pregnancy relative to nonpregnant controls[58] or in the postpartum period.[135]

Whereas neutrophil function appears to be enhanced during pregnancy, there is further evidence that neutrophils are inhibited in the presence of pregnancy sera or plasmas. For example, the sera of pregnant women have been reported to inhibit bacterial killing[18] by granulocytes from nonpregnant donors, or phagocytosis.[140] However, not all the reports are consistent, and pregnancy sera have also been shown to increase the phagocytosis of immune complexes.[157]

There are no reports of altered granulocyte counts in preeclampsia, but it has been proposed that the neutrophils are abnormally activated.[59] This concept is based on the observation that, although neutrophil elastase immunoreactivity in peripheral blood plasma is increased in normal pregnancy, it is significantly higher in preeclampsia, but not in proportion to the clinical grading of the condition. The same authors suggest that neutrophil activation could lead to endothelial damage, the putative mechanism of end-stage preeclampsia suggested by Roberts et al.[153]

7.4. Serum Immunoglobulins

Normal pregnancy is associated with reduced serum concentrations of IgG and IgA,[14,173,183] but increases in IgD.[105,114,183] Serum IgM concentrations have been reported to fall during the second trimester but return to normal levels toward term,[16] but others have not confirmed this pattern.[173,183]

The glycosylation of immunoglobulins alters in pregnancy. A higher proportion of the serum IgG is asymmetrically glycosylated on one of the two Fab chains, which hinders antigen binding sterically, and makes the antibody functionally monovalent. Such asymmetric antibodies would act as blocking antibodies if they had antipaternal activity.[20]

Maternal serum concentrations of IgG but not IgA are significantly reduced in preeclampsia.[14,183] The pattern with respect to IgM is inconsistent, but its concentration is unaccountably increased in the cord sera of infants born to preeclamptic or eclamptic women.[204] There are single reports of significantly reduced IgD[183] and increased IgE[4] concentrations in preeclamptic sera. The fall in IgG has been ascribed to losses in urine associated with proteinuria,[183] but this cannot account for the different patterns of changes in serum IgA and IgE. A full explanation of the mechanisms and relevance of what is observed has yet to be given.

7.5. HLA Antibodies

The hypothesis that lymphocytotoxic HLA antibodies might stimulate rejection of the fetal allograft is now known to be inappropriate; but the functions of maternal HLA antibodies as blocking antibodies have been emphasized, and an absolute or relative deficiency postulated when pregnancy fails, such as with recurrent abortions or preeclampsia. Most investigators have examined the occurrence of lymphocytotoxic antibodies, rather than B cell antibodies or noncomplement fixing antibodies. In preeclampsia, increased,[29,191] unchanged,[49,68] or reduced[91] levels have been reported. In only one study have HLA-DR antibodies been examined,[11] showing no differences between preeclamptic and normal women. It is most probable that these antibodies are formed sporadically, as a result of fetomaternal bleeding, usually at delivery, and have no significance. They do not affect the fetus for two reasons: because trophoblast does not express the relevant HLA antigens and because after they are transported across the trophoblast barrier, they are absorbed within the "placental sponge".[42,85]

7.6. Other Antibodies

Since HLA antibodies are not involved, abnormal antibodies generated directly against trophoblast or other components of the placenta have been sought as evidence of a breakdown of immune homeostasis. If present, they could generate circulating immune complexes which might account for some of the features of preeclampsia, or render trophoblast cells susceptible to lysis by K cells. Such antibodies have been detected but none of the reports has been confirmed. For example, preeclampsia has been associated with maternal antibodies to placental polysaccharides,[98] to a placental microsomal fraction,[54] to trophoblast cells,[81,115] to retroviral antigens contained within the placenta,[189] or to placental basement membrane.[17]

An alternative approach is that at least some aspects of the preeclampsia syndrome may be caused by autoantibodies. It is well known, for example, that autoimmunity is a predisposing factor particularly when associated with systemic lupus erythematosus and either the lupus anticoagulant or antiphospholipid antibodies,[22] although such antibodies are not found in the majority of cases.[186] It has already been mentioned that anti-endothelial autoantibodies have also been detected significantly more often than normal in preeclampsia,[147] but whether this is primary or secondary is unknown. An increased prevalence of autoantibodies to laminin,[50] smooth muscle,[4] or platelets[160] in preeclamptic women has also been reported.

7.7. Immune Complexes in Preeclampsia

Circulating immune complexes may activate blocking or aggressive immune mechanisms and their possible presence in the blood of either normal or preeclamptic pregnant women is therefore of some interest. Unfortunately, there is no agreement between different investigators on this issue. Many cannot detect immune complexes in either normal or preeclamptic sera.[12,57,107,146] However, increased levels in normal pregnancy sera compared with nonpregnant controls[124] or in preeclamptic sera compared with normal pregnant controls[3,134,163,179,180,198] have been claimed. In preeclampsia deposits of immune complexes have been found in skin[80] and renal biopsies,[141,196] but the renal histology is not consistent, nor comparable to that seen in unequivocal immune complex disease.[102,174] Likewise, changes in the complement system do not suggest activation, as would be expected with immune complex disorders.

7.8. The Complement System

Changes in the serum concentrations of components of the complement system would be expected in an illness with highly disturbed coagulation function and diffuse endothelial dysfunction. Total hemolytic complement and C1q concentrations remain unchanged.[45,104,145,187] Plasma C3 concentrations are normal[204] or increased[190] and there are increases in the products of its activity—C3a and C5a.[62] The plasma concentration of C3D—the other main product of C3 activity—may[123] or may not[8] be increased, depending on who you believe. This may depend on the severity of the illness at the time when the measurements are made; in women with the HELLP syndrome—an acute terminal presentation of preeclampsia with disseminated intravascular coagulation, microangiopathic hemolysis, and widespread organ dysfunction, particularly involving the liver—not only are the plasma concentrations of anaphylatoxins (C3a/C3a desArg and C5a/C5a desArg) significantly higher than normal, but those of terminal C5b-9 complement complexes are increased at the time of delivery relative to one and seven days later; this indicates that the terminal part of the complement cascade has been activated.[63] However, the changes do not precede the onset of the clinical syndrome.[64] Serum concentrations of C4 are reduced relative to normal,[74,79] as they are in conditions such as active lupus erythematosus, but not to the same extent except in exceptional cases, but once again not all investigators find this change.[134] It may or may not be relevant that the activity of the enzyme, kininase I, which inactivates the anaphylotoxins C3a, C4a, and C5a is increased in the sera of preeclamptic women;[87] the enzyme may be of placental origin.[86] Clearly, more detailed investigation is needed.

8. SUMMARY

The first-pregnancy preponderance and apparent partner specificity of preeclampsia suggest that it might have an immune etiology. The pathogenesis of preeclampsia is undefined, although it is clear that it is a placental disorder. The maternal syndrome appears to be mediated by placental ischemia secondary to spiral artery insufficiency. This leads to a hypothesis that preeclampsia is a two-stage disease. The first comprises processes that limit the size of the spiral arteries (poor placentation) or obstruct them (acute atherosis). Either or both may have immunological causes, although there is no direct evidence. Factors limiting placentation could involve maternal immune intolerance of the fetal allograft, which in their most extreme expression could lead to immunologically mediated abortion. Thus, preeclampsia may be part of a wider spectrum of pregnancy loss secondary to poor maternal immune accommodation of the genetically disparate fetus.

The second stage involves the consequences of the ensuing placental ischemia. The syndrome is currently tentatively ascribed to diffuse maternal endothelial dysfunction. There is less reason to invoke immunological mechanisms in the second stage although neutrophil activation could explain generalized endothelial damage.

It should be clear that these conclusions are provisional and that the greatest need is for more investigation to eliminate the uncertainty that clouds our concepts.

REFERENCES

1. **Abitbol, M. M.,** Production of experimental toxemia in the pregnant dog, *Obstet. Gynecol.,* 48, 537–548, 1976.
2. **Alanen, A. and Lassila, O.,** Deficient natural killer cell function in preeclampsia, *Obstet. Gynecol.,* 60, 631–634, 1982.
3. **Alanen, A., Kekomaki, R., Kero, P., Lindstrom, P., and Wager, O.,** Circulating immune complexes in hypertensive disorders of pregnancy, *J. Reprod. Immunol.,* 6, 133–140, 1984.
4. **Alanen, A.,** Serum IgE and smooth muscle antibodies in preeclampsia, *Acta Obstet. Gynaecol. Scand.,* 63, 581–582, 1984.
5. **Altshuler, G., Russell, P., and Ermocilla, R.,** The placental pathology of small-for-gestational age infants, *Am. J. Obstet. Gynecol.,* 121, 351–359, 1975.
6. **Altshuler, G. and Russell, P.,** The human placental villitides: a review of chronic intrauterine infection, *Curr. Topics Pathol.,* 60, 63–112, 1975.
7. **Alvarez, H., Medrano, C. V., Sala, M. A., and Benedetti, W. J.,** Trophoblast development gradient and its relationship to placental hemodynamics, *Am. J. Obstet. Gynecol.,* 114, 873–878, 1972.
8. **Armstrong, N. P. I., Teisner, B., Redman, C. W. G., Westergaard, J. G., Folkersen, J., and Grudzinkas, J. G.,** Complement activation, circulating protease inhibitors and pregnancy-associated proteins in severe pre-eclampsia, *Br. J. Obstet. Gynaecol.,* 93, 811–814, 1986.
9. **Assali, N. S., Longo, L. D., and Holm, L. W.,** Toxemia-like syndromes in animals: spontaneous and experimental, *Obstet. Gynecol. Surv.,* 15, 151–181, 1960.
10. **Baird, J. N.,** Eclampsia in a lowland gorilla, *Am. J. Obstet. Gynecol.,* 141, 345–346, 1981.
11. **Balasch, J., Ercilla, G., Vanrell, J. A., Vives, J., and Gonzalez-Merlo, J.,** Effects of HLA antibodies on pregnancy, *Obstet. Gynecol.,* 57, 444–446, 1981.
12. **Balasch, J., Mirapeix, E., Borche, L., Vives, J., and Gonzalez-Merlo, J.,** Further evidence against preeclampsia as an immune complex disease, *Obstet. Gynecol.,* 58, 435–437, 1981.
13. **Bardeguez, A. D., McNerney, R., Frieri, M., Verma, U. L., and Tejani, N.,** Cellular immunity in preeclampsia: alterations in T-lymphocyte subpopulations during early pregnancy, *Obstet. Gynecol.,* 77, 859–862, 1991.
14. **Benster, B. and Wood, E. J.,** Immunoglobulin levels in normal pregnancy and pregnancy complicated by hypertension, *J. Obstet. Gynaecol. Br. Commonw.,* 77, 518–522, 1970.
15. **Berger, M. and Boucek, R. J.,** Irreversible uterine and renal changes induced by placental ischemia (rabbit), *Am. J. Obstet. Gynecol.,* 89, 230–240, 1964.
16. **Best, J. M., Bannatvala, J. E., and Watson, D.,** Serum IgM and IgG responses in postnatally acquired rubella, *Lancet,* ii, 65–68, 1969.
17. **Bieglmayer, C., Rudelstorfer, R., Bartl, W., and Janisch, H.,** Detection of antibodies in pregnancy serum reacting with isolated placental basement membrane collagen, *Br. J. Obstet. Gynaecol.,* 93, 815–822, 1986.

18. **Bjorksten, B., Soderstrom, T., Damber, M. G., Schoultz, B., and Stigbrand, T.,** Polymorphonuclear leukocyte function during pregnancy, *Scand. J. Immunol.,* 8, 257–262, 1978.

19. **Bolis, P. F., Bianchi, M. M., La Fianza, A., Franchi, M., and Belvedere, M. C.,** Immunogenetic aspects of pre-eclampsia, *Biol. Res. Prog.,* 8, 42–45, 1987.

20. **Borel, I., Gentile, T., Angelucci, J., Pividori, J., Guala, M. del C., Binaghi, R. A., and Margni, R. A.,** IgG asymmetric molecules with anti-paternal activity isolated from sera and placenta of pregnant human, *J. Reprod. Immunol.,* 20, 129–140, 1991.

21. **Brain, P., Marston, R. H., and Gordon, J.,** Immunological responses in pregnancy, *Br. Med. J.,* 4, 468, 1972.

22. **Branch, D. W., Andres, R., Digre, K. B., Rote, N. S., and Scott, J. R.,** The association of antiphospholipid antibodies with severe preeclampsia, *Obstet. Gynecol.,* 73, 541–545, 1989.

23. **Brocklehurst, J. C. and Ross, R.,** Familial eclampsia, *J. Obstet. Gynaecol. Br. Emp.,* 67, 971–974, 1960.

24. **Brosens, I. and Renaer, M.,** On the pathogenesis of placental infarcts in pre-eclampsia, *J. Obstet. Gynaecol. Br. Commonw.,* 79, 794–799, 1972.

25. **Brosens, I., Robertson, W. B., and Dixon, H. G.,** The physiological response of vessels of the placental bed to normal pregnancy, *J. Pathol. Bacteriol.,* 93, 569–579, 1967.

26. **Brosens, I. A., Robertson, W. B., and Dixon, H. G.,** The role of the spiral arteries in the pathogenesis of pre-eclampsia, in *Obstetrics and Gynecology Annual,* Wynn, R. M., Ed., Appleton-Century-Crofts, New York, 177–191, 1972.

27. **Bulmer, R. and Hancock, K. W.,** Depletion of circulating T lymphocytes in pregnancy, *Clin. Exp. Immunol.,* 28, 302–305, 1977.

28. **Campbell, D. M. and MacGillivray, I.,** Pre-eclampsia in second pregnancy, *Br. J. Obstet. Gynaecol.,* 82, 131–140, 1985.

29. **Carretti, N., Chiaramonte, P., Pasini, C., Zanetti, M., and Fagiolo, U.,** Association of anti-HLA antibodies with toxemia in pregnancy, in *Immunology in Obstetrics and Gynecology,* Centaro, A., Carretti, N., and Addison, G. M., Eds., Excerpta Medica, Holland, 1974, 221–225.

30. **Cavanagh, D., Rao, P. S., Tsai, C. C., and O'Connor, T. C.,** Experimental toxemia in the pregnant primate, *Am. J. Obstet. Gynecol.,* 128, 75–85, 1977.

31. **Cheney, R. T., Tomaszewski, J. E., Raab, S. J., Zmijewski, C., and Rowlands, D. T.,** Subpopulations of lymphocytes in maternal peripheral blood during pregnancy, *J. Reprod. Immunol.,* 6, 111–120, 1984.

32. **Chesley, L. C. and Cooper, D. W.,** Genetics of hypertension in pregnancy: possible single gene control of preeclampsia and eclampsia in the descendants of eclamptic women, *Br. J. Obstet. Gynaecol.,* 93, 898–908, 1987.

33. **Chng, P. K.,** Occurrence of pre-eclampsia in pregnancies to three husbands. Case report, *Br. J. Obstet. Gynaecol.,* 89, 862–863, 1982.

34. **Chua, S., Wilkins, T., Sargent, I., and Redman, C.,** Trophoblast deportation in pre-eclamptic pregnancy, *Br. J. Obstet. Gynaecol.,* 98, 973–979, 1991.

35. **Chun, D., Braga, C., Chow, C., and Lok, L.,** Clinical observations on some aspects of hydatidiform moles, *J. Obstet. Gynaecol. Br. Commonw.,* 71, 180–184, 1964.

36. **Clements, P., Yu, D. T. Y., Levy, J., and Pearson, C. M.,** Human lymphocyte subpopulations: the effect of pregnancy, *Proc. Soc. Exp. Biol. Med.,* 152, 664–666, 1976.

37. **Cooper, D. W. and Liston, W. A.,** Genetic control of severe pre-eclampsia, *J. Med. Genet.,* 16, 409–416, 1979.

38. **Cornfield, D. B., Jemcks, J., Binder, R. A., and Rath, C. E.,** T and B lymphocytes in pregnant women, *Obstet. Gynecol.,* 53, 203–206, 1979.

39. **Curzen, P., Jones, E., and Gaugas, J. M.,** Maternal-fetal mixed lymphocyte reactivity in pre-eclampsia, *Br. J. Exp. Pathol.,* 58, 500–503, 1977.

40. **D'Amelio, R., Bilotta, P., Pachi, A., and Aiuti, F.,** Circulating immune complexes in normal pregnant women and in some conditions complicating pregnancy, *Clin. Exp. Immunol.,* 37, 33–37, 1979.

41. **De Wolf, F., Brosens, I., and Renaer, M.,** Fetal growth retardation and the maternal arterial supply of the human placenta in the absence of sustained hypertension, *Br. J. Obstet. Gynaecol.,* 87, 678–685, 1980.

42. **Doughty, R. W. and Gelsthorpe, K.,** Some parameters of lymphocyte antibody activity through pregnancy and further eluates of placental material, *Tissue Antigens,* 8, 43–48, 1976.

43. **El-Maallem, H. and Fletcher, J.,** Impaired neutrophil function in pregnancy, *Br. J. Haematol.,* 44, 375–381, 1980.

44. **Ellis, S.,** HLA G: at the interface, *Am. J. Reprod. Immunol.,* 23, 84–86, 1990.

45. **Fadel, H. E., Soliman, M. D. E., and El-Mehairy, M. M.,** Serum complement activity in pre-eclamptic pregnancies, *Int. J. Gynaecol. Obstet.,* 12, 6–9, 1974.

46. **Feeney, J. G. and Scott, J. S.,** Pre-eclampsia and changed paternity, *Eur. J. Obstet. Gynecol. Reprod. Biol.,* 11, 35–38, 1980.

47. **Feeney, J. G., Tovey, L. A. D., and Scott, J. S.,** Influence of previous blood transfusions on incidence of pre-eclampsia, *Lancet,* i, 874–877, 1977.

48. **Ferris, T. F., Herson, P. B., Dunnill, M. S., and Lee, M. R.,** Toxemia of pregnancy in sheep: a clinical, physiological and pathological study, *J. Clin. Invest.,* 48, 1643–1655, 1969.

49. **Fingleton, A. M.,** Leucocytoxic antibodies and pre-eclampsia of pregnancy, *Transplantation,* 12, 319–321, 1971.

50. **Foidart, J. M., Hunt, J., Lapiere, C.-M., Nusgens, B., De Rycker, C., Bruwier Labotte, R., Bernard, A., and Mahieu, P.,** Antibodies to laminin in preeclampsia, *Kidney Int.,* 29, 1050–1057, 1986.

51. **Fox, H.,** The placenta in maternal disorders, in *Pathology of the Placenta,* W. B. Saunders, London, 1978, 214–222.

52. **Fox, H.,** Effect of hypoxia on trophoblast in organ culture, *Am. J. Obstet. Gynecol.,* 107, 1058–1064, 1970.

53. **Garcia, A. G. P.,** Placental morphology of low-birth-weight infants born term, *Contrib. Gynecol. Obstet.,* 9, 100–112, 1982.

54. **Gaugas, J. M. and Curzen, P.,** Complement fixing antibody against solubilized placental microsomal fraction in pre-eclampsia sera, *Br. J. Pathol.,* 55, 570–573, 1974.

55. **Gill, T. J.,** Immunogenetics of spontaneous abortion in humans, *Transplantation,* 35, 1–6, 1983.

56. **Gille, J., Williams, J. H., and Hoffman, C. P.,** The feto-maternal lymphocyte interaction in pre-eclampsia and in uncomplicated pregnancy, *Eur. J. Obstet. Gynecol. Reprod. Biol.,* 7, 227–238, 1977.

57. **Gleicher, N., Theophilopoulos, A. N., and Beers, P.,** Immune complexes in pregnancy, *Lancet,* ii, 1108, 1978.

58. **Gleicher, N., Beers, P., Kerenyi, T. D., Cohen, C. J., and Gusberg, S. B.,** Leukocyte migration enhancement as an indicator of immunologic enhancement. I. Pregnancy, *Am. J. Obstet. Gynecol.,* 136, 1–4, 1980.

59. **Greer, I. A., Haddad, N. G., Dawes, J., Johnstone, F. D., and Calder, A. A.,** Neutrophil activation in pregnancy-induced hypertension, *Br. J. Obstet. Gynaecol.,* 96, 978–982, 1989.

60. **Gusdon, J. P., Heise, E. R., Quinn, K. J., and Matthews, L. C.,** Lymphocyte subpopulations in normal and preeclampsia pregnancies, *Am. J. Reprod. Immunol.,* 5, 28–31, 1984.

61. **Gyongyossy, A. and Kelentey, B.,** An experimental study of the effect of ischaemia of the pregnant uterus on the blood pressure, *J. Obstet. Gynaecol. Br. Emp.,* 65, 617–624, 1958.

62. **Haeger, M., Bengstson, A., Karlsson, K., and Heideman, M.,** Complement activation and anaphylatoxin (C3a and C5a) formation in preeclampsia and by amniotic fluid, *Obstet. Gynecol.,* 73, 551–556, 1989.

63. **Haeger, M., Unander, M., and Bengtsson, A.,** Enhanced anaphylatoxin and terminal C5b-9 complement complex formation in patients with the syndrome of hemolysis, elevated liver enzymes, and low platelet count, *Obstet. Gynecol.,* 76, 698–702, 1990.

64. **Haeger, M., Unander, M., and Bengtsson, A.,** Complement activation in relation to development of preeclampsia, *Obstet. Gynecol.,* 78, 46–49, 1991.

65. **Halbrecht, I. G. and Komlos, L.,** Mixed wife-husband leukocyte cultures in disturbed and pathological pregnancies, *Isr. J. Med. Sci.,* 10, 1100–1105, 1974.

66. **Harlap, S. and Davies, A. M.,** Maternal blood group A and pre-eclampsia, *Br. Med. J.,* 3, 171–172, 1974.

67. **Harris, J. W. S. and Ramsey, E. M.,** The morphology of human uteroplacental vasculature, *Contrib. Embryol. Carnegie Inst.,* 38, 43–58, 1966.

68. **Harris, R. E. and Lordon, R. E.,** The association of maternal lymphocytotoxic antibodies with obstetric complications, *Obstet. Gynecol.,* 48, 302–304, 1976.

69. **Hertig, A. T.,** Vascular pathology in the hypertensive albuminuric toxemias of pregnancy, *Clinics,* 4, 602–614, 1945.

70. **Hill, J. A., Hsia, S., Doran, D. M., and Bryans, C. I.,** Natural killer cell activity and antibody dependent cell-mediated cytotoxicity in preeclampsia, *J. Reprod. Immunol.,* 9, 205–212, 1986.

71. **Hodari, A. A., Bumpus, F. M., and Smeby, R.,** Renin in experimental "toxemia of pregnancy", *Obstet. Gynecol.,* 30, 8–15, 1967.

72. **Hodgkinson, C. P., Hodari, A. A., and Bumpus, F. M.,** Experimental hypertensive disease of pregnancy, *Obstet. Gynecol.,* 30, 371–380, 1967.

73. **Hoff, C., Stevens, R. G., Mendenhall, H., Peterson, R. D. A., and Spinnato, J. A.,** Association between risk for preeclampsia and HLA DR4, *Lancet,* 335, 660–661, 1990.

74. **Hofmeyr, G. J., Wilkins, T., and Redman, C. W. G.,** C4 And plasma protein in hypertension during pregnancy with and without proteinuria, *Br. Med. J.,* 302, 218, 1991.
75. **Holland, E.,** Recent work on the etiology of eclampsia, *J. Obstet. Gynaecol. Br. Emp.,* 16, 255–273, 1909.
76. **Holland, E.,** Recent work on the etiology of eclampsia. II, *J. Obstet. Gynaecol. Br. Emp.,* 16, 325–337, 1909.
77. **Holland, E.,** Recent work on the etiology of eclampsia. II, *J. Obstet. Gynaecol. Br. Emp.,* 16, 384–400, 1909.
78. **Horvath, J. S., Phippard, A. F., Gillin, A. G., Thompson, J. F., Duggin, G. G., and Tiller, D. J.,** A model of pre-eclampsia, including renal histology, in the baboon (Abstr.), in VII World Congress of Hypertension in Pregnancy, Perugia, Italy, 1990, 88.
79. **Houwert-de Jong, M. H., Claas, F. H. J., Gmelig-Meyling, F. H. J., Kalsbeek, G. L., Valentin, R. M., te Velde, E. R., and Schuurman, H. J.,** Humoral immunity in normal and complicated pregnancy, *J. Reprod. Immunol.,* 19, 205–214, 1985.
80. **Houwert-de Jong, M. H., Te Velde, E. R., Nefkens, M. J. J., and Schuurman, H. J.,** Immune complexes in skin of patient with pre-eclamptic toxaemia, *Lancet,* ii, 387, 1982.
81. **Hulka, J. F. and Brinton, V.,** Antibody to trophoblast during early postpartum period in toxemia pregnancy, *Am. J. Obstet. Gynecol.,* 86, 130–134, 1963.
82. **Hustin, J., Foidart, J. M., and Lambotte, R.,** Maternal vascular lesions in pre-eclampsia and intrauterine growth retardation: light microscopy and immunofluorescence, *Placenta,* 4, 489–498, 1983.
83. **Hustin, J. and Gaspard, U.,** Comparison of histological changes seen in placental tissue cultures and in placentae obtained after fetal death, *Br. J. Obstet. Gynaecol.,* 84, 210–215, 1977.
84. **Ikedife, D.,** Eclampsia in multiparae, *Br. Med. J.,* 280, 985–986, 1980.
85. **Innes, A., Stewart, G. M., Thomson, M. A. R., Cunningham, C., and Catto, G. R. D.,** Human placenta—an antibody sponge?, *Am. J. Reprod. Immunol.,* 17, 57–60, 1988.
86. **Ito, M., Mizutani, S., Kurauchi, O., Kasugai, M., Narita, O., and Tomoda, Y.,** Purification and properties of microsomal carboxypeptidase N (kininase I) in human placenta, *Enzyme,* 42, 8–14, 1989.
87. **Ito, Y., Mizutani, S., Nomura, S., Kurauchi, O., Kasugai, M., Narita, O., and Tomoda, Y.,** Increased serum kininase I activity in pregnancy complicated by pre-eclampsia, *Horm. Metab. Res.,* 22, 252–255, 1990.
88. **Jaameri, K. E. U., Koivuniemi, A. P., and Carpen, E. O.,** Occurrence of trophoblasts in the blood of toxaemic patients, *Gynaecologia,* 160, 315–320, 1965.
89. **Jeffcoate, T. N. A. and Scott, J. S.,** Some observations on the placental factor in pregnancy toxemia, *Am. J. Obstet. Gynecol.,* 77, 475–489, 1959.
90. **Jenkins, D. M., Need, J. A., Scott, J. S., Morris, H., and Pepper, M.,** Human leukocyte antigens and mixed lymphocyte reaction in severe preeclampsia, *Br. Med. J.,* 1, 542–544, 1978.
91. **Jenkins, D. M., Need, J. A., and Rajah, S. M.,** Deficiency of specific HLA antibodies in severe pregnancy pre-eclampsia/eclampsia, *Clin. Exp. Immunol.,* 27, 485–486, 1977.

92. **Johnson, N., Moodley, J., and Hammond, M. G.,** Human leucocyte antigen status in African women with eclampsia, *Br. J. Obstet. Gynaecol.,* 95, 877–879, 1988.
93. **Johnson, P. M., Barnes, R. M., Hart, C. A., and Francis, W. J. A.,** Determinants of immunological responsiveness in recurrent spontaneous abortion, *Transplantation,* 38, 280–284, 1984.
94. **Jones, C. J. P. and Fox, H.,** An ultrastructural and ultrahistochemical study of the human placenta in maternal pre-eclampsia, *Placenta,* 1, 61–76, 1980.
95. **Joy, J. E.,** Pregnancy toxaemia in a multiparous chimpanzee at Dallas zoo, *Int. Zoo Yearb.,* 11, 239–241, 1969.
96. **Juberg, R. C., Gaar, D. G., Humphries, J. R., Cenac, P. L., and Zambie, M. F.,** Sex ratio in the progeny of mothers with toxemia of pregnancy, *J. Reprod. Med.,* 16, 299–302, 1976.
97. **Kajii, T. and Ohama, K.,** Androgenetic origin of hydatidiform mole, *Nature,* 268, 633–634, 1977.
98. **Kaku, M.,** Placental polysaccharide and the aetiology of the toxaemia of pregnancy, *J. Obstet. Gynaecol. Br. Emp.,* 60, 148–156, 1953.
99. **Khong, T. Y., Pearce, J. M., and Robertson, W.,** Acute atherosis in preeclampsia maternal determinants and fetal outcome in the presence of the lesion, *Am. J. Obstet. Gynecol.,* 157, 360–363, 1987.
100. **Khong, T. Y., Liddell, H. S., and Robertson, W. B.,** Defective haemochorial placentation as a cause of miscarriage: a preliminary study, *Br. J. Obstet. Gynaecol.,* 94, 649–655, 1987.
101. **Kilpatrick, D. C., Liston, W. A., Jazwinska, E. C., and Smart, G. E.,** Histocompatibility studies in pre-eclampsia, *Tissue Antigens,* 29, 232–236, 1990.
102. **Kincaid-Smith, P. and Fairley, K. C.,** The differential diagnosis between pre-eclamptic toxemia and glomerulo-nephritis in patients with proteinuria during pregnancy, in *Hypertension in Pregnancy,* Lindheimer, M. D., Katz, A. I., and Zuspan, F. P., Eds., John Wiley & Sons, New York, 1976, 157–168.
103. **Kitzmiller, J. L. and Benirschke, K.,** Immunofluorescent study of placental bed vessels in pre-eclampsia of pregnancy, *Am. J. Obstet. Gynecol.,* 115, 248–251, 1973.
104. **Kitziller, J. L., Stoneburner, L., Yelenosky, P. F., and Lucas, W. E.,** Serum complement in normal pregnancy and pre-eclampsia, *Am. J. Obstet. Gynecol.,* 117, 312–315, 1973.
105. **Klapper, D. G. and Mendenhall, H. W.,** Immunoglobulin D concentration in pregnant women, *J. Immunol.,* 107, 912–915, 1971.
106. **Klonoff-Cohen, H. S., Savitz, D. A., Cefalo, R. C., and McCann, M. F.,** An epidemiologic study of contraception and preeclampsia, *JAMA,* 262, 3143–3147, 1989.
107. **Knox, G. E., Stagno, S., Volanakis, J. E., and Huddleston, J. F.,** A search for antigen-antibody complexes in preeclampsia: further evidence against immunologic pathogenesis, *Am. J. Obstet. Gynecol.,* 132, 87–89, 1978.
108. **Knox, W. F. and Fox, H.,** Villitis of unknown aetiology: its incidence and significance in placentae from a British population, *Placenta,* 5, 393–402, 1984.

109. **Kumar, D.,** Chronic placental ischemia in relation to the toxemias of pregnancy, *Am. J. Obstet. Gynecol.,* 84, 1323–1329, 1962.

110. **Kvarstein, B. and Gjonnaess, H.,** The influence of pregnancy and contraceptive pills upon oxygen consumption during phagocytosis by human leukocytes, *Acta Obstet. Gynaecol. Scand.,* 60, 505–506, 1981.

111. **Labarrere, C. A., Alonson, J., Manni, J., Domenichini, E., and Althabe, O.,** Immunohistochemical findings in acute atherosis associated with intrauterine growth retardation, *Am. J. Reprod. Immunol.,* 7, 149–155, 1985.

112. **Labarrere, C. and Althabe, O.,** Chronic villitis of unknown aetiology and decidual maternal vasculopathies in sustained chronic hypertension, *Eur. J. Obstet. Gynecol. Reprod. Biol.,* 21, 27–32, 1986.

113. **Labarrere, C., Althabe, O., and Telenta, M.,** Chronic villitis of unknown aetiology in placentae of idiopathic small for gestational age infants, *Placenta,* 3, 309–317, 1982.

114. **Leslie, G. A.,** Structure and biologic functions of human IgD. II. Alterations of serum IgD levels during pregnancy, *Proc. Soc. Exp. Biol. Med.,* 144, 741–743, 1973.

115. **Levanon, Y. and Rossetini, S. M. O.,** Presence of circulating placental antigens and antibodies in toxemic and normal pregnancy patients, *Z. Immun.,* 136, 178–186, 1968.

116. **Lichtig, C., Deutsch, M., and Brandes, J.,** Immunofluorescent studies of the endometrial arteries in the first trimester of pregnancy, *Am. J. Clin. Pathol.,* 83, 633–636, 1985.

117. **Lichtig, C., Deutsch, M., and Brandes, J.,** Vascular changes of endometrium in early pregnancy, *Am. J. Clin. Pathol.,* 81, 702–707, 1984.

118. **Little, W. A.,** Placental infarction, *Obstet. Gynecol.,* 15, 109–130, 1960.

119. **Ljunggren, H.-G. and Karre, K.,** In search of "missing self": MHC molecules and NK cell recognition, *Immunol. Today,* 11, 237–244, 1990.

120. **MacGillivray, I.,** Some observations on the incidence of pre-eclampsia, *J. Obstet. Gynaecol. Br. Commonw.,* 65, 536–539, 1958.

121. **MacLennan, A. H., Sharp, F., and Shaw-Dunn, J.,** The ultrastructure of human trophoblast in spontaneous and induced hypoxia using a system of organ culture, *J. Obstet. Gynaecol. Br. Commonw.,* 79, 113–121, 1972.

122. **Marti, J. J. and Herrman, U.,** Immunogestosis. A new concept of "essential" gestosis, with special consideration of the primigravid patient, *Am. J. Obstet. Gynecol.,* 128, 489–493, 1977.

123. **Massobrio, M., Benedetto, C., Bertini, E., Tetta, C., and Camussi, G.,** Immune complexes in preeclampsia and normal pregnancy, *Am. J. Obstet. Gynecol.,* 152, 578–583, 1985.

124. **Masson, P. L., Delire, M., and Cambiaso, C. L.,** Circulating immune complexes in normal human pregnancy, *Nature,* 266, 542–543, 1977.

125. **McFarlane, A. and Scott, J. S.,** Pre-eclampsia/eclampsia in twin pregnancies, *J. Med. Genet.,* 13, 208–211, 1976.

126. **McKay, D. G., Hertig, A. T., Adams, E. C., and Richardson, M. V.,** Histochemical observations on the human placenta, *Obstet. Gynecol.,* 12, 1–36, 1958.

127. **Mills, J. A., Klebanoff, M. A., Graubard, B. I., Carey, J. C., and Berendes, H. W.,** Barrier contraceptive methods and preeclampsia, *JAMA,* 265, 70–73, 1991.

128. **Mitchell, G. W., Jacobs, A. A., Haddad, V., Paul, B. B., Strauss, R. R., and Sbarra, A. J.,** The role of phagocyte in host-parasite interactions. XXV. Metabolic and bactericidal activities of leukocytes from pregnant women, *Am. J. Obstet. Gynecol.,* 108, 805–813, 1970.

129. **Moore, M. P., Carter, N. P., and Redman, C. W. G.,** Lymphocyte subsets defined by monoclonal antibodies in human pregnancy, *Am. J. Reprod. Immunol.,* 3, 161–164, 1983.

130. **Moore, M. P., Carter, N. P., and Redman, C. W. G.,** Lymphocyte subsets in normal and preeclamptic pregnancies, *Br. J. Obstet. Gynaecol.,* 90, 326–331, 1983.

131. **Musci, T. J., Roberts, J. M., Rodgers, G. M., and Taylor, T. N.,** Mitogenic activity is increased in the sera of preeclamptic women before delivery, *Am. J. Obstet. Gynecol.,* 159, 1446–1451, 1988.

132. **Need, J. A., Bell, B., Meffin, E., and Jones, W. R.,** Pre-eclampsia in pregnancies from donor inseminations, *J. Reprod. Immunol.,* 5, 329–338, 1983.

133. **Okamura, K., Furakawa, K., Nakkakuki, M., Yamada, K., and Suzuki, M.,** Natural killer cell activity during pregnancy, *Am. J. Obstet. Gynecol.,* 149, 396–399, 1984.

134. **Okerengwo, A. A., Williams, A. I., and Abeziako, P. A.,** Immunological studies on pre-eclampsia in Nigerian women, *Int. J. Gynaecol. Obstet.,* 33, 121–125, 1990.

135. **Ostensen, M., Revhaug, A., Volden, G., Berge, L., Husby, G., and Giercksky, K. E.,** The effect of pregnancy on functions of inflammatory cells in healthy women and in patients with rheumatic disease, *Acta Obstet. Gynaecol. Scand.,* 66, 247–253, 1987.

136. **Page, E. W.,** The relation between hydatid moles, relative ischemia of the gravid uterus, and the placental origin of eclampsia, *Am. J. Obstet. Gynecol.,* 37, 291–293, 1939.

137. **Page, E. W.,** Placental dysfunction in eclamptogenic toxemias, *Obstet. Gynecol. Surv.,* 3, 615–628, 1948.

138. **Pearson, M. G. and Pinker, G. D.,** ABO Blood groups and toxaemia of pregnancy, *Br. Med. J.,* i, 777–778, 1956.

139. **Penrose, L. S.,** On the familial appearances of maternal and foetal incompatibility, *Ann. Eugenics,* 13, 141–145, 1947.

140. **Persellin, R. H. and Thoi, L. L.,** Human polymorphonuclear leukocyte phagocytosis in pregnancy. Development of inhibition during gestation and recovery in the postpartum period, *Am. J. Obstet. Gynecol.,* 134, 250–254, 1979.

141. **Petrucco, O. M., Thomson, N. M., Lawrence, J. R., and Weldon, M. W.,** Immunofluorescent studies in renal biopsies in pre-eclampsia, *Br. Med. J.,* 1, 473–476, 1974.

142. **Pitkin, R. M. and Witte, D. L.,** Platelet and leukocyte counts in pregnancy, *JAMA,* 242, 2696–2698, 1979.

143. **Plum, J., Thiery, M., and Sabre, L.,** Distribution of mononuclear cells during pregnancy, *Clin. Exp. Immunol.,* 31, 45–49, 1978.

144. **Pollak, V. E. and Nettles, J. B.,** The kidney in toxemia of pregnancy: a clinical and pathologic study based on renal biopsies, *Medicine,* 39, 469–526, 1960.

145. **Prall, R. H. and Kantor, F. S.**, Serum complement in eclamptogenic toxemia, *Am. J. Obstet. Gynecol.*, 95, 530–533, 1966.

146. **Pudifin, D. J., Moodley, J., and Duursma, J.**, Pre-eclamptic toxaemia is not associated with elevated levels of circulating immune complexes, *S. Afr. Med. J.*, 63, 304–305, 1983.

147. **Rapaport, V. J., Hirata, G., Yap, H. K., and Jordan, S. C.**, Anti-vascular endothelial cell antibodies in severe preeclampsia, *Am. J. Obstet. Gynecol.*, 162, 138–146, 1990.

148. **Redman, C. W. G.**, Hypertension in pregnancy, in *Textbook of Obstetrics*, Turnbull, A. C. and Chamberlain, G. V. P., Eds., Churchill Livingstone, London, 1989, 515–541.

149. **Redman, C. W. G., Sargent, I. L., and Sutton, L.**, Immunological aspects of human pregnancy and its disorders, in *Immunological Aspects of Reproduction in Mammals*, Crighton, D. B., Ed., Butterworths, London, 1984, 219–250.

150. **Redman, C. W. G.**, Does immune abortion exist? Are there immunologically mediated mechanisms? If so, which mechanisms, *Res. Immunol.*, 141, 169–175, 1990.

151. **Redman, C. W. G., Bodmer, J. G., Bodmer, W. F., Beilin, L. J., and Bonnar, J.**, HLA Antigens in severe pre-eclampsia, *Lancet*, ii, 397–399, 1978.

152. **Redman, C. W. G.**, The fetal allograft, *Fetal Med. Rev.*, 2, 21–43, 1990.

153. **Roberts, J. M., Taylor, R. N., Musci, T. J., Rodgers, D. M., Hubel, C. A., and McLaughlin, M. K.**, Preeclampsia: an endothelial cell disorder, *Am. J. Obstet. Gynecol.*, 161, 1200–1204, 1989.

154. **Robertson, W. B., Brosens, I., and Dixon, H. G.**, The pathological response of the vessels of the placental bed to hypertensive pregnancy, *J. Pathol. Bacteriol.*, 93, 581–592, 1967.

155. **Robertson, W. B., Brosens, I., and Dixon, G.**, Uteroplacental vascular pathology, *Eur. J. Obstet. Gynecol. Reprod. Biol.*, 5, 47–65, 1975.

156. **Rodgers, G. M., Taylor, R. N., and Roberts, J. M.**, Preeclampsia is associated with a serum factor cytotoxic to human endothelial cells, *Am. J. Obstet. Gynecol.*, 159, 908–914, 1988.

157. **Rosenthal, M.**, Enhanced phagocytosis of immune complexes in pregnancy, *Clin. Exp. Immunol.*, 28, 189–191, 1977.

158. **Ruschoff, J., Boger, A., and Zwiens, G.**, Chronic placentitis—a clinico-pathological study, *Arch. Gynecol.*, 237, 19–25, 1985.

159. **Russell, P.**, Inflammatory lesions of the human placenta. III. The histopathology of villitis of unknown aetiology, *Placenta*, 1, 227–244, 1980.

160. **Samuels, P., Main, E. K., Tomaski, A., Mennuti, M. T., Gabbe, S. G., and Cines, D. B.**, Abnormalities in platelet antiglobulin tests in preeclamptic mothers and their neonates, *Am. J. Obstet. Gynecol.*, 157, 109–113, 1987.

161. **Sargent, I. L., Redman, C. W. G., and Stirrat, G. M.**, Maternal cell-mediated immunity in normal and pre-eclamptic pregnancy, *Clin. Exp. Immunol.*, 50, 601–609, 1982.

162. **Sargent, I. L., Wilkins, T., and Redman, C. W. G.**, Maternal immune responses to the fetus in early pregnancy and recurrent miscarriage, *Lancet*, ii, 1099–1104, 1988.

163. **Schena, F. P., Manno, C., Selvaggi, L., Loverros, G., Bettocchi, S., and Benomo, L.,** Behaviour of immune complexes and the complement system in normal pregnancy and in pre-eclampsia, *J. Clin. Lab. Immunol.,* 7, 21–26, 1982.

164. **Schmorl, G.,** Quoted by Chesley, L. C., in *Hypertensive Disorders of Pregnancy,* Appleton-Century-Crofts, New York, 1978, 582.

165. **Scott, J. S.,** Pregnancy toxaemia associated with hydrops foetalis, hydatidiform mole and hydramnios, *J. Obstet. Gynaecol. Br. Emp.,* 65, 689–701, 1958.

166. **Seidl, D. C., Hughes, H. C., Bertolet, R., and Lang, C. M.,** True pregnancy toxemia (preeclampsia) in the guinea pig (Cavia porcellus), *Lab. Animal Sci.,* 29, 472–478, 1979.

167. **Seidman, D. S., Ever-Hadani, P., Stevenson, D. K., and Gale, R.,** The effect of abortion on the incidence of pre-eclampsia, *Eur. J. Obstet. Gynecol. Reprod. Biol.,* 33, 109–114, 1989.

168. **Shanklin, D. R. and Sibai, B. W.,** Ultrastructural aspects of pre-eclampsia. I. Placental bed and uterine boundary vessels, *Am. J. Obstet. Gynecol.,* 161, 735–741, 1989.

169. **Sheppard, B. L. and Bonnar, J.,** The ultrastructure of the arterial supply of the human placenta in pregnancy complicated by fetal growth retardation, *Br. J. Obstet. Gynaecol.,* 83, 948–959, 1976.

170. **Shibuya, T., Izuchi, K., Kuroiwa, A., Okabe, N., and Shirakawa, K.,** Study on nonspecific immunity in pregnant women: increased chemiluminescence response of peripheral blood phagocytes, *Am. J. Reprod. Immunol.,* 15, 19–23, 1987.

171. **Simon, P., Fauchet, R., Pilorge, M., Calvez, C., Le Fiblec, B., Cam, G., Ang, K. S., Genetet, B., and Cloup, B.,** Association of HLA-DR4 with the risk of recurrence of pregnancy hypertension, *Kidney Int.,* 34(Suppl.), 125–128, 1988.

172. **Sinha, D., Wells, M., and Faulk, W. P.,** Immunological studies in human placentae: complement components in pre-eclamptic chorionic villi, *Clin. Exp. Immunol.,* 56, 175–184, 1984.

173. **Song, C. S., Merkatz, I. R., Rifkind, A. B., Gillette, P. N., and Kappas, A.,** The influence of pregnancy and oral contraceptive steroids on the concentration of plasma proteins, *Am. J. Obstet. Gynecol.,* 108, 227–231, 1970.

174. **Spargo, B. H., Lichtig, C., Luger, A. M., Katz, A. I., and Lindheimer, M. D.,** The renal lesion in pre-eclampsia, in *Hypertension in Pregnancy,* Lindheimer, M. D., Katz, A. I., and Zuspan, F. P., Eds., John Wiley & Sons, New York, 1976, 129–137.

175. **Sridama, V., Pacini, F., Yang, S.-L., Moawad, A., Reilly, M., and DeGroot, L. J.,** Decreased levels of helper T cells. A possible cause of immunodeficiency in pregnancy, *N. Engl. J. Med.,* 307, 352–356, 1982.

176. **Sridama, V., Yang, S.-L., Moawad, A., and DeGroot, T. J.,** T-cell subsets in patients with preeclampsia, *Am. J. Obstet. Gynecol.,* 147, 566–569, 1983.

177. **Stevenson, A. C., Say, B., Ustaoglu, S., and Durmus, Z.,** Aspects of pre-eclamptic toxaemia of pregnancy, consanguinity and twinning in Ankara, *J. Med. Genet.,* 13, 1–8, 1976.

178. **Stevenson, A. C., Davison, B. C. C., Say, B., Ustuoplus, L. D., Einen, M. A., and Toppozada, H. K.,** Contribution of fetal/maternal incompatibility to aetiology of pre-eclamptic toxaemia, *Lancet,* ii, 1286–1289, 1971.

179. **Stimson, W. H., McAdam, A., and Hutchinson, R. S.,** An assay for antigen-antibody complexes in human sera using C1q-enzyme conjugates, *J. Clin. Lab. Immunol.,* 5, 129–131, 1981.

180. **Stirrat, G. M., Redman, C. W. G., and Levinsky, R. J.,** Circulating immune complexes in pre-eclampsia, *Br. Med. J.,* 1, 1450–1451, 1978.

181. **Stout, C. and Lemmon, W. B.,** Glomerular capillary endothelial swelling in a pregnant chimpanzee, *Am. J. Obstet. Gynecol.,* 105, 212–215, 1969.

182. **Strickland, D. M., Guzick, D. S., Cox, K., Gant, N. F., and Rosenfeld, C. R.,** The relationship between abortion in the first pregnancy and development of pregnancy-induced hypertension in the subsequent pregnancy, *Am. J. Obstet. Gynecol.,* 154, 146–148, 1986.

183. **Studd, J. W. W.,** Immunoglobulins in normal pregnancy, pre-eclampsia and pregnancy complicated by nephrotic syndrome, *J. Obstet. Gynaecol. Br. Commonw.,* 78, 786–790, 1971.

184. **Sunder-Plassmann, G., Derfler, K., Wagner, L., Stockenhuber, F., Endler, M., Nowotny, C., and Balcke, P.,** Increased serum activity of interleukin-2 in patients with pre-eclampsia, *J. Autoimmun.,* 2, 203–205, 1989.

185. **Tallon, D. F., Corcoran, D. J. D., O'Dwyer, E. M., and Greally, J. F.,** Circulating lymphocyte subpopulations in pregnancy: a longitudinal study, *J. Immunol.,* 132, 1784–1787, 1984.

186. **Taylor, P. V., Skerrow, S., and Redman, C. W. G.,** Pre-eclampsia and anti-phospholipid antibody, *Br. J. Obstet. Gynaecol.,* 98, 604–606, 1991.

187. **Tedder, R. S., Nelson, M., and Eisen, V.,** Effects of serum complement of normal and pre-eclamptic pregnancy and of oral contraceptives, *Br. J. Exp. Pathol.,* 56, 389–395, 1975.

188. **Tedesco, F., Radillo, O., Candussi, G., Nazzaro, A., Mollnes, T. E., and Pecorari, D.,** Immunohistochemical detection of terminal complement complex and S protein in normal and pre-eclamptic placentae, *Clin. Exp. Immunol.,* 80, 236–240, 1990.

189. **Thiry, L., Yane, F., Sprecher-Goldberger, S., Cappel, R., Bossens, M., and Neuray, F.,** Expression of retrovirus related antigen in pregnancy. II. Cytotoxic and blocking specificities in immunoglobulins eluted from the placenta, *J. Reprod. Immunol.,* 2, 323–330, 1981.

190. **Thomson, N. C., Stevenson, R. D., Behan, W., Sloar, D., and Horne, C.,** Immunological studies in pre-eclamptic toxaemia, *Br. Med. J.,* 1, 1307–1309, 1976.

191. **Tiilikainen, A.,** Fetomaternal histocompatibility in toxemia of pregnancy, in *Human Anti-Human Gammaglobulins,* Grubb, R. and Samuelsson, G., Eds., Pergamon Press, Oxford, 1971, 223–227.

192. **Toder, V., Eichenbrenner, I., Amit, S., Serr, D., and Nebel, L.,** Cellular hyperreactivity to placenta in toxemia of pregnancy, *Eur. J. Obstet. Gynecol. Reprod. Biol.,* 9, 379–384, 1979.

193. **Toder, V., Blank, M., Gleicher, N., Voljovich, I., Mashiah, S., and Nebel, L.,** Activity of natural killer cells in normal pregnancy and edema-proteinuria hypertension gestosis, *Am. J. Obstet. Gynecol.,* 145, 7–10, 1983.

194. **Toivanen, P. and Hirvonen, T.,** Sex ratio of newborns: preponderance of males in toxemia of pregnancy, *Science,* 170, 186–187, 1970.

195. **Tominaga, T. and Page, E. W.,** Accommodation of the human placenta to hypoxia, *Am. J. Obstet. Gynecol.,* 94, 679–685, 1966.

196. **Tribe, C. R., Smart, G. E., Davies, D. R., and Mackenzie, J. C.,** A renal biopsy study in toxaemia of pregnancy, *J. Clin. Pathol.,* 32, 681–692, 1979.

197. **Vandenbeeken, Y., Vlieghe, M. P., Delespesse, G., and Duchateau, J.,** Characterization of immunoregulatory T cells during pregnancy by monoclonal antibodies, *Clin. Exp. Immunol.,* 48, 118–120, 1982.

198. **Vasquez-Escobosa, C., Perez-Medina, R., and Gomez-Estrada, H.,** Circulating immune complexes in hypertensive disease of pregnancy, *Obstet. Gynecol.,* 62, 45–48, 1982.

199. **Wallenburg, H. C. S., Stolte, L. A. M., and Janssens, J.,** The pathogenesis of placental infarction. I. A morphologic study in the human placenta, *Am. J. Obstet. Gynecol.,* 116, 835–840, 1973.

200. **Wardle, E. N. and Wright, N. A.,** Role of fibrin in a model of pregnancy toxemia in the rabbit, *Am. J. Obstet. Gynecol.,* 115, 17–26, 1973.

201. **Wentworth, P.,** Placental infarction and toxemia of pregnancy, *Am. J. Obstet. Gynecol.,* 99, 318–326, 1967.

202. **Wilton, A. N., Cooper, D. W., Brennecke, S. P., Bishop, S. M., and Marshall, P.,** Absence of close linkage between maternal genes for susceptibility to pre-eclampsia/eclampsia and HLA DR beta, *Lancet,* 336, 653–657, 1990.

203. **Woods, L. L.,** Importance of prostaglandins in hypertension during reduced uteroplacental perfusion pressure, *Am. J. Physiol.,* 257, R1558–R1561, 1989.

204. **Yang, S.-L., Kleinman, A. M., and Wei, P.-Y.,** Immunologic aspects of term pregnancy toxemia. A study of immunoglobulins and complement, *Am. J. Obstet. Gynecol.,* 122, 727–731, 1973.

205. **Young, J.,** The aetiology of eclampsia and albuminuria and their relation to accidental haemorrhage (an anatomical and experimental investigation), *J. Obstet. Gynaecol. Br. Emp.,* 26, 1–28, 1914.

206. **Zeek, P. M. and Assali, N. S.,** Vascular changes in the decidua associated with eclamptogenic toxemia of pregnancy, *Am. J. Clin. Pathol.,* 20, 1099–1109, 1950.

Chapter

14

Immunological Processes of Abortion

James F. Mowbray, Jennifer L. Underwood, and
Gholam R. Jalali
Department of Immunopathology
St. Mary's Hospital Medical School
London, England

The case for an immunological cause of some repeated abortions in man, and the occurrence of resorption of a large proportion of murine fetuses, must be considered in the light of both animal and human evidence. The current state of understanding of the phenomenon in mice is high, and it would be the appropriate starting point. At the outset it should, however, be noted that resorption of fetuses in mice is akin to a missed abortion or anembryonic pregnancy in man, and that espulsion of a dead fetus does not occur in rodents. The term abortion should then be restricted to the damage and death of an embryo accompanied by its expulsion by the onset of uterine contractions. This terminal event does not occur in mice before the normal end of the murine pregnancy, whereas in man, the death of the fetus is usually fairly rapidly followed by the onset of labor. If there is no fetus present, as in an anembryonic pregnancy, the remaining sac alone does not always cause the onset of labor and a missed abortion occurs. To a large extent this appears to be the consequence of very early damage to the

8868-6/93/$0.00 + $.50

conceptus so that the fetal pole is not developed, or even becomes incorporated in the trophectoderm layer.

Embryo resorption in mice can be initiated in several ways, by interference with the hormone control of pregnancy using the progesterone receptor blocker RU 486,[12] or by administration of endotoxin, or occurring spontaneously in some mating combinations.[1] There are probable analogies for these in human pregnancy, where there is also another recognizable group in which the abortions probably occur from genetic defects, as, for example, the high rate of spontaneous abortion seen in trisomy 21. There are differences in the changes which occur in the last group compared with spontaneous abortion which may be of immunological origin.

In the murine pregnancy where the rate of intrauterine resorption is low, it can be induced by the administration of endotoxin.[11] In several strain combinations there is a high rate of resorption, compared with that found in the parental strains.[4] With advancing female age, irrespective of parity, the resorption rate tends to rise. Thus, a useful model can be found in older females mating in a CBA × BALB/c combination. The resorption rate in the reverse mating is lower. Obviously, whatever part of the genome is required for the phenomenon, the mother is homozygous for all genes, and the fetus is heterozygous. It should also be noted that the phenomenon in mice is not of *recurrent* resorption, it is of a large fraction of the fetuses in *one* pregnancy. Indeed, there is evidence that the high rate of absorption of F1 matings is abrogated by deliberate immunization of the females with cells from the paternal strain.[2] Thus, the condition in mice could be considered to be self-resolving, although the normal process of study is to kill the mouse at the end of pregnancy and count the number of normal and resorbed fetuses. This is in contradistinction to the phenomenon which occurs in about 20% of recurrent aborting women, when the first pregnancy is successful and subsequent pregnancies abort.

The mechanisms of fetal death and resorption in mice have been studied largely by depletion of an intact immune response. From this the pathway is found to involve:

1. Asialo-GM1-positive natural killer (NK) cells
2. Tumor necrosis factor (TNF)
3. Natural killer (NK) activity

It may be induced, even in syngeneic matings, by administration of endotoxin. It is prevented by:

1. Depletion of asialo-GM1-positive cells
2. Polyclonal rabbit antibody against TNF-α
3. Administration of granulocyte macrophage colony-stimulating factor (GM-CSF)

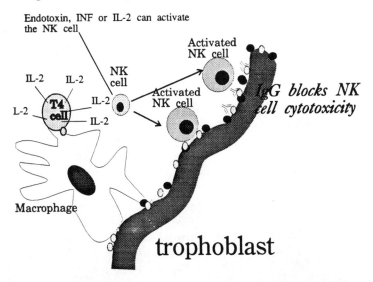

Figure 1. Mechanism of immunological damage to trophoblasts. Cytokine-dependent activation of NK cells results in attachment of the NK cell to the target antigen of trophoblast. Normally IgG antibody bound to the target antigen prevents attachment or killing.

4. Prevention of release of TNF and interleukin-1 (IL-1) by oxypentifylline
5. Immunization of the female with paternal-strain lymphoid cells (*vide supra*)
6. Passive transfer of IgG from mice immunized against the paternal strain to the pregnant females

The apparent mode of attack induced in allopregnancy or by endotoxin is shown in Figure 1. The common pathway is amenable to blocking by the methods outlined above, with the assumption that antibody is able to block the attachment site of NK or lymphokine-activated killer (LAK) cells to trophoblast. Antigen of trophoblast origin would, in the allopregnancy model, stimulate macrophages, cause presentation to T lymphocytes, and hence production of IL-2. A nonspecific immune reactant, activated NK or LAK cells may thus be generated by a specific antigenic response. It is of interest to note that Clark has shown that transforming growth factor (TGF)-β is a competitive antagonist of IL-2 for stimulation of lymphocytes induced by concanavalin A (ConA).[3] This might be an important control mechanism if IL-2-induced activation of NK cells was necessary to produce trophoblast damage. There is, however, a little evidence that LAK killing is less important than NK attack in the murine resorption model. TNF Production by NK cells is part of the mechanism of damage to target cells. It appears that, after NK cells are activated, anti-TNF antibody may be ineffective in preventing resorption.[17] This is not positive proof that local TNF production is not responsible for the NK attack, as the intimate production of TNF at the two cell surfaces may prevent the antibody being able to inactivate the cytokine.

How then can we fit this together into an integrated hypothesis? It would seem that stimulation of a macrophage population to produce TNF may occur spontaneously in some strain combinations, but may, of course, be induced with endotoxin. The TNF then activates NK cells to attack targets on the conceptus which are assumed to be external, that is trophoblast, in nature. What is the possible nature of the NK target surface component? NK Cells have specificity for tumor cell surface components, possibly of fetal type. It may be that the trophoblast plasma membrane possesses NK receptor molecules by virtue of being a fetal tissue. This alone would not explain the relative absence of resorption in most matings, and its appearance in a few allogeneic matings. It is easier to understand why immunization with alloantigenic determinants may prevent the attack, by the development of antibody which may block such NK target sites, than to see how an alloantigen could elicit directly NK cell attack which is, perforce, a "nonspecific" immune mediator.

It may be necessary to study the possibility that alloantigens interact early in the sequence and are in fact fundamental to the local NK activation necessary to produce the TNF response. In man there is trophoblast directly accessible within the maternal circulation, and hence remote macrophage activation would be easier than in the murine system, where the reaction is probably much more confined to the uterus.

At this stage, we should consider the genetic factors that are associated with resorption and recurrent abortion. In the mouse combinations, obviously, the fetuses possess half the paternal antigens, and the fathers are homozygous for all antigens. Whatever gene products in the paternal strain are responsible for the production of protective maternal immunity, they are present in all the fetuses. The presence of alloantigens in the fetus different from those of the mother may elicit protective immunity and explain why an antigen nonspecific attack (NK cell mediated) may be prevented. It may also be the reason for the finding that endotoxin-induced abortion is easier to produce in syngeneic than in semiallogeneic pregnancies.[1] Thus, it is not necessarily true that abortion or resorption is induced by sensitization by alloantigens, although it is genetically determined. The ability of a strain combination to induce resorption of a large fraction of fetuses may be due to a genetically controlled environment that allows the development of activated NK cells in the neighborhood of trophoblast. In the mouse this is within the uterus, but in man, the villous trophoblast is in contact with circulating cells and antibodies. Could there be a situation in which the nonspecific NK killing mechanism is set up by a genetically controlled situation, and that artificially produced alloimmunization results in antibody, which blocks the attachment site of NK cells?

TABLE 1.

Reaction of 5 Eluted IgG Preparations (AB) with 5 Antigen Preparations (VA) Prepared from the Same Placentas* and Used to Coat Well

	VA1	VA2	VA3	VA4	VA5
	(cpm** Bound to Well)				
AB 1	1469	548	825	200	733
AB 2	759	1548	851	209	690
AB 3	725	591	1152	346	445
AB 4	190	188	284	969	126
AB 5	1107	841	633	397	1667

Note: A solid-phase RIA was used to show the binding of the IgG to each IgG preparation to each 80-kDa antigen preparation. The antigen was prepared from the vesicle, after acidification to remove the IgG, by digestion with trypsin, followed by gel filtration. Each antibody binds to its own antigen specifically (underlined). The IgG bound to the antigen on the plate was measured by the addition of radiolabeled protein A (8000 cpm per well). Results are mean of duplicates, and background values are subtracted.

*   No. is 5 placentas, 1 IgG, and 1 VA from each.
** cpm is counts per minute.

In the human situation we have shown that in all successful pregnancies studied, even first pregnancies, there is IgG antibody bound to the syncytio-trophoblast.[8] This is bound to an 80-kDa antigen which is highly polymorphic (Table 1). There are considerable analogies with the 80-kDa cell membrane protein to which a monoclonal antibody was derived,[9] that prevented killing of human, mouse, or parasitic cells by activated NK cells. The antigen we have studied is also present on mature peripheral B-lymphocytes, but not T lymphocytes or platelets. This is a probable very important component in the NK pathway; the protein in target cell membranes appears to be necessary for NK killing, which is blocked by the monoclonal antibody to the protein. The analogy with the syncytiotrophoblast is considerable where the protein is bound to IgG antibody, and evidence is accumulating that removal of the antibody uncovers reactivity of the target cell membrane.

In our experience, about 20% of aborting couples show a single successful, first pregnancy, followed by abortion of all successive pregnancies (Table 1). The other immunologically modifiable group aborts all pregnancies. One might consider that if the father is heterozygous for the sensitizing gene product, not all first pregnancies would be affected, and yet there would be a good chance that after alloimmunization had been set up, all pregnancies in that woman would be affected. Immunization with paternal antigens then produces protective antibodies which block the attachment site of NK cells.

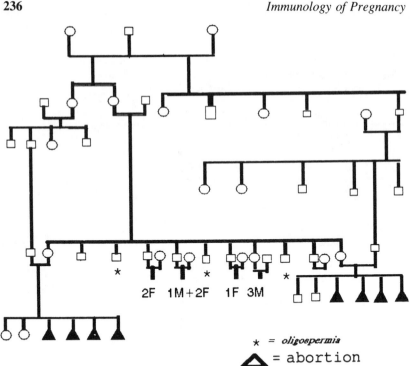

Figure 2. Inheritance of spontaneous abortion and infertility in a family with cousin marriages. This shows a pattern seen in Arab families. Half the pregnancies of women marrying cousins abort and half of their brothers have oligospermia.

That the phenomenon of abortion in man and resorption in mice is genetically controlled is shown by the following features:

- Man

    1. Abortion occurs with one partner, but not with another
    2. Repeated abortion may occur in several generations of a family

- Mice

    1. High levels of resorption occur in matings between inbred strains
    2. Endotoxin-induced abortion is difficult to produce in allogeneic matings

There is obviously a possibility that some of these events may be due to lethal recessive genes which produce one of three types of inherited abortion (Figures 2, 3, and 4). The variety with which we are concerned now, however, is treatable by immunization, and the offspring born are normal. Similarly, in mice there is an apparently nonimmunological pregnancy failure

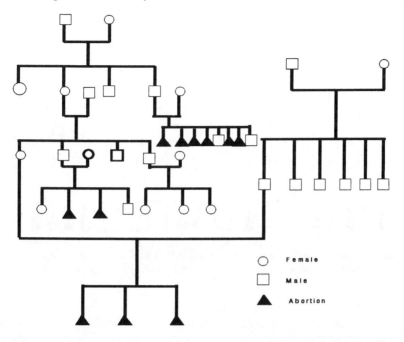

Figure 3. Apparent dominant autosomal inheritance of abortion. This European family shows abortion which skips a generation. It is passed on both by males and females, precluding a possible Surani effect.

in the *Mus musculus/Mus caroli* combination. When the fetus is invested with a trophectoderm syngeneic with the mother, the conceptus survives;[6] the problem is evidently one of the contact of the trophoblast of the one species with the decidua of another, rather than immunological attack on the trophoblast.

In this group of couples, or inbred-strain murine matings, the observed frequencies of abortion would depend on whether the gene product was needed in the trophoblast or the inner cell mass, and to some extent whether inheritance was from the father or the mother. This is because of the phenomenon of gene imprinting first described by Surani et al.[16] It is now accepted that, at least early in development, the paternal genes only are expressed in the trophoblast, and maternal ones in the developing inner cell mass. This may explain the apparently strange modes of inheritance of abortion sometimes seen in families. An example is shown in Figure 4, where there is known abortion of male fetuses, and transmission occurs through females, with one exception. Apparent recessive recurrent abortion from a presumed lethal gene is found in inbred human families. The Islamic world provides good examples of this, seen in Figure 2. It will be seen that abortion occurs in about half of the sisters in a sibship if they marry within the family, and with low frequency if they marry outside. It should be noted

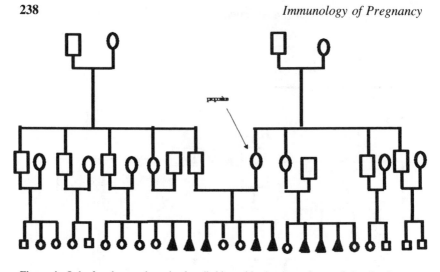

Figure 4. Only females are born in the sibships with abortions. Some of the abortions are known to have been males.

that the loss of all fetuses in one couple is not seen, and this distinguishes it from the commoner kind of abortion which is amenable to immunization treatment discussed above. Abortion in these couples is uninfluenced by immunization of the wife with paternal cells, and the absence of antibodies to paternal cells or the receptors for them found in the immunologically modifiable group are found quite often in the families discussed here.

This group of recurrent abortion is thus largely separable from other groups, but must be remembered when undertaking any review of recurrent abortion overall in populations to study the immunological varieties. Do murine equivalents occur? As already mentioned, the cross-species mating of *Mus musculus* and *Mus caroli* represents an example, and possibly the difficulties observed when trying to establish new inbred lines may be further demonstrations. To date, no one has shown the production of animals homozygous for a particular gene to be associated with recurrent resorption, nor is there an example of gene imprinting producing an apparent dominant effect of a lethal gene in mice. This may in large part be a consequence of the use of syngeneic murine lines, rather than study of outbred populations, which in man so far have yielded the best evidence.

Occam's razor would suggest that it is more likely that a number of events occurring together are explained by one, rather than more than one cause. In terms of the genetics, however, it seems most likely that two independent events are occurring.

A single antigen theory would suggest that most women will not respond to an antigen by developing a response, but if they do, it is nonspecific and damaging. The protection against it is possible again only by deliberate immunization. The fundamental genetic determinant of the condition would be that a woman was homozygous for the absence of the surface component and able to recognize it as one against which to mount an NK response. Again, this lacks the ability to explain the endotoxin effect in inbred strains.

Abortion is instituted, sometimes after the end of the first, normal pregnancy and it continues. This means that fetuses with different haplotypes of paternal genes all abort. The phenomenon in both mice and men is partner specific. Thus, a nonspecific process occurs which is genetically determined. The easiest way to consider this would be to suggest that there is an innate ability to respond to an antigen of paternal origin present on trophoblast, leading to NK cell generation and damage to the trophoblast by direct attack. The development of a protective antibody response is, however, against different alloantigens of paternal origin, which vary from pregnancy to pregnancy.

The ability of endotoxin to initiate resorption in inbred strains suggests that the NK target on trophoblast is present in all/most strains. The inbred strain does not normally do anything, presumably because the system is not armed. In the allogeneic situation activation may occur, but usually this is blocked by the development of protective, blocking IgG antibodies. In those strain combinations which do not do this, antibody production may be weak, and may only be elicited by iatrogenic immunization rather than by fetal antigens, *or* the antigen is present on lymphocytes and not in the fetal trophoblast, or fetal cells migrating to the mother. This has an air of recombinance about it—a recombinant in the male might mean that for either haplotype, the protective response is always in the wrong fetus. Immunization with the whole paternal antigen set would, however, result in the production of protective antibodies! This would be an elegant explanation of the ability of paternal cells to immunize, but not of either fetal haplotype. Such a possibility of recombinant paternal genes implies that the two loci are normally in linkage disequilibrium on the same chromosome.

The position that requires explanation is, thus, that there are two separate phenomena occurring, sensitization and immunization. The first results in production of activated NK cells and potentially LAK cells as well, by an alloimmune reaction leading to TNF- and sometimes IL-2-induced activation of NK cells. Attack on trophoblast can be inhibited by the immunization of the mother by another set of antigens to produce antibody. The antibody produced can be shown to protect the mouse, although no direct evidence for the protective activity of antibody, rather than other components of the immune response, is available in the human case.

The phenomena associated with recurrent human abortion are explicable if it is assumed that sensitization and protective immunization are independent. Thus, the woman who has a normal first pregnancy and then aborts all subsequent pregnancies may be sensitized by the fetal transfusion at the time of placental separation, but without the simultaneous production of protective antibody.

An explanation would be needed that would produce a setup for abortion of all fetuses, although they were not genetically identical. If sensitization

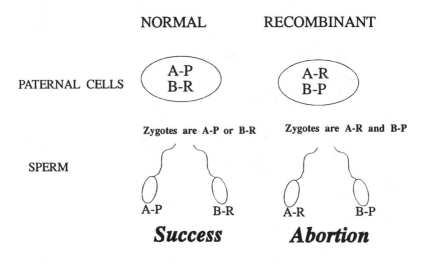

Figure 5. Possible mechanism of immunological loss of all fetuses despite paternal heterozygosity. Sensitization by A is blocked by antibodies to antigen P; sensitization by B is blocked by antibodies to antigen R. The hypothesis requires two linked loci, one of which produces maternal sensitization by alleles A or B. The other locus product immunizes to provide cross-reacting antibody to A or B. If recombination occurs, the sensitizing antigen is always associated with the wrong protective antibody. Thus ALL pregnancies can fail.

and protection are caused by different gene products, and if they are, as they must be, polymorphic, the protection afforded by the immunogen may be specific for the sensitizing antigen. Figure 5 shows a possible way that such protection may, rarely, go wrong. If the two genes are on the same chromosome, there would be a preservation of the linkage disequilibrium, as dissociation of the two would run a serious risk of abortion, and hence loss of the genetic arrangement. If, as seen in Figure 5, there is a crossover such that a recombinant in a male is such that the specific sensitizing antigen is now associated with the protective antigen being on the other chromosome, whichever haplotype is transmitted to the fetus, sensitization without protection will occur.

Sensitization might occur with an epitope that would react to produce macrophage and T cell activation, without the necessary "carrier" epitope(s) being present, this being necessary for presentation of the epitope to a B lymphocyte. It could even be that there was, for antibody production, the necessity for the presence of the allogeneic epitope and major histocompatibility complex (MHC) determinants, to produce the phenomenon. Either hypothesis is testable in the human or rodent models.

Having, over some years, considered the conundrum of the immunogenetics of the immunologically modifiable form of recurrent abortion, we are attracted by the crossover concept. It is the only way we can easily explain the loss of all fetuses before immunization, combined with the efficacy of paternal cell immunization in prevention of subsequent abortion. It is important, however, to recognize that a poorly responsive mother, or maternal strain, might fail to be immunized by antigens present in any fetus, and hence abort all. This possibility would not, however, show a partner-specific effect of the kind normally observed in man, and the infrequency of the phenomenon in F_1 matings between murine inbred strains.

What would be the nature of the genetics of the woman that makes her respond to the sensitizing stimulus? Obviously, she will not respond to an antigen which she possesses, so that she is assumed not to have either of the paternal sensitizing antigens. Immunization with paternal cells would, however, result in her obtaining the missing immune responses, although this simple model would suggest that if enough pregnancies have occurred, she would have been immunized by the other haplotype, and should then not abort. It is our finding that rather the reverse occurs. As first noted by Cowchock et al.,[5] the "primary aborter" with a large number of abortions (in our series more than 6) is unlikely to be protected by immunization with paternal cells. If the model is correct, protective immunization is uncommon in the absence of the sensitizing antigen, or does not persist into the next pregnancy.

A problem of the model is that, while it is agreed that the woman will only respond to either antigen if she does not possess it herself, this requires the absence of both alleles of the antigen from the woman. One assumes that absence of one antigen will be commoner than absence of both. Thus, there would be expected a frequency of abortion of half the fetuses more commonly than of both. It is our assumption that this does not happen, but investigation of the situation in 850 couples with recurrent abortion of all kinds shows that loss of some but not all pregnancies is common in the relatives of the "primary aborter" (Table 2). The true frequency of this group may be underestimated, since the family is completed on average by 1.6 live births. Thus, if a 50% pregnancy loss occurs randomly, the expected number of abortions found in an affected couple would be 0.80, with 1.6 live children. These would probably be dismissed as the single, randomly distributed abortions, due primarily to disjunctional faults, found in any group of breeding couples. Thus, it may be that the model will fit quite well the observed distribution of abortion seen in our populations, but that in other societies where large families and inbreeding are the rule, there would be an increase in the fraction of aborting women who had approximately 50% abortion over those with 100% abortion. When we take the ratios of 50% and 100% abortion in Arab couples, who normally have large families, we see a distribution in favor of this. Overall, it does then seem that the model would give us some confidence that it is worthy of further study.

To investigate the above possibility, it would be necessary to know something more about the genes involved, and their localization in the

TABLE 2.
Incidence of Abortion in Separate Pregnancies in Recurrent
Aborting Women

Type of aborter	No Family History % (No. of couples %)	Abortions in Family of Wife (No. of couples %)	Husband	Both
Unrelated Families				
All abortions	60 (55)	30 (27)	12 (11)	8 (7)
Live and abortions	12 (33)	12 (33)	6 (17)	6 (17)
2 Live and abortions	6 (100)	0	0	0
>2 Live and abortions	2 (50)	2 (50)	0	0
Arab Families				
All abortions	10 (71)	4 (29)	0	0
Live and abortions	6 (60)	3 (30)	0	1 (10)
2 Live and abortions	1 (25)	2 (50)	0	1 (25)
>2 Live and abortions	3 (100)	0	0	0

genome. Although it was once popular to believe that HLA sharing might explain unresponsiveness of a woman to paternal antigens that might be required for protection,[13] this hypothesis of a trophoblast lymphocyte cross-reacting (TLX antigen) which was MHC linked[10] has fallen into disrepute. Nevertheless, some large studies of HLA sharing[14] have shown that there is a weak effect seen in recurrent abortion, albeit more with class II than class I. If one were looking for other gene loci which might still be in linkage disequilibrium with HLA, this might be seen. Using the standard explanation of sharing and maternal unresponsiveness, the observed sharing could only directly explain about 5% of the abortions. Instead, it might indicate that the sensitizing and protective antigens lay on the same chromosome as the MHC. The hypothesis outlined would *not* show an effect of sharing of the antigens involved in the production of abortion. The low, but statistically significant, degree of excess HLA sharing in the large study of recurrent abortion of Reznikoff-Etievant et al.[15] is explained by about 5% of the couples showing excess sharing. If there is, as Gill has proposed,[7] an MHC-linked lethal gene in man akin to the grc in rats or t-locus in mice, then the 5% might be of couples with a lethal gene cause, whereas in the majority of immunologically modifiable abortion, excess HLA sharing would not occur.

REFERENCES

1. **Chaouat, G., Menu, E., Kinsky, R., and Brezin, C.,** Immunologically mediated abortions, one or several pathways, *Res. Immunol.,* 141, 188–195, 1990.
2. **Chaouat, G., Clark, D. A., and Wegmann, T. G.,** Genetic aspects of the CBA × DBA/2 and B10 × B10A models of murine pregnancy failure and its prevention by lymphocyte immunisation, in *Early Pregnancy Loss, Mechanisms and Treatment,* Beard, R. W. and Sharp, F., Eds., Peacock Press, Ashton-Under-Lyme, U.K., 1988, 89–102.
3. **Clark, D. A., Falbo, M., Rowley, R. B., Banwatt, D., and Stedronsk-Clark, J.,** Active suppression of host-versus-graft reaction in pregnant mice. IX. Soluble suppressor activity obtained from all pregnant mouse decidua that blocks the cytolytic effector response to interleukin 2 is related to TGF-β, *J. Immunol.,* 141, 3833–3840, 1988.
4. **Clark, D. A., McDermott, M., and Sczewzuk, M. R.,** Impairment of the host-versus-graft reaction in pregnant mice. II. Selective suppresion of cytotoxic cell generation correlates with soluble suppressor activity and with successful allogeneic pregnancy, *Cell. Immunol.,* 52, 106–110, 1980.
5. **Cowchock, F. S., Smith, J. B., David, S., Scher, J., Batzer, F., and Corson, S.,** Paternal mononuclear cell immunisation therapy for repeated miscarriages: predictive variables for pregnancy success, *Am. J. Reprod. Immunol.,* 22, 12–17, 1990.
6. **Croy, B. A., Rossant, J., and Clark, D. A.,** Histological and immunological studies of postimplantation death of Mus caroli embryos in Mus musculus uterus, *J. Reprod. Immunol.,* 4, 277–293, 1982.
7. **Gill, T. J.,** Genetic factors in fetal loss, *Am. J. Reprod. Immunol. Microbiol.,* 15, 133–137, 1987.
8. **Jalali, G. R., Underwood, J. L., Mowbray, J. F.,** IgG on normal human placenta is bound both to antigen and Fc receptors, *Transplant. Proc.,* 81, 572–574, 1989.
9. **Jaso-Friedmann, L., Evans, D. L., Grant, C. C., St. John, A., Harris, D. T., and Koren, H. S.,** Characterisation by monoclonal antibodies of a target cell antigen complex recognized by nonspecific cytotoxic cells, *J. Immunol.,* 8, 2861–2868, 1988.
10. **McIntyre, J. A. and Faulk, W. P.,** Trophoblast antigens in normal and abnormal human pregnancy, *Clin. Obstet. Gynecol.,* 29, 976–998, 1986.
11. **Parant, M.,** Possible mediators in endotoxin-induced abortion, *Res. Immunol.,* 141, 164–168, 1990.
12. **Szekeres-Bartho, J., Chaouat, G., and Kirsty, R.,** A progesterone-induced blocking factor corrects high resorption rates in mice treated with anti-progesterone, *Am. J. Obstet. Gynecol.,* 163, 1320–1322, 1990.
13. **Taylor, C. and Faulk, P. W.,** Prevention of recurrent abortion with leucocyte transfusion, *Lancet,* 2, 68–69, 1981.
14. **Reznikoff-Etievant, M. F., Durieux, I., Hutchet, J., Salmon, C., and Netler, A.,** Recurrent spontaneous abortion, HLA antigen sharing and anti-paternal immunity. Immunotherapeutic assay, in *Reproductive Immunology: Materno-Fetal Relationship,* Chaouat, G., Ed., Colloque Inserm, Paris, 1987, 187–202.

15. **Reznikoff-Etievant, M. F., Durieux, I., Hutchet, J., Salmon, C., and Netler, A.,** Human MHC antigens and paternal leucocyte injections in recurrent spontaneous abortions, in *Early Pregnancy Loss. Mechanisms and Treatment,* Beard, R. W. and Sharp, F., Eds., Peacock Press, Ashton-Under-Lyme, U.K., 1988, 275–384.

16. **Surani, M. A., Barton, S. C., and Norris, M. L.,** Influence of parental chromosome on spartial specificity in the androgenetic pathogenetic chimeras of the mouse, *Nature,* 326, 395–397, 1987.

17. **Wegmann, T.,** personal communication.

Chapter 15

Birth Control Vaccines: Principles, Procedures, and Prospects

Raj Raghupathy and Gursaran P. Talwar
National Institute of Immunology
Shahid Jit Singh Marg
New Delhi, India

1. INTRODUCTION

As the population of this planet, and of some countries in particular, keeps rising inexorably, one realizes that there is an unmistakable need for improved and reliable methods for birth control that are available more easily now more so than ever. Safe, effective, and reversible birth control vaccines would be a great addition to currently available methods and, in fact, may turn out to be superior in some respects.[25] Thus, while the need for better methods for birth control in developing countries is obvious, such methods would find much use in developed countries as well.

Vaccines are traditionally meant to deal with external entities—bacteria, toxins, viruses, and parasites. The idea of using selected target antigens that are from within, or ''self'' antigens as immunogens is, on the one hand, still relatively novel, but on the other hand, is an idea which has been actively pursued by a number of investigators over the last two decades. That birth control can be brought about by immunological means is evidenced by naturally occurring immunologic infertility and by experimental data. While this chapter will review the latter, a brief mention can be made about natural immunologic infertility, of which a large number of authenticated cases have been reported over the years in subjects in whom all other causative factors, genetic, anatomic, and endocrinological, have been clearly ruled out.[116] Agglutinating and immobilizing anti-sperm antibodies are the best documented causative factors of immunologic infertility.[14,39,42] The work of Shaha and colleagues,[100,101] described later in this chapter, has demonstrated "natural" immunologic infertility in an experimental system in a convincing manner. They have used anti-sperm antibodies from infertile subjects to isolate specific sperm antigens which, when used as immunogens, resulted in infertility in animals. Another line of evidence for immune infertility comes from studies on vasectomized men; vasectomy often results in the production of anti-sperm antibodies. These antibody levels sometimes persist even after reanastomoses (ligation of the vas deferens), with a concurrent persistence of infertility (reviewed by Raghupathy et al.[90]). Such "natural" cases implicate anti-sperm antibodies in infertility and provide a logical framework for the belief that infertility can be accomplished by immunological means (reviewed by Alexander[5]).

2. POSSIBLE SITES OF IMMUNE INTERVENTION OF FERTILITY

Theoretically, a number of vaccines are feasible for the control of fertility, since the reproductive process is interceptible at a number of points. A brief review of the processes leading to successful reproduction would be relevant at this point. Successful pregnancy is the culmination of a complex cascade of events that starts with the production and maturation of gametes, and the fertilization of the female gamete by the male gamete. This results in the formation of an embryo which then has to develop through gestation. The development of gametes is under the control of two gonadotropins made by both the male and the female, follicle stimulating hormone (FSH) and luteinizing hormone (LH), which travel from the pituitary to the gonads via the blood stream. The gonadotropins, FSH and LH, act on the male gonads to generate sperm and testosterone; in the female, they stimulate follicular development, ovulation, and the production of female sex hormones. These gonadotropins are in turn under the control of the hypothalamic hormone, gonadotropin releasing hormone (GnRH). The fertilized egg and early embryo secrete factors such as chorionic gonadotropin which enable the sustenance of the corpus luteum and make possible the establishment and maintenance of pregnancy during early stages of gestation. It is clear, therefore, that multiple sites are available for interception by immune effectors (Figure 1)

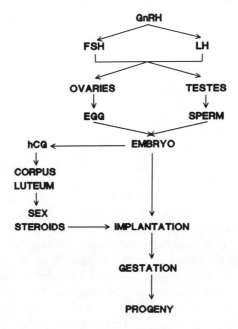

Figure 1. The process of mammalian reproduction: multiple sites are available for immune intervention.

and thus a variety of potential vaccines can be developed for the control of fertility.

The principle underlying birth control vaccines is basically simple: pregnancy can be blocked by the generation of immune effectors that can inactivate a hormone playing an indispensable role in reproduction, or counteract a gamete antigen crucial for gamete development and/or fertilization. These immune effectors have traditionally been antibodies, but it is conceivable that cellular effectors can also be induced to block fertility.

The primary prerequisite of an antifertility vaccine is that the antigen should be unique to the reproductive system and should have a fertility-related function that can be blocked. The ideal vaccine would not interfere with the processes of ovulation and sex hormone function. Oral contraceptives inhibit the hypothalamic-pituitary-gonadal axis and this is certainly not a desirable feature. The attractiveness of birth control vaccines stems at least partially from its lack of effect on this axis. Perhaps one of the most attractive features of a birth control vaccine is that it is relatively free from the risk of user failure. Condoms, for instance, suffer from this risk; failure to comply with this simple method often results in unplanned pregnancies. In underdeveloped countries this is a particularly important feature: if immunization and subsequent monitoring is done by local clinics, one would not have to depend on the user for maintenance of birth control. Moreover, immunization involves the injection of small amounts of the immunogen, in far, far fewer doses than contraceptive pills. This would spare the body from constant drugging with synthetic compounds and this particular feature makes vaccines an attractive method even for people in developed countries. Vaccines are under development against human chorionic gonadotropin (hCG), GnRH, FSH, sperm, and egg antigens.

3. hCG VACCINES

Human chorionic gonadotropin (hCG) happens to be the first antigen targeted for development of birth control vaccines and is also in the most advanced stages of testing and development. hCG is a pregnancy-specific hormone produced by the trophectoderm of the early embryo and is essential to the maintenance of pregnancy. The principle of hCG vaccines is to induce antibodies that can bind to hCG and render it biologically inactive. hCG plays a vital role in the rescue of the corpus luteum and in the continued secretion of progesterone, which is essential for the sustenance of the endometrium by preventing menstrual shedding and for preparing the uterus for implantation of the embryo. Thus, hCG is indispensable, therefore, for the maintenance of pregnancy in the first 6 to 8 weeks before the trophoblast assumes the role of synthesizing progesterone. It is clear, therefore, that the inactivation of hCG would result in the nonestablishment of pregnancy, without any repercussions on normal ovulation and levels of sex hormones.

Indeed, this is borne out by passive and active immunization studies with hCG. Early studies by Talwar and colleagues[117] showed that the administration of anti-hCG antibodies to pregnant baboons results in a rapid decline in the levels of progesterone and these animals subsequently aborted. Active immunization of rodents,[41] baboons,[109,110,115] and marmosets[32] with hCG prevents pregnancy. hCG is composed of two subunits, α and β. The α-subunit is highly homologous to the α-subunit of LH, FSH, and thyroid stimulating hormones (TSH). Hence attention has been focused on the hCG-specific unit, the β-subunit. βhCG, being a "self" molecule, is poorly immunogenic in humans; however, presentation to the immune system of βhCG linked to a nonself carrier[68] bypasses the necessity of T cells specific for hCG because carrier-specific T cells presumably stimulate βhCG-specific B cells to proliferate and secrete antibodies.

The prototype vaccine consisted of βhCG linked covalently to tetanus (TT) (βhCG-TT);[22,103,125] the ability of this conjugate to induce anti-hCG antibodies was confirmed in probing clinical trials in India, Finland, Sweden, Brazil, and Chile.[47,68,102,125] This vaccine evoked the production of antibodies in 61 out of the 63 women immunized, and the antibodies generated were bioeffective in neutralizing hCG *in vivo* and *in vitro*.[22] Careful analyses employing several different parameters confirmed that there were no signs of altered pituitary, ovarian, or kidney function.[23,68] The alum-absorbed vaccine retains its potency for one year at room temperature.[3] One limitation of this vaccine became obvious when the sera were assayed for anti-hCG antibodies; there was a large variation in antibody responses from individual to individual, and those with low antibody titers became pregnant.[102]

Efforts were then directed at enhancing the immune response and minimizing individual variability. Two new vaccine formulations were developed and found to be much more immunogenic. In these formulations, the β-subunit of ovine LH (βoLH) was included as part of the immunogen and cholera toxin chain B (CHB) was also tested for its suitability as a carrier. One formulation consisted of a mixture of βhCG-TT/CHB and βoLH-TT/CHB; such a mixture of βhCG and αoLH produces a higher antibody titer than βhCG alone, in monkeys.[122] Another formulation takes advantage of the fact that βhCG can specifically form dimers with not just αhCG but also with heterospecies αLH.[113] This vaccine consists of a heterospecies dimer (HSD) of βhCG and αoLH, linked to TT or CHB. This HSD has a higher steroidogenic potency than the native hCG molecule, is more immunogenic in monkeys and rats, and it elicits antibodies with superior bioneutralizing capacity.[83,121]

Phase I clinical trials, designed to investigate vaccine efficacy and possible side effects, on tubectomized women showed that the mixed and HSD formulations were superior to the older βhCG vaccine.[119] Of the 105 women inducted in this trial, aimed at evaluating the immunogenicity of the vaccine formulations and at investigating any possible side effects, it was found that all the immunized women produced anti-hCG antibodies.[82] These antibodies were devoid of cross-reaction with hFSH and hTSH, but as expected cross-reacted with hLH. No abnormal side effects of this immunization procedure was noticed. Menstrual regularity was maintained in about 90% of the cycles and there was no correlation between the length of the cycles and anti-hCG antibody titers.[46] Hematological and clinical chemistry analyses indicated that this vaccine did not have any adverse reactions. Extensive immunopathology studies showed that there were no autoantibodies to nuclear antigens, DNA, parietal cells, smooth muscles, islet cells, adrenal cortex, thyroid, thyroglobulin, and C-reactive protein. Extensive teratology studies with the hCG vaccine conducted in pregnant rats and monkeys showed that there were no developmental abnormalities in the offspring. Long-term studies in monkeys showed that when immunization was discontinued, antibody titers declined and the animals regained fertility. Of the 12 baboons and 64 bonnet monkeys subsequently rendered pregnant, normal healthy infants were born; none of these offspring had any anthropometric and developmental abnormalities.[124]

There was some indication of local hypersensitivity reactions in some women due to the use of the same carrier (TT) throughout the immunization schedule. When diphtheria toxoid (DT) was used alternatively with TT as carrier in subsequent Extended Phase I trials, none of the women manifested hypersensitivity to the vaccine. This "alternate carrier approach" has the added advantage of stimulating a response in subjects hyporesponsive to the first carrier[29,124] and possibly in subjects showing a suppressed response due to preexposure to the carrier (see below).

Extended Phase I trials confirmed previous observations; all women in this trial made anti-hCG antibodies and no adverse effects were observed on clinical parameters, ovulation, and pathology. The anti-hCG antibodies so generated are effective in neutralizing the bioactivity of hCG *in vitro*. hCG challenge tests *in vivo* demonstrated the ability of these antibodies to scavenge exogenously administered hCG, thereby preventing sustained progesterone production. This study also helped clinch the choice of the annealed αoLH-βhCG heterospecies dimer as the optimal vaccine preparation. The all-important Phase II clinical trials began in late 1990 in three different centers in India; about 750 **unprotected** cycles are to be screened. These trials are designed to indicate the threshold of anti-hCG antibodies required for prevention of pregnancy, and the outcome of these trials is awaited.

What is interesting and important is that the αoLH does not induce antibodies cross-reactive to hFSH and hTSH.[121] Fears that anti-oLH antibodies might be detrimental[13,45] have been discounted. A reassuring verdict on the lack of deleterious side effects has come from chronic toxicology studies in monkeys conducted by Thau and colleagues.[57,127,128] They have shown that hyperimmunization of 63 rhesus monkeys with oLH in complete Freund's adjuvant (CFA) for a period of 5 to 7 years gave rise to antibodies that reacted with LH and hCG, but did not cause any pathological effects on the pituitaries, kidneys, or other organs. The animals continued to ovulate and to have regular menstruation despite the presence of anti-LH antibodies; this is possibly because the affinity of ovarian receptors for LH is greater than the affinity of the antibody for LH.[57]

Another approach to an hCG-based vaccine comes from the work of Stevens and his group.[109,110,112] This method, adopted by the WHO Task Force on Birth Control Vaccines, utilizes a C-terminal fragment of βhCG, linked to DT. The 37-amino acid carboxy-terminal peptide (CTP) is used, on the grounds that it does not cross-react with βhLH.[111] We have used the whole βhCG because it is a much better immunogen than the CTP, presumably because it has more than one immunogenic epitope, giving rise to better coverage in terms of immune responsiveness. The antibodies produced to CTP are of lower affinity and poorer bioneutralization capacity than βhCG itself.[121] Previous attempts from our own and other laboratories to use carboxy-terminal peptides linked as immunogens showed that these are quite unsatisfactory and that the bioefficacy and affinity of anti-βhCG antibodies are superior to anti-CTP antibodies.[19,53,81,89,97] The titers of anti-hCG antibodies are about 10- to 20-fold higher than those obtained with CTP immunization.[111] Hence our choice of βhCG as the immunogen in our vaccines.

The CTP vaccine designed by Stevens and co-workers consists of a synthetic peptide spanning residues 109 to 145 of βhCG and is linked to DT. It is used with a water-soluble synthetic adjuvant and a saline-oil emulsion vehicle consisting of squalene and Arlacel A. After efficacy trials in baboons and routine toxicological and immunosafety studies in baboons, this vaccine has undergone Phase I clinical trials in humans without any adverse reactions being recorded.[45] What the CTP vaccine does achieve is the generation of antibodies without cross-reactivity to hLH.[111] An unexpected finding with this vaccine is the cross-reaction of anti-CTP antibodies with striated muscle tissue and with somatostatin-secreting cells in pancreatic islets.[91] These antibodies were absorbable with CTP, but not with the carrier, indicating that these antibodies are indeed elicited by the peptide itself. Even though there was no indication of a resultant autoimmune disease,[91] the fact that these autoantibodies were produced is worrisome. Antibodies generated by the βhCG vaccines do not manifest any such autoreactivity. The fact that this vaccine is based on a synthetic peptide is indeed attractive, as it would be easily amenable to economic production. Phase II trials are planned and further developments on it are eagerly awaited.

What makes hCG an attractive candidate immunogen? It is essential for the maintenance of pregnancy, it is pregnancy specific, and it is produced very early in pregnancy in amounts that can easily be neutralized by antibodies. It is also the most advanced among the birth control vaccines and much is expected of research and development in this area.[63]

4. A RECOMBINANT hCG VACCINE

The vaccinia virus has been extremely useful for the expression of foreign genes of interest, due to its ability to accommodate a large amount of foreign DNA without loss of infectivity and with proper processing and posttranslational modification.[106] Thus, vaccinia vectors have been considered for their potential as vehicles for immunogens of interest.[107] In a series of studies, Chakrabarti and colleagues[18] first reported two vaccinia constructs, one containing the gene for βhCG and another the gene for αoLH; coinfection of cell lines with these recombinant viruses resulted not only in the expression of immunoreactive peptides, but in the association of a bioactive dimer with gonadotropic properties.[50]

This was followed by a report describing the construction of recombinant viruses containing genes coding for α- and βhCG. Infection with these recombinant viruses separately results in the expression of subunit proteins and coinfection with these recombinant viruses results in the production of bioactive hCG secreted into the culture medium.[18] However, these were found to be unsatisfactory as immunogens in experimental animals. A recent accomplishment has been the production of a construct which anchors βhCG to the cell membrane of the infected cell. The construct was made by incorporating a membrane anchor sequence of 49 amino acids.[108] Immunization with this vaccinia-hCG construct generated consistently high anti-hCG responses in rats. Intradermal injection of bonnet monkeys with this construct results in high levels of antibody production in 8 out of 8 monkeys, and the antibodies so generated are capable of neutralizing the bioefficacy of hCG *in vitro*. A recombinant vaccine such as this one would be cheap to produce, the immunization procedure is simple, and the regimen may require fewer doses than the conventional approach using antigen and adjuvants.

5. GnRH VACCINE

The gonadotropin releasing hormone (GnRH) plays a crucial and indispensable role as a master molecule initiating the cascade of events leading to the maintenance of fertility in males and females. It is a decapeptide synthesized and secreted by the hypothalamus and it stimulates the secretion of FSH and LH (Figure 1). Thus, inactivation of GnRH by antibodies would result in infertility in both males and females, as GnRH is an identical molecule in males and females and plays key roles in both sexes. Loss of GnRH results in interruption of normal estrous cycles, suppression of gonadal steroids, gonadal atrophy, and block of gestation in mammals. The administration of monoclonal anti-GnRH antibodies results in the blocking of ovulation in rats and suppression of estrous cycle in dogs.[118] In baboons, monoclonal anti-GnRH antibodies are abortifacient.[21]

Like hCG, GnRH is essentially a self peptide, and a hapten in addition. It has to be linked to a foreign carrier such as bovine serum albumin (BSA), keyhole limpet hemocyanin (KLH), TT, or DT, to render it immunogenic.[104,105] Fraser[26] demonstrated that the immunization of monkeys with GnRH linked to BSA, in CFA, results in a decline in sex steroids and a reduction in fertility. Similar findings were reported in marmosets.[40] It must be noted that these experiments were done with CFA as the adjuvant. We found that immunization with GnRH-carrier conjugates with alum as adjuvant[126] and TT as carrier[104] gave substantial anti-GnRH antibody titers and, thus, paved the way for a potential vaccine. Immunization of bonnet monkeys and baboons with GnRH linked to TT (GnRH-TT) elicits long-lasting antibodies of a titer high enough to block cyclicity and ovulation.[126] Immunization of males with GnRH results in decreased testicular size, cessation of spermatogenesis,[17] and a reduction in testosterone levels.[26,27,98] Work on GnRH-based vaccines for use in males is now focused on inducing infertility while ensuring the maintenance of libido using exogenous androgen, without at the same time restoring spermatogenesis. Immunization of male rats with GnRH with provision of supplemental testosterone resulted in a reversible block in fertility in all immunized rats, with no effect on sexual behavior.[48,49] Supplementation with higher doses of testosterone, however, brings about restoration of sperm production, thus indicating, first, that this vaccination effect is reversible, and second, that the dosage of androgen supplemented is critical.[11]

A need has been felt for the development of a reliable, acceptable, and easily administrable method of contraception that is nonsteroidal, has no biological effect on the infant, and does not interfere with the production of milk during the lactational period. The postpartum anovulatory period can be prolonged by intercepting the bioactivity of GnRH. For instance, the daily intranasal administration to women of a GnRH agonist prevents ovulation throughout the period of lactation without side effects or changes in nursing behavior.[28] This observation substantiates the idea that blocking GnRH action is an acceptable method for postpartum contraception; preliminary evidence suggests that the GnRH vaccine may achieve the same objective without any of the problems associated with daily administration of large amounts of GnRH agonists. Experiments in monkeys show that immunization of female monkeys shortly after delivery extends the period of suppressed ovulation without affecting the production of milk.[137] The immunization results in prolongation of the nonovulatory period even after weaning, while control nonimmunized animals start ovulating shortly after weaning. This gives hope that a GnRH-based vaccine will be useful as a contraceptive in the postpartum period. Toxicology studies have been approved and this vaccine is currently undergoing Phase I/II clinical trials in India and under the South-to-South Collaborative Programme in Population Sciences and Reproductive Health in other countries.

Our own focus has shifted into another interesting arena. Immunization with GnRH does lead to a significant reduction of testes size, but, interestingly enough, is accompanied by a significant decline in the weights of all accessory reproductive organs. The effect on the prostate gland is dramatic, with a significant proportion of immunized rats and monkeys showing a marked atrophy of the prostate.[43] These observations have prompted us to think in terms of an approach for nonsurgical immunotherapy against hormone-dependent prostatic hypertrophy. Toxicological studies on this vaccine have been completed and drug regulatory agencies have cleared it for clinical trials in patients of prostate carcinoma. Phase I/II safety-cum-efficacy trials have been initiated in two centers in India and in two clinics abroad under the South-to-South Collaborative Programme in Population Sciences and Reproductive Health. Early results indicate that this vaccine induces anti-GnRH antibodies in humans; as the antibody titers increase, there is a concurrent decline in LH, FSH, and testosterone levels. Preliminary results of clinical studies and ultrasound analyses indicate clinical improvement and a decrease in prostate size, but more data are awaited before unequivocal conclusions can be drawn. One encouraging feature is that no adverse side effects have been noticed. Similarly, it is possible that the GnRH vaccine might be useful for therapy in sex hormone-dependent breast cancer and for control of precocious puberty.

6. CARRIER-INDUCED SUPPRESSION—AN IMPORTANT CONSIDERATION IN HAPTEN-CARRIER CONJUGATE VACCINES

During Phase I clinical trials on the αoLH-βhCG vaccine, it was observed that some of the subjects failed to manifest a clear booster anti-hCG response upon secondary immunization with the vaccine, even though they had initially developed substantial anti-hCG titers after primary immunization. Antibody responses in these women was restored by immunization with the same αoLH-βhCG dimer linked to an alternate carrier.[29] We speculated that this form of hyporesponsiveness may be related to the phenomenon of "epitope-specific suppression" initially described by Herzenberg[33a] and colleagues (1983) and subsequently extended by others.[24a,44,97a] These studies have confirmed that preimmunization with a carrier (such as TT) often results in an inhibitory effect on the production of antibodies to new epitopes or ligands linked to the same protein.

In experiments designed to investigate the effects of carrier preimmunization on anti-βhCG and anti-αoLH levels after subsequent immunization with the αoLH-βhCG dimer conjugated to TT, we immunized four different strains of mice once with TT and subsequently with αoLH-βhCG-TT. We found that presensitization with TT inhibits anti-βhCG responses in some, but not all, mouse strains tested.[10] Interestingly, enough, this hyporesponsiveness is directed only at βhCG and not against αoLH, even though both these ligands are presented in a composite manner, conjugated to the same carrier, TT. It is possible that in strains other than those included in this study, responses to αoLH could also be affected. This indicates that carrier-induced suppression specifically affects only some determinants and not others and that, too, in a strain-specific manner.[10] These inferences from our experiments on mice, when extended to our observations in the human clinical trials with this vaccine, suggest that the decline in anti-hCG titers after secondary immunization in some of the vaccinees may be attributable to the HLA haplotype distribution in the population.

We have also been able to devise a strategy to circumvent carrier-induced hyporesponsiveness; we have found that preimmunization does *not* result in a suppression of anti-hapten responses when subsequent immunization is done with a synthetic T-helper epitope as carrier.[10] This offers the possibility of "bypassing" the suppressive effect of carrier preimmunization. The peptide that we selected is MHC-restricted; it may be possible to devise a bypass protocol using MHC nonrestricted T-helper epitopes. Panina-Bordignon et al.[85] have identified a so-called "universal" or "promiscuous" epitope in tetanus toxin; this peptide is not MHC restricted and can conceivably be used as a universally stimulatory helper epitope, provided, of course, that this peptide has the ability to bypass the suppressive effect of TT.

Another strategy that helps overcome carrier-induced suppression is to use an alternate carrier like diphtheria toxoid (DT);[29,95] however, we have found that DT can also induce similar strain-dependent suppressive effects on haptens linked to it.[96] In experiments designed to assess the influence of the carrier on antibody responses to GnRH, we found that preimmunization with a carrier (diphtheria toxoid and tetanus toxoid) results in a strain-dependent inhibition of anti-GnRH responses in mice. We find that responses to GnRH are suppressed by carrier presensitization in some strains, with no effect in some others and an actual enhancement of responses in yet other strains.[96] The data thus indicate that the generation of epitope-specific suppression is not a universal phenomenon; it is strain dependent and carrier dependent.

It is important, therefore, that every hapten-carrier conjugate vaccine be studied from this perspective individually and this is particularly important when these conjugates are being developed as potential vaccines in humans, where one aims for an efficacy rate of over 90%.

7. FSH VACCINE

The principle behind the use of follicle stimulating hormone (FSH) as a candidate contraceptive immunogen is based on the necessity of FSH for spermatogenesis[15] and for the maintenance of fertility in adult males.[65]

Passive immunization with anti-FSH antiserum leads to a drastic reduction in the quantity and quality of ejaculated sperms and results in infertility.[67] Active immunization with FSH results in either acute oligospermia or azoospermia. For active immunization studies, Moudgal[64] has evolved the use of ovine FSH (oFSH) as it cross-reacts with human FSH and is immunogenic by itself, without need for conjugation with carriers. The adjuvant used in Alhydrogel, which is approved for human use. Bonnet monkeys immunized with FSH for over 9 years had low sperm counts with infertility when in oligospermic state and a decrease in viability and motility of sperm.[64] However, Nieschlag and Wickings[79] report that spermatogenesis was initially suppressed after immunization with FSH but that spermatogenesis returned to normal levels three years later, despite continued active immunization. This might detract from the usefulness of this vaccine.[80]

Moudgal reports that no apparent side effects were noted as a result of oFSH immunization.[66] Preclinical toxicology studies to elucidate immunopathological effects of anti-FSH antibodies have been awaited. These toxicology studies are now reported to be complete and Phase I clinical trials are being planned.[138]

8. SPERM ANTIGEN VACCINES

It is interesting that the earliest leads for an immunological approach for the control of fertility came from "natural" situations of anti-sperm immunity in infertile men and women. The possibility of inducing antibodies against sperm by deliberate immunization was demonstrated as early as almost a century ago by Landsteiner and by Metchnikoff. Spermatozoa carry a number of auto- and isoantigens; males are not immunologically tolerant to sperm and testicular antigens, because sperm and testes develop long after immunocompetence (and tolerance to self antigens) are established (reviewed by Raghupathy et al.[90]). A significant proportion of infertile subjects have circulating anti-sperm antibodies, and these antibodies have been shown to be responsible for reduction in fertility in a large number of men (reviewed by Alexander[5]). These antibodies are capable of agglutinating, immobilizing, and/or killing sperm; anti-sperm antibodies from infertile women can also block penetration of human zona pellucida by human sperm,[129] as also the fertilization of zona-free hamster oocytes by human sperm.[20] Agglutinating and immobilizing antibodies are associated with decreased sperm motility and this in turn results in a reduction of the penetration of cervical mucus by sperm.[58] Cytotoxic anti-sperm antibodies from the serum and seminal plasma of infertile men reduce sperm survival and motility.[56]

Among the most dramatic results in sperm antigen-based birth control vaccines come from the laboratory of Primakoff and co-workers. They identified a 64-kDa antigen, PH-20, an integral membrane protein on both the plasma membrane and the inner acrosomal protein of guinea pig spermatozoa. Immunization of male and female guinea pigs with this antigen, in CFA, results in a 100% block of fertility.[88] Over time, the antibody titers declined and the animals regained fertility. This antigen plays an essential role in sperm adhesion to the zona pellucida of the egg and antibodies to it presumably block fertilization *in vivo;* indeed antisera from immunized (and infertile) female guinea pigs block sperm adhesion to zona pellucida *in vitro.*[87] Primakoff et al. suggest that a human analog of PH-20 would be a suitable candidate for effective immunocontraception.

Other purified sperm antigens that have been considered for use as contraceptive immunogens include lactate dehydrogenase C4 (LDH-c_4), an isoenzyme of lactate dehydrogenase specific to male sperm and testis. LDH-c_4 is the best characterized sperm antigen in terms of its sequence, structure, physicochemical properties, etc.[30] It is an internal antigen that presumably leaks out to the plasma membrane of sperm, thereby exposing it to sperm antibodies. Active immunization of female rabbits, mice, and baboons with LDH-c_4 reduces fertility significantly. Sperm-agglutinating anti-LDH antibodies were found within the female reproductive tract. In primates, the infertility effect was reversible, in that when antibody titers declined, females became pregnant and delivered offspring. This particular vaccine candidate has not reached very high efficacy levels; fertilization is suppressed by 40 to 60% in mice,[51] by 70% in rabbits, and by 63% in baboons.[30] Goldberg and colleagues have defined some of the antibody-stimulating determinants on LDH-c_4;[30] selected peptides (chosen on the basis of recognition by antibodies) were conjugated to BSA and DT as carriers and one such conjugate gave a 71% reduction in fertility in baboons.

Using monoclonal antibodies, Naz and co-workers have identified two interesting sperm antigens, GA-1 (for germ cell antigen) and FA-1 (for fertilization antigen).[76] GA-1 is a glycoprotein expressed on the plasma membrane of sperm and makes its appearance at the spermatocyte stage in the testis. Initially identified in the rabbit,[72] cross-reacting antigens were subsequently demonstrated on mouse, bull, monkey, and human sperm as well.[70] Immunization of female rabbits and mice with GA-1 resulted in a significant reduction in fertility.[74] Antibodies to GA-1 appear to act postfertilization, probably by inhibiting early embryonic development. A human sperm-specific monoclonal antibody has helped in the identification and isolation of the FA-1 antigen[72] that cross-reacts with antigens on mouse, rabbit, bull, and rhesus monkey sperm. A significant proportion of female rabbits immunized with purified FA-1 became infertile, and the antibodies raised appear to inhibit the fertilization process itself.[70] Interestingly enough, anti-FA-1 antibodies are found in several immunoinfertile couples,[71] thus providing "natural" evidence for the immunogenicity (and possible efficacy) of FA-1 in humans. Antigens such as FA-1 would make interesting candidates for birth control vaccines.

A rational and logical approach to identifying sperm antigens relevant to fertility is to tap nature's experiments on fertility, i.e., to exploit the presence of circulating antibodies from subjects with immune infertility. This is precisely the approach adapted by Shaha and colleagues, and it has proven to be a particularly rewarding one. Using a rabbit antiserum to human spermatozoa, Shaha et al.[99] first identified human sperm-specific molecules of which some cross-react with a molecule in the testis of laboratory animals. One such antiserum, for instance, cross-reacts with antigens in the acrosome of human, monkey, rabbit, hamster, rat, and mouse sperm. In Western blots the antiserum recognizes a major band with an apparent molecular weight of 40 kDa on human sperm extracts and 24 kDa on rat testicular cytosol. This antiserum produces strong agglutination of human sperm and prevents the attachment of mouse sperm to mouse oocytes *in vitro* and reduces the fertility rate in female mice. Shaha et al.[101] then showed that this antigen is recognized by sera from infertile human subjects, indicating a possible relationship between infertility in these individuals and the presence of antibodies to this molecule.

A monoclonal antibody raised against this antigen mimicked the infertile human sera and rabbit antiserum in its immunofluorescence staining patterns on human, guinea pig, rat, mouse, and hamster sperm, and in its ability to agglutinate human sperm. This antibody was able to block significantly the attachment of hamster sperm to the zona pellucida of hamster oocytes, indicating that the physiological action of this antibody is probably at the level of this first step in fertilization, i.e., sperm-zona binding.[100] The purified 24-kDa rat testicular protein is immunogenic and can elicit high antibody titers in rats and monkeys, if adjuvants permissible for human use are used. Over 80% of the immunized rats became infertile and remained infertile for over 3 months in one study. Monkeys of proven fertility became infertile during the period when antibody levels were adequate and animals regained fertility when antibody titers declined. Sera from immunized monkeys are negative for auto-antibodies; antibodies to parietal cells, islet cells, smooth muscle tissue, and nuclear antigens.

The fact that the 40-kDa human sperm antigen cross-reacts with monkey and rat sperm is a particularly attractive feature; it makes possible safety and efficacy studies in animals and also provides a source of the antigen for characterization and for use as immunogen; until such time this antigen can be obtained by the recombinant expression route, for which experiments are underway.

This group has also looked at the possibility of devising strategies for oral immunization, as it has the advantage of stimulating the production of antibodies at multiple sites.[1] Immunization with sperm by the oral route[60] and by the intragastric route[6] results in lowered fertility rates in animals. Suri et al.[114] have shown that oral immunization with the 24-kDa sperm antigen described above resulted in the appearance of anti-sperm antibodies in genital tract secretions. These antibodies were of the agglutinating type and could recognize sperm in immunofluorescence assays and could bind to the 24-kDa antigen in Western blots. What is particularly encouraging is that all but one immunized rat in one study became infertile over a 3-month period of continuous mating; the rat that proved to be an exception had low titers of IgA anti-sperm antibodies in reproductive tract secretions.

Among the first of the products and processes emanating from research in this area to actually reach the market is a single injection procedure for the sterilization or castration of male animals. This approach, developed at the National Institute of Immunology, takes advantage of the fact that the testis is immunologically sequestered by the blood-testis barrier; at any such time that this barrier is compromised the formation of anti-sperm antibodies takes place. We have demonstrated that an intratesticular injection of bacillus Calmett-Guérin (BCG) in moderate concentrations causes the degeneration of the blood-testis barrier, which results in the infiltration of mononuclear cells into the testes. This finally leads to a block in spermatogenesis.[77,78] Levels of testosterone in animals rendered aspermic are normal. BCG given as a homogeneous suspension leads to reversible azoospermia; in the course of time, the blood-testis barrier is restored and spermatogenesis resumes.[78]

A reversible anti-fertility vaccine has merit for human contraception, but for animal usage a permanent or quasi-permanent method is acceptable and even desirable. A single intracaudal injection results in aspermatogenesis without loss of libido, while an intratesticular injection causes the destruction of Leydig cells. BCG has been substituted with a mycobacterial extract which is homogeneous and stable at room temperature. The only side effect noted is a transient local inflammation. This product, TALSUR, is 100%

efficacious in all mammals tested, e.g., dogs, cats, bulls, goats, rams, monkeys, etc. This procedure is 100% effective and has been approved for animal use based on extensive safety studies. TALSUR has applications in the creation of "teaser" bulls capable of identifying females in heat and at the same time curbing the proliferation of scrub animals of low genetic quality. It is also being applied to the control of stray dog populations in cities.

9. EGG ANTIGENS

The zona pellucida has received a lot of attention, as it is an excellent site for immunological intervention of fertility; the zona is a noncellular sheath that surrounds the mammalian oocyte and the pre-implantation embryo and has sperm-binding functions during the fertilization process. Zona pellucida antigens are attractive vaccine candidates because even low levels of antibodies may be effective in blocking fertility due to the small number of mature eggs present at any given time. Spermatozoa have to first traverse the zona in order to reach and fertilize the oocyte, and the zona has several specific antigens of interest.[84]

Anti-zona antibodies are capable of preventing fertilization of oocytes *in vitro*.[130] Anti-zona antibodies inhibit sperm attachment and penetration *in vitro*.[2,93] Passively transferred antibodies to zona cause infertility in mice.[92]

These *in vitro* and *in vivo* observations stimulated a great deal of interest in the pursuit of zona antigens as possible vaccine candidates. A fortuitous development was the observation that human zona pellucida antigens cross-react with porcine zona; pig oocytes are available in sufficiently large quantities and this makes for easy availability of the appropriate immunogens. Active immunization with porcine zona antigens results in dramatic inhibitory effects on fertility in dogs,[54] monkeys,[31] and rabbits.[135] The downside of these otherwise encouraging experiments was that there was a severe disruption of normal ovarian follicular development and differentiation. Ovarian function was adversely affected. However, recent findings in monkeys provide hope and go a long way towards dispelling the doubts generated by the initial active immunization studies. In marmosets, bonnet monkeys, and squirrel monkeys, these effects are less severe than those in rabbits,[94] and only a temporary and generally mild disruption of ovarian function was observed after active immunization with a purified zona pellucida antigen, ZP3.[94] These studies suggest that the disruption of ovarian function may not be a common feature of all species studied and that the use of purified antigens may obviate, or at least reduce, such deleterious effects.

The problem of disruption of ovarian function has also been solved by the use of appropriate, milder adjuvants. Animals receiving CFA as an adjuvant along with antigen showed a marked reduction in ovarian follicles, but animals injected with the sodium phthalyl derivative of lipopolysaccharide

(SPLPS) contained normal follicles at all stages of development, indicating normal ovulation and cyclic ovarian activity.[133] SPLPS was as good an adjuvant as CFA, in terms of anti-zona antibody titers. The immunization of female bonnet monkeys with purified zona pellucida, along with adjuvants approved for human use such as SPLPS and muramyl dipeptide (MDP), results in a block in fertility that lasts for about one year. The regularity of cycles was not affected, progesterone profiles suggested the occurrence of ovulation, and ultrasonography revealed the presence of growing follicles and corpora lutea.[124] MDP as an adjuvant appears to elicit titers that are as high as those elicited with CFA.[94] These studies indicate that the choice of appropriate adjuvants is an important consideration for zona immunization and that if better immunization regimens are developed, then the zona pellucida might indeed be an attractive vaccine candidate.

Most promising among the zona pellucida antigens is the ZP3 macromolecules, immunization with which results in an impressive block in fertility but which at the same time results in a transient effect on ovarian function. Efforts are therefore now directed at identifying subunits of this molecule for use either as synthetic peptide vaccines or recombinantly engineered peptides. It is hoped that the use of smaller immunogenic peptides may help circumvent the problem of ovarian dysfunction, while at the same time bringing about infertility.[86,94]

10. FUTURE PERSPECTIVES

An ideal birth control vaccine should induce sustained immunity in over 90% of the vaccinees and this is perhaps one of the most formidable tasks facing workers in this field today. How does one stimulate effective and sustained immunity over a substantial period of time, while at the same time reducing a number of administrations of the vaccine? While biochemical procedures have helped unravel the nature of the immunogens involved, basic immunobiology will help us better understand the nature of immune response to self antigens, hapten/ligand-carrier conjugates, T cell epitopes (both helper and suppressor), secretory immunity, etc.[134] Recombinant DNA technology comes to the rescue in (1) identifying antigens of interest via cDNA libraries; (2) large-scale production of antigens by recombinant bacteria or by insect cells using baculovirus vectors; and (3) the use of vaccinia vectors as immunogen vehicles. An ideal vaccine is one that is producable in large quantities at reasonable cost; recombinant DNA technology will certainly play a critical role in this regard.

It is obvious that serious and persistent attention needs to be paid to the development of better and more effective adjuvants with superior immunopotentiating attributes, which can boost responses to weak immunogens and which can reduce the necessity for frequent injections.[24] In developing countries, the last is particularly important, as repeated available of subjects is not always feasible. Another approach to achieving the goal of high efficacy is to use polyvalent vaccines, i.e., vaccine formulations containing more than one immunogen, targetting the same site or multiple sites for intervention, thereby increasing the range of receptivity.[7] The wide distribution of HLA haplotypes in human populations makes for a wide disparity of immune responses, and a wide range of high and low responders to given antigens. A polyvalent vaccine would ensure that most members of a given population would respond to at least some of the immunogens in a polyvalent formulation, thereby ensuring that infertility is induced by one or the other mechanism.

Human monoclonal antibodies may be useful for short-term passive immunocontraception by intrauterine administration of antibodies, for instance, particularly as a back up during the period that antibody titers are being boosted by active immunization or when antibody titers decline over time.

While one of the attractive features of birth control vaccines is that they are free from the risk of user failure, the downside of that is that subjects have to be monitored for antibody titers on a regular basis. In some countries, this might be difficult. Still, this is not really an insurmountable problem, if simple, easy-to-perform assays are developed for measuring antibody levels and if concerted efforts are made for regular monitoring and providing booster injections when needed.

The next few years ought to see much attention focused on cell-mediated immune mechanisms directed at achieving infertility. Hill and Anderson have elegantly characterized the intricate effects of cell-mediated immunity on gametes and embryonic cells.[8,9,35,36,37] It is clear that, except for a few scattered reports,[61] we know far less about cellular immune effects on fertility than we do about humoral immunity. It may be fruitful to consider evolving strategies for the induction of local cell-mediated immunity against fertility, as this may have dramatic effects on fertility.[8,9] Cytokines and related factors released by activated lymphocytes and macrophages significantly decrease the motility of sperm and can also arrest embryonic development.[36] A novel approach to the induction of cell-mediated immune effectors against fertility has been devised by Upadhyay and colleagues. The intrauterine administration of extracts from the seeds of the herb *Azardichta indica* has been found to activate local cellular immune responses, resulting in a long-term, reversible block in fertility in rats,[132] mice, rabbits, and bonnet monkeys.[131] In rats, a single intrauterine application blocks fertility for 4 to 6 months without affecting ovulation and other ovarian functions.

Much more attention needs to be focused on local secretory immunity with the aim of inducing immunity by intrauterine administration of by intragastric or oral immunization.[4] Since oral administration is one of the easiest modes of administrating drugs or vaccines, there is a need for optimization of oral immunization procedures.[114]

INDEX

studies with hemochorial placentation, 73–74

Antiasialo-GM1 antibody, and fetal resorption, 144

Anti-β human chorionic gonadotropin (βhCG), 254

Antibodies in preeclampsia, 216–217

Antibody-mediated theory, 5–6

Anti-carboxy-terminal peptide (CTP) antibodies, 250–251

Anti-cardiolipin antibodies (ACL), 180

Anti-endothelial autoantibodies, 217

Antifertility vaccine, primary prerequisite of, 247–248; see also Birth control vaccines

Antigen-presenting cell-dependent immunoregulation, decidual, 107–108

Antiglucocorticoids, activity of, 159

Antihormones, in immunoregulation, 159

Anti-human chorionic gonadotropin (hCG) antibodies, 248, 250

Anti-idiotypic antibodies, role of in pregnancy, 6

Anti-interleukin-2 receptor antibodies, abrogation of LAK cells and cytotoxic T lymphocytes, 190

Antipaternal antibodies, 5

Antipaternal cytotoxic lymphocytes, 41

Antiphospholipid antibodies, 180, 217

Antiprogestational steroid, abortificient effect of, 159

Anti-Rho antibodies, 180

Antisperm antibodies
agglutinating and immobilizing of, 246
effect on early embryonic development, 116
in genital tract secretions, 258

Anti-TLX immunity, 4

Anti-zona antibodies, 259, 260

Asialo-GM1⁺ cells
in animal pregnancy, 84–85
and resorbing pregnancies, 72

Atherosis, acute, 209–210

Autoantibodies
natural, discovery of, 1–2
in preeclampsia, 217

Autoimmunity, in fetal abortion, 180

Azardichta indica, 261

B

B cell antibodies, in preeclampsia, 216

B cell growth factor (BCGF), inhibitory effect on embryo development, 117

B cell-stimulating factor-2 (BSF-2), protein inhibiting, 101

B lymphocytes
in nonpregnant endometrium, 68
in term decidua, 67

Bacillus Calmett-Guerin (BCG), 258

Beta human chorionic gonadotropin, 248

Beta human chorionic gonadotropin vaccine, 248–249

Beta integrins, 66

Beta-lactoglobulin homolog (βLG/PP14), immunosuppressive activity of, 119

Beta-lactoglobulin secretory protein family, 105

Beta 2M protein, 48

Birth control vaccines, 245–246
by carrier-induced suppression, 254–255
EGG antigen, 259–260
follicle stimulating hormone, 255
future perspectives on, 260–262
gonadotropin releasing hormone, 252–253
human chorionic gonadotropin, 248–251
possible sites of intervention in, 246–248
recombinant human chorionic gonadotropin, 251–252
sperm antigen, 255–259

Blastocoel, MHC negative status of, 3

Blastocyst culture supernatant, immunosuppressive effect of, 40

Blastocyst stage, immunosuppressive activity produced in, 37

Blocking antibodies, elicitation by placental antigens, 24

Blocking factors, pregnancy-associated, 4

Blood transfusion protective against preeclampsia, 207

Bm mutant major histocompatibility complex antigens, 55

Bovine serum albumin (BSA), 252

Breast cancer, following DMBA exposure, 25

C

C3 concentrations, in preeclampsia, 217–218

C4 concentrations, in preeclampsia, 218

c-fms protooncogene

G

H